LIFE EXTENDERS AND MEMORY BOOSTERS!

Incorporating the Research and Contributions of
*Hans Kugler, Ph.D., President, National Health Federation
*Earl Mindell, R.Ph., Ph.D., Author, Vitamin Bible
*Joe Weissman, M.D., Clinical Assistant Professor, University of California at Los Angeles Medical School
*Joan Priestley, M.D., Center for 21st Century Medicine, Los Angeles
*Richard Passwater, Ph.D., Author, The New Supernutrition
*Ronald DiSalvo, Ph.D., Director of Research and Product Development John Paul Mitchell Systems
*Murray Susser, M.D., Author, Solving the Puzzle of Chronic Fatigue Syndrome
*Cynthia Watson, M.D., Clinical Faculty Instructor, University of Southern California
*Megan Shields, M.D., Diplomate, American Board of Family Practice
*Ronald Peters, M.D., American College of Advancement in Medicine
*Victor Contreras, M.D., Occupational Medicine
*Kaj Alvestrand, Nutritional Consultant, Sweden
*Benjamin Friedrich, Geriatric Institute of Romania

Health Quest Publications ■ Reno, Nevada

Disclaimer

The material presented herein is for informational purposes only. We *strongly advise* people who wish to begin a supplement program to consult with a well qualified medical professional prior to beginning. We are in no way offering medical diagnoses that apply to individuals and no information in this book should be construed in such manner.

Copyright 1993 by Health Quest Publications

All rights reserved under International and Pan-American Copyright Conventions. Published in the United States by Health Quest Publications, Reno, Nevada.

Library of Congress Catalog Card Number: 93-091382

ISBN: 1-883201-00-4

Edited and Compiled by David Steinman

Illustrations by Terri Steinman

Photos by Steven Foster

Manufactured in the United States of America

First Health Quest Publications Edition: April 1993

Second Health Quest Publications Revised Edition: January 1994

10   9   8   7   6   5   4   3

Contents

Foreword

Have you ever admired a classic car? Just one glance and you know it's been lovingly cared for. Routinely serviced to keep it running smoothly. Washed and waxed frequently to keep it looking beautiful. Restored inside and out to maintain its youthful glow and performance. If only we took such good care of ourselves.

If only we didn't worry so much about health plans that covered us while we're in the hospital and cared more about a health plan designed to keep us out of the hospital.

If only we were better informed to ask questions of those in whose hands we trust our lives. "Is chemo and radiation my only choice for cancer therapy?" "How can I avoid prostate cancer?" "What does my lab test really mean?" "Can heart disease be prevented?" "Will natural herbs really make me smarter?"

It's never too early or too late to get healthier. As long as you're still breathing, there is hope.

Hope to live longer than you ever imagined. Hope to be in far better health than you ever dreamed. Science is grabbing a hold on aging and reversing its process. Youth rejuvenating hormones show promise helping the elderly regain their youthful qualities. DHEA, a major natural hormone, is gaining worldwide attention that is part of this revolutionary research.

As we get older, we get fat, get cancer, develop heart disease, our cholesterol goes up—all the things that DHEA combats in animal models. Science fiction has become science fact. Respected professionals such as Temple University's Dr. Arthur Schwartz, best selling author Dr. Earl Mindell, biochemist Dr. Norman Applezweig, University of Kentucky neuroscientist Philip Landfield, all of them, and many more, are unraveling the secrets of this youth hormone.

The quest for longevity is gaining impressive momentum. Richard Cutler, Ph.D., a research chemist and gerontologist at the National Institute of Aging, estimates the current human lifetime potential is 110 to 115 years. According to reports in the Chicago Tribune, studies in Stockholm, Sweden have shown that chemical pathways which desstroy brain cells can be blocked. Extraordinary discoveries like this can help prevent degenerative brain diseases such as Alzheimer's, Parkinson's, epilepsy, stroke and others.

Everything that happens to our bodies affects our aging. You have the wherewithal to control it, rather than succumb to it. You can live longer, look better, delay the major degenerative diseases of aging including stroke, heart disease, breast cancer, osteoporosis, arthritis—even improve your memory, I.Q. and your sex life. You can do it. Simply. Easily. Naturally. Not 10 or 20 years from now. Not next month. But today.

Whether you're in perfect health or bad health; old or young; rich or poor, you can have a new life, a better life, a longer life. There's a pot of gold awaiting you. It is filled with health and vitality.

It's yours for the taking. Researchers have discovered more about aging in the last five years, than in the entire history of civilization. But what does it all mean? How do you use this knowledge day after day? How can you take advantage of the latest breakthroughs in longevity research? You start now.

Not only will you feel and act younger, you can also look younger. An exciting breakthrough in natural beauty care is wild yam skin cream. *Dioscorea villosa* (wild yam) is one of the most important raw sources of progesterone. There is a world of difference between naturally derived progesterone from wild yam and synthetic progestins. In a remarkable natural wild yam skin cream, progesterone precursors, called diosgenins, are delivered through the skin. They are more potent than progesterone so are effective in smaller doses. Prescription progesterones, taken internally, can effect cholesterol build-up, salt build-up, fluid retention and blood sugar imbalances. Researchers have noted that the adverse effect of synthetic progestins were eliminated by using natural progesterone (Hargrove 1989).

Wild yam skin cream offers beauty pluses that may help alleviate dry skin, dry hair, puffiness and bags around the eyes and a sagging look in the face.

Living better, living smarter means knowing how to replace dangerous synthetic substances with benefit-enhancing natural ones. Why even risk the side effects when they can altogether be avoided?

Surgery, chemotherapy and radiation are prime examples. One in two Americans are expected to be stricken with cancer by the year 2,000; yet we seem to be taking one step forward and two steps back. Unfamiliar avenues deserve to be explored. Luckily, there are those who dare to break away from the pack. From their pioneering work comes one of the most important disease prevention breakthroughs in medical history: shark cartilage and its use in the prevention and treatment of cancer.

The fantastic, highly documented story unfolded through the personal dedication of Dr. I.W. Lane. (So important, *60 Minutes* devoted a prime time segment to it.) Dr. Lane has brought the use of shark cartilage in cancer therapy to the general public. The story is an incredible adventure in healing. A grapefruit-size tumor shrunk to the size of a walnut. Terminally ill cancer patients given a second chance.

In case after case tumors dried up and ceased to exist. It was a result of a process known as antiangiogenesis, or the blockage of the formation of new blood vessels. Without the replacement of new blood vessels, a tumor is unable to grow, and it eventually dies. Pure shark cartilage is not merely offering hope; it seems to be saving lives.

We have just scratched the surface of what alternative medicine holds in store for us. No longer can we make believe such choices do not exist. No longer can we close our eyes and ears to the daily news of promising non-toxic therapies designed to strengthen a person's immune system and quality of life.

Powerful antioxidants, like vitamin A, C and E, can help prevent cancer and heart disease. In a group of twenty patients with coronary heart disease, just one gram of vitamin C every eight hours for ten days significantly reduced the tendency for blood platelets to stick together and adhere to arterial walls (Passwater 1991). Beta Carotene, a non-toxic precursor of vitamin A, provides strong protection against lung disease caused by cigarette smoke and pollution. Low vitamin E levels in the blood are a better predictor of heart disease development than any other parameter (Passwater 1991).

It goes on and on. Vitamins, natural hormones, plant substances, ...nature abounds with a virtual endless supply of what we need to stay healthy and live longer. The more you know, the more you can enjoy your life.

Can you imagine a "fat drug" that lets you eat normally and lose weight at the same time? They're called medium chain triglycerides, they occur naturally in your body and you'll learn all about them on the following pages.

Want to reinvigorate your sex life? Then you'll want to know about a miraculous tree in South America whose bark is used specifically as an aphrodisiac. Unfounded? Wait until you read about the clinical research conducted by Dr. Walter Lewis from Washington University and senior botanist at Missouri Botanical Garden.

Need help for prostate problems? Come with us on a trip to the high plateaus of South Africa where the Pygeum (Pygeum africanum) tree grows upwards of 100 feet. Its therapeutic history dates back well before the 18th century where tribes used the bark to make a medicinal tea. Today, it has come under scientific scrutiny as research has proven it useful for chronic inflammation of the prostate and for benign prostatic hypertrophy. Pygeum contains beta-sistosterol, part of a group of common plant compounds known as phytosterols. Beta-sistosterol in Pygeum is reported to reduce the swelling and inflammation of the prostate. And the existence of linear alcohols helps lower cholesterol levels within the prostate gland. Pygeum is far less costly than drugs and has no reported side effects.

Vitamins and herbs that can keep your body healthy can do the same for your mind. They can improve memory loss, prevent brain aging and may even increase your intelligence.

We're not talking about designer drugs. Foods as common as anchovies and sardines tend to be considered by many as "brain food." If you find that bit of information hard to swallow, you'll want to know about DMAE, found abundantly in the aforementioned fish. Scientifically known as dimethylaminoethonol, DMAE has been labeled the "brain stimulant". It appears to alter the levels of acetylcholine, an important neurotransmitter involved in learning and memory. Results from the use of DMAE have shown that it elevates mood, improves memory and learning, increases intelligence, and extends lifespan. DMAE is a free radical scavenger attacking the scourge of aging. It also fights degenerative brain dysfunctions such as Alzheimer's disease.

When it comes to brain stimulants, it's important to think about plants. The *Ginkgo biloba* tree species is 100 to 300 million years old, depending on the source. Its leaves provide a substance that can improve short-term memory, ease symptoms of aging, and are effective against a wide variety of brain disorders such as Alzheimer's disease and dementia. Ginkgo biloba extract supplies blood and oxygen to the brain and is beneficial in increasing mental alertness.

Many of these ideas and practices may be new to you. Yet, as we discover how much we really do not know, we simultaneously discover how long these "alternative" methods have been part of man's vital existence. The use of cayenne pepper as a folk remedy dates back to 7000 B.C. The idea that hot and spicy foods create ulcers may be exactly conversely true. They may actually heal. Cultures that eat curries, and specifically spicy foods with cayenne pepper, have a very low incidence of peptic ulcers.

There is growing evidence that capsicum, a form of cayenne pepper, actually has a mild, stimulating, anti-inflammatory, and antibiotic effect on the stomach. The healing properties come from a compound in capsicum called capsaicin. Laboratory animal studies have shown that capsaicin *stimulates* the mucosal blood flow in the stomach (Limlomwongse 1979). This mucosal production helps protect the stomach lining from ulcer formation. If you think chili peppers can do a healing job on your ulcers, wait until you read about the power of ginger, fenugreek seeds and bromelain from pineapple.

No matter what your present age, you can achieve enthusiastic results through an optimal nutritional supplement program. One of the most common diseases of aging is arthritis. More and more evidence is being amassed that supports the correlation between natural substances and arthritic relief.

In the highly regarded journal, *Science*, researchers discovered the powerful immune response capabilities of type II collagen. Type II collagen is a fibrous protein which is the chief constituent of connective tissue. In a double blind study, (one in which neither the researcher nor participant knows who is using the substance being tested), patients suffering from severe rheumatoid arthritis who were adminstered collagen experienced a decrease in the number of swollen and tender joints after only three months. The placebo group experienced no change. Unlike drugs, collagen is an easily administered non-toxic treatment for rheumatoid arthritis.

Natural substances can indeed offer substantial relief to the problems of aging. But an ounce of prevention is worth a pound of cure. There are simple, inexpensive measures you can take to enjoy a life freer of illness.

Along with a routine exercise program, the right nutrition and the right nutritional supplements are at the top of the list. Today, it is not good enough to simply eat a "well balanced diet." Those old nutritional dictates are old news. Eating from the four basic food groups each day with no supplemental nutritional regimen in place will leave your body only partially capable of fighting the life-long war against pollution, free radicals, cancer, stress, aids and the degenerative diseases of aging.

Many physicians are ill equipped in nutritional education. There is, however, the exception—medical doctors and health professionals who are vigorously committed to alternative techniques that promise a better quality of life. Many of these dedicated men and women have assisted in the creation of this book.

Such luminaries as Dr. Linus Pauling, world renowned best selling author of *Vitamin C and the Common Cold* and two-time Nobel Prize winner; Dr. Earl Mindell, R.Ph., Ph.D., author of the multi-million copy and international best seller *Earl Mindell's Vitamin Bible;* Dr. Richard Passwater, Ph.D., distinguished biochemist, author of the best selling classic *The New Supernutrition* and recipient of the nutrition industry's prestigious Achievement Award; Dr. Hans Kugler, Ph.D., author of numerous books on nutrition and longevity and President of the National Health Federation; Dr. Cynthia Watson, M.D., clinical university instructor, author, and recognized expert on aphrodisiacs... these are just a few of the people who make up a valuable list of those who believe that a vibrant, long life may sometimes mean taking the road less travelled.

Vitamins are cheaper than drugs. Prevention smarter than treatment. When a health problem does occur, one of the prime incentives toward turning to nutrition and nutritional supplements is that nutrients are safer than prescription drugs.

This book will open your mind and provoke you to think. Today, it's just not enough to depend on your doctor for all the answers. He or she doesn't know them. It's up to you to be informed, to know what questions to ask, and to know you have every right to ask them.

Poor knowledge, misinformation, outdated evidence, and sheer guesswork on the part of many medical professionals can lead you down a road of sheer confusion or inappropriate advice.

Be alert. Practicing physicians haven't enough time in their day to study the complex and often voluminous material on the awesome variety of medical topics.

The plethora of information on anti-aging and optimal health is overwhelming, often technical, and can be uncomfortably intimidating.

This book changes all that. It's an exciting wake-up call that touches upon virtually every aspect of longevity and health via a natural pathway. It takes you to the newest frontiers of the turn of the century's nutritional breakthroughs. Scientists and trained physicians have scoured the medical journals and scientific literature to create a source that is packed with cutting edge news, information, and research the average person is unable to acquire on their own. The chapters that follow contain a concise, simplified, easy-to-follow format on health and nutrition that virtually everyone can understand and enjoy learning. Start now. This is your indispensable reference book for the good life. Put it to good use. Your life will truly change for the better for having done so.

Megan Shields, M.D.
Los Angeles, California

Introduction

*"Scientists have launched a search for the right combina-
tion of vitamins, minerals, other nutrients, and exercise
necessary to keep life's mainspring tightly wound," reports
the Chicago Tribune. "Findings already show how to boost
the body's immunity to disease with selenium and vitamins C
and E; head off osteoporosis with calcium, exercise and
estrogen replacement therapy; improve memory with iron and
zinc; and perk up mental function with vitamin B-6, to name
just a few"* (Kotulak 1991).

If I were to present to you a new group of miracle drugs that could
protect you against diseases like cancer, heart attack, stroke, diabetes,
Alzheimer's, arthritis and even the perils of old age itself, this discovery
would become headline news on TV, radio stations, newspapers and maga-
zines throughout the world.

The results would be obvious:
•People would live longer, healthier, happier lives.
•Our nation and senior citizens would no longer live in fear of being
financially destroyed by costly, unnecessary medical procedures.

•Our perception of aging would become much more positive.
•We could enjoy two careers--perhaps three, four or more!
•Think of all the amazing historic events we could witness!

The truth is that these miracle substances are available.

They're inexpensive, readily available—and the key to living a longer and healthier life than ever before in the history of human kind. These miracle substances should be part of every optimal nutrition program. But they aren't drugs.

They're dietary supplements.

Even the most mainstream researchers and organizations in America are jumping on the optimal nutrition band wagon and spreading the word that nutritional supplementation is virtually essential—that optimal nutrition can help prevent cancer and the other major killing diseases of Americans today—helping people live longer, healthier lives.

In the last few months, front page stories in the *Los Angeles Times* have reported that the federal Centers for Disease Control recommend that women's diets be supplemented with folic acid during pregnancy to help prevent birth defects, and that chromium picolinate may well extend human life span. Meanwhile, *Lancet*, the prestigious British medical journal, reports that broad-based multi-vitamin and mineral supplements can cut in half the number of sick days suffered by the elderly.

"If you eat well and take moderate supplements of vitamins A,C, E, and selenium you could dramatically reduce your risk of cancer," says Dr. R. Lee Clark, president emeritus of the M.D. Anderson Hospital and Tumor Institute in Houston.

Dietary supplements "can cut your risk of cancer by 50 percent," says Dr. Heinrich Wrba, head of the Cancer Research Institute at Austria's University of Vienna.

Indeed the good news is spreading like wild fire.
•*Time* magazine reported in April 1992 that nutritional supplements are a key to increasing human life span and that they can help us double our vital

years. "Antioxidants," reports *Time*, "may one day revolutionize health care." For example, says the magazine, "Doctors at Harvard Medical School, who have been following 22,000 male physicians as part of a 10-year health study, have made a stunning discovery about beta carotene. They found that men with a history of cardiac disease, who were given beta carotene supplements of 50 milligrams every other day, suffered half as many heart attacks, strokes and deaths as those popping [only] placebo pills."

•The pioneering studies of Dr. Bess Dawson-Hughes, chief of the Tufts Calcium and Bone Metabolism Laboratory, have shown that calcium supplements not only build new bone in postmenopausal women, they reduce fracture rates. That's important news when you consider that thinning bones cause 1.2 million fractures annually. "It's time to increase our calcium intake," Dr. Dawson-Hughes told the *Chicago Tribune* recently. "No more hedging. No more excuses. No more nothing. Just get the calcium intake up."

•*How about adding an additional 35 healthy years to your life?* "By the proper intakes of vitamins and other nutrients and

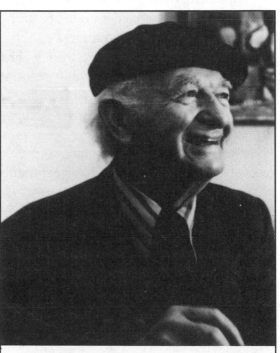

Linus Pauling, Ph.D., is one of the leading researchers and proponents of optimal nutrition. His research has focused on the ability of optimal nutrients to help prevent and fight off disease states including oxidative stress and aging. Dr. Pauling's own supplement program consists of some 18 grams daily of vitamin C, in addition to other nutrients. At 93, he is as active as ever—living proof of the powers of optimal nutrition.

by following a few other healthful practices from youth or middle age on, you can, I believe, extend your life and years of well-being by twenty-five or even thirty-five years," says Dr. Linus Pauling in his wonderful book *How to Live*

Longer and Feel Better. Dr. Pauling strongly advocates optimal nutritional habits including the daily use of dietary supplements. Indeed, Pauling is living proof that vitamin and mineral supplements help prolong life. The two time Nobel Prize laureate, now 92, continues to work long hours daily—and he supplements his diet with an array of dietary nutrients, including 18 grams of vitamin C daily mixed with his morning orange juice.

•Other experts agree with Dr. Pauling. Professor Emeritus of Medicine and Biochemistry at the University of Nebraska Denham Harman, the founder of the free radical theory on aging, says that antioxidants in an optimal nutrition program are the key to extending life. *The same supplements readily available to you and which you are going to learn about have been shown in experimental studies to have the potential to add 25 to 30 vital years to your life, Dr. Harman says.* In one such study, experimental mice were fed the free radical-fighting substance 2-mercaptoethylamine and their life span increased by 30 percent. *"This increase," Dr. Harman says, "is equivalent to raising the human life span from 73 to 95 years."*

•A year long study of senior citizens, conducted by Dr. Ranjit Chandra of the Memorial University of Newfoundland in St. John's, found that those people who received daily vitamin and mineral supplements had 40 to 50 percent fewer days of illness as compared to seniors who got only placebos.

•Following the results of worldwide studies associating optimal blood levels of vitamin E with lower risk for heart disease, the World Health Organization has begun advising European men and women to supplement their diets with vitamin E to help them prevent cardiovascular illnesses.

•University of California researchers say their studies of more than 11,000 men and women show that *supplementing your diet with vitamin C alone can add as much as six healthy years of life for men and a smaller number of years for women.*

These remarkable breakthroughs in longevity—and the extension of vitality into what was considered old age—are only the tip of the iceberg. People are getting the message and they're feeling empowered, using nutritional supplements as a means of keeping themselves healthy well into their golden years.

It seems that we Americans are catching on that good health and a long life can be ours—with the help of optimal nutrition. And that means taking our supplements daily!

The *Chicago Tribune* reports, "One of the most profound discoveries to date is that our diet not only supplies our bodies with energy and protein, it also is key to determining how well our genes manage life processes— whether, for instance, they putt along, or shut down, or perform like Olympic athletes."

Beyond Vitamins & Minerals

The excitement isn't being fanned simply by vitamins and minerals.

Many researchers report that their most important and promising discoveries go beyond the simple ABCs of nutritional supplementation that some of us learned about in our high school health courses. Nutritional detectives today are discovering the longevity, anti-disease potential of a new class of youth-enhancing nutrients that appear to have the power to improve our gene performance. Called *phytochemicals*, these nutrients are being uncovered in foods such as alfalfa, garlic, lemon and licorice—all sorts of fruits, vegetables and grains. The substances being isolated are known technically as anthocyanosides, limonoids, glucarates, phenolic acids, flavonoids, coumarins, polyacetylenes and carotenoids, and scientists believe that they will prove to be more potent than even vitamins and minerals (Kotulak 1991). Phytochemicals are neither vitamins nor minerals, yet they are equally potent and vital to the healthy functioning of our bodies. The name phytochemical is derived from the Greek word *phyto*, meaning plant, and very simply means a plant substance.

It isn't surprising that researchers have found key phytochemicals in a host of both rare and common plants. After all, many of our most important drug therapies, from aspirin, which was derived from willow bark, to the newly discovered anti-cancer medication taxol whose source is the Pacific yew tree, were isolated from nature's drug store. In the case of other lesser known but no less important phytochemicals—they have been demonstrated to have strong potential for palliating the physical effects of stress, improving our body's overall immunity as well as helping prevent the major killing diseases of Americans today like atherosclerosis, cancer, diabetes, high blood pressure, and stroke.

One example of the multiple capabilities of the phytochemicals is *Echinacea* which contains substances that destroy the germs of infection directly, and bolster the body's defenses by magnifying the white blood cell count (Mowrey 1986).

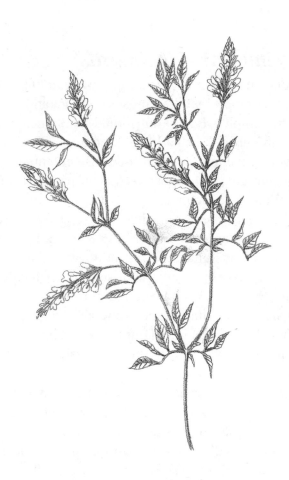

Medicago sativa has been shown to protect again radiation, reduce cholesterol, and act much like a natural antibiotic against bacterial illness. It is only one of many herbal medicines Nature has provided us with to keep our bodies and minds strong and healthy.

Meanwhile *Medicago sativa* (alfalfa) is known to contain an array of important substances including several saponins, many sterols, flavonoids, coumarins, alkaloids, acids, sugars, proteins and trace elements. Saponins in *Medicago sativa* have been shown to inhibit increases in blood cholesterol levels by 25 percent when high cholesterol diets are fed to monkeys, rats and rabbits (Malinow 1976, 1977, 1979; Cookson 1967, 1968). French scientists have shown that *Medicago sativa* can reduce tissue damage caused by radiotherapy (De Froment 1974), while other researchers note that it possesses antibacterial action against gram negative bacteria such as *Salmonella typhi* (Gestetner 1971) and contains at least one protein with known anti-tumor activity (Tyihak 1970). *Medicago sativa* is also a fiber which has been shown, along with bran and pectin, to bind and neutralize various types of agents carcinogenic to the colon (Smith-Barbaro 1981). Finally, some work suggests that *Medicago sativa* inactivates dietary chemical carcinogens in the liver and small intestine before they have a chance to do the body any harm (Wattenberg 1975).

Many more sources of dynamic phytochemicals are found in nature's drug store and we can use them to achieve a long healthy life through optimal nutrition:

•Animal and human research has established *Allium sativum*'s ability to lower blood serum cholesterol levels (Kritchevsky 1975, Bordia 1973).

•Liver damage from exposure to carbon tetrachloride has been mitigated in experimental animal subjects with use of *Angelica sinensis*.

•Kelp contains antioxidant, anticarcinogenic and anti-toxic properties and has been demonstrated to help prevent breast cancer in women (Hirayama 1978, Wynder 1979, Kagawa 1978, Fujimoto 1979, Nomura 1978).

We are perched on the edge of virtual eternity. Longer periods of youthfulness can be ours. Why is this important?

Think about your youth, counsels Dr. Pauling in his writings. For many people, the years of their youth are times of not only joy but misery and unhappiness, he says, adding: It is only when people reach their thirties—sometimes their forties—that they truly learn how to enjoy life and derive sustained happiness. But just as this happiness is settling in, for all too many people physical infirmities follow—heart disease, arthritis, senility. If people are destined to lose their physical health by the time they reach their late fifties, sixties or seventies, that period of sustained happiness will be shortened. On the other hand, through optimal nutritional habits—and other health practices that we are going to detail—you can sustain the golden, happy years of life for a much longer period than ever before. You will retain your youth, vigor and vitality. For most people who use optimal nutrition habits, when they retire at age 65, the party is only just beginning.

Nobody in America has ever lived to die of old age. People die of cancer, heart disease, Alzheimer's disease or some other condition long before they die of old age. These are afflictions of a diseased state—not old age. No human has made it to old age. "Aging is written into our species script; how long we can potentially live is called our maximum life-span, which is currently considered to be about one hundred and twenty years," writes Dr. Jeffrey Fisher, M.D. in his book *Rx 2000* (Simon & Schuster 1992). "Since average life expectancy at birth is not even eighty years, this leaves a lot of years to add to our expectations. Given all the advances we're going to see in controlling and alleviating the diseases of aging, achieving theoretical maximum life span is beginning to be a realistic hope. And once we achieve it, we'll push it further—to one hundred fifty and beyond."

"Aging research is still in its infancy, but what's already certain is that one of the causes of aging that we *will* be able to do something about is in our genes."

By the year 2000 medical science will have decoded virtually the entire human genome. "Maybe there are major genes in humans that, if we alter [them], could project a longer human life span," molecular biologist Thomas Johnson told the *Los Angeles Times*. "This would be an absolutely tremendous sociological finding. It would . . . affect every aspect of the way we live our lives if we all of a sudden had average life spans of 120 years instead of 70 years" (Stolberg 1992).

The *Times* describes Johnson's work as on the "cutting edge" of a fascinating scientific sojourn—a modern-day quest for the legendary Fountain of Youth. "He is among a growing corps of 2,000 molecular biologists, geneticists, immunologists and other researchers across the United States who are trying to unlock the secrets of aging," reports the *Los Angeles Times.*

"They are tinkering with genes, human growth hormones and new drugs, and with strategies of diet, nutrition and exercise . . . . Their strides in recent years have been so significant that a startling new body of thought has emerged, one that says humans may one day live much longer than anyone dreamed possible. Some go so far as to say that the maximum life span, now at 120 years, and average life expectancy, about 75 years in the United States, could double or triple."

"The ideal of all of our work is sometime in the future, we would take pills that would slow or postpone our aging," University of California at Irvine biologist Michael Rose told the *Los Angeles Times.*

Already researchers are exploring the use of human growth hormone and an endocrine rejuvenator, known by its acronym DHEA, to reverse signs of aging such as the shrinking of certain organs and increased fatty deposits.

And if you take care of your body today, who knows what miracles the future will bring to sustain your health for more years than you can even imagine?

Are you ready for one of the most incredible journeys of your life?

The information contained in the following pages is your key to health and longevity. These are the modern nutritional breakthroughs proven to extend life and promote optimal health.

1. The RDAs

*Is it possible that the primates in a science laboratory are
better fed than the average American man or woman?
You bet!*

We've all seen nutritional labels attached to food product containers.
And many of us have noticed that the amounts of vitamins and minerals shown
on the labels are usually expressed as a percentage of the U.S. Recommended
Dietary Allowance.

Experts advising the federal government created the RDA concept many
years ago. In 1941, the Food and Nutrition Board of the National Research
Council of the Academy of Sciences was established by the government to
safeguard public health, explains Dr. Earl Mindell, R.Ph., Ph.D., author of
Vitamin Bible (Warner Books 1991). "They are not meant to be optimal intake,
nor are they recommendations for an ideal diet," says Dr. Mindell. Essentially
the RDA for each vitamin and mineral is the Food and Nutrition Board's
estimate of the *minimum* amount of that vitamin or mineral a person needs on
a daily basis to prevent nutrient-deficiency diseases such as scurvy in the case
of inadequate vitamin C intake or the scaly dermatitis condition known as
pellagra which occurs in the absence of nicotinic acid, one of the B vitamins.

Making sure that you meet the RDA for each vitamin and mineral is all very well and good--and even adequate--if you're living in a Third World nation where nutritional deficiencies are common. But here in one of the richest, most agriculturally and technologically advanced nations in the world, nutritional deficiencies, while important, are no longer the only concern of nutritionists.

"If you look at most conventional doctors, they are of the opinion that vitamins are necessary to prevent diseases like beri beri, scurvy, and pellagra," says Joseph Weissman, M.D., a board-certified immunologist, author of *Choose to Live* and clinical assistant professor at the University of California at Los Angeles School of Medicine. "These three are very obvious diseases of deficiency, and certainly you can get enough vitamins and other nutrients in your foods to prevent those conditions. But when it comes to most conventional doctors' recommendations on the intake of antioxidants, they are fighting a war with bows and arrows instead

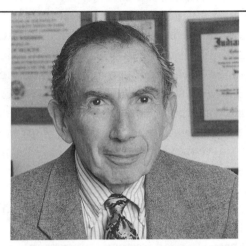

Joseph Weissman, M.D., discovered the need for optimal nutrition through a tragedy in his own family. When he went on to author *Choose to Live*, Dr. Weissman discovered that the *X Factor* is a major cause of illness, and that supplementation with antioxidants and other important protective substances can help deter the damage caused by exposure to environmental pollution.

of high-tech electronic equipment. They completely ignore the need of antioxidants to prevent disease through their ability to attack free radicals. I disagree with such doctors who tell you that you don't need to supplement."

"When I wrote *Choose To Live* in 1989," continues Dr. Weissman, "I detailed the pervasive rise of chemical and physical pollution that today threatens our health. Under these modern day circumstances with so much pollution exposing us to what I call the *X Factor*, what is in the diet is just not enough. It may have been enough two hundred years ago. But you need more protection in this day and age. Our environment is polluted, as are our foods, and drinking water, and you need all the protection you can get. It is important that people be aware that they need to take antioxidants of all types and in large amounts."

This emphasis Dr. Weissman puts today on supplementation, especially with antioxidants, represents a shift in his own thinking. "If we go back ten years ago, I was a very traditional physician. I found the thought of taking vitamins to be personally repugnant. I would never recommend them to patients. It was my feeling that the vitamins and minerals in your foods were adequate. But a tragedy in our own family changed my belief in medicine as I practiced it then. My son-in-law died at a very young age of a heart attack."

That was when he began research for *Choose To Live* and he discovered the history of all our major illnesses and how they were extremely rare before the industrial revolution, and how they are so prevalent today.

Once that thought came to mind, he knew the next step would be to learn what people should do to protect their health. "In order for people to be healthy today, I now realize, they *must* make a major reassessment of their lifestyle," says Dr. Weissman.

"There is a need for more antioxidants than are available in the diet. They are going to neutralize these chemicals and other substances that produce free radicals. Although I am not certain of the amount that should be taken, I tend to err on the side of taking high doses."

Today, the real action in nutritional science is finding out how much more than the RDAs is needed for peak nutrition—for the kind of winning, optimal nutritional habits that can add years to your life and life to your years!

RDA Represents Minimal Nutritional Needs

The RDA estimates were created many years ago and are based on experimental animal studies in which one vitamin, mineral or other nutrient is removed from the diet of mice or rats to purposely make them sick. Researchers gradually return small, measured amounts of the nutrient to their diet until the animals are able to reproduce and show no clinical disease symptoms. In other words if you consume no more than the RDA you will be consuming the absolute bare minimum amount of nutrients required for minimal health maintenance. You will not suffer from diseases linked with nutritional deficiencies. But that's all. An analogy would be like buying or building a house with walls, floor, and roof but nothing else. Sure, you own a house and it will protect you from the rain and the heat of the burning sun—but not much else. In the same way, simply maintaining the RDAs will keep you from dying of nutritional deficiency but will not provide you with the maximum benefits to be derived from *optimal* nutrition.

Who's Healthier?

Yet, evidence is mounting that there is a great deal of vitality and health that we can gain from nutrients when we include them in our diet at levels exceeding the RDAs. Ironically, laboratory animals may enjoy more nutritious diets than some people. Two-time Nobel Prize winner Linus Pauling (1986) says he's "impressed" by the fact that the Committee on the Feeding of Laboratory Animals of the U.S. National Academy of Sciences-National Research Council (NAS-NRC) recommends far more vitamin C for monkeys than the Food and Nutrition Board of the same NAS-NRC recommends for human beings.

Dr. Pauling goes on to say he is quite certain that, "the first committee has worked hard to find the *optimum* intake for the monkeys, the amount that puts them in the best of health." Yet, he's very critical of the dietary recommendations for humans made by the same organization. The NAS-NRC Food and Nutrition Board which determines human nutritional needs, he says, "has not made any effort to find the optimum intake of vitamin C or of any other vitamin for the American people."

In fact, says Dr. Pauling, "In its Recommended Daily Allowances, so well publicized that they are referred to on breakfast-cereal boxes by the initials RDA, the committee rations the vitamins at not much above the minimum daily intake required to prevent the particular deficiency disease that is associated with each of them."

Why is this? Dr. Pauling (1986) observes that FDA's antipathy towards nutrient supplements, "is the result of ignorance, bias, misunderstanding of the nature of vitamins and other orthomolecular substances, and lack of hope or visio—they seem to have the conviction that nothing new can be discovered."

It's troubling to leading edge nutritional experts that all too many apparently well-intentioned physicians, dietitians, and nutritionists are telling the lay public that simply meeting the RDA requirements is enough. Indeed we know of one well known media personality who is busy telling the American public that they can obtain all the nutrients they need from the average diet and that using optimal nutritional strategies will produce nothing more than expensive urine!

That kind of misinformed hype may sound good on a 30 second bite on a television news program but the information itself simply flies in the face of the thousands of nutritional studies conducted in this country that have found that the general public often cannot even meet the minimal requirements of the RDAs—as a result of lifestyles that may include fast food meals, overly processed foods, and foods robbed of their nutrition by overcooking, poor storage and the depleted soils in which they've been grown.

People who believe these assertions—put forward by well-meaning but poorly informed health professionals—are depriving themselves of the opportunity to live healthy long lives well into their nineties and beyond. Indeed, these people spreading such fallacious information ultimately may be doing themselves or the people they advise a great deal of harm. People who disparage dietary supplements may well end their days finding themselves having totally lost their independence and laying in hospital beds undergoing heart bypass surgery, chemotherapy or surgery for hip replacements. That's the current progression for all too many Americans who're meeting those self-same RDAs!

We can do better!

Minimal nutrition simply is not enough for sustained longevity and health. As Dr. Pauling (1986) says so clearly, "No evidence compels the conclusion that the minimum required intake of any vitamin comes close to the optimum intake that sustains good health."

In fact, to the contrary, there's a tremendous body of evidence that optimal nutrition goes far beyond the minimal RDAs set by the federal Government.

What Is The 'Ideal' Amount of Vitamins?

How much higher above the RDAs should people supplement their diets?

That's a key question and it's the question that Emanuel Cheraskin, M.D., D.M.D., posed more than 30 years ago. Professor Emeritus at the University of Alabama Medical School, Dr. Cheraskin has published more than 460 medical papers and has some 210 citations to his credit in the National Library of Medicine. Dr. Cheraskin decided to find a large group of the absolutely healthiest people around and to see what nutrients they were consuming and in what amounts.

He mailed two nationally recognized survey forms—the Cornell Medical Index and the Standard Food Frequency Questionnaire to several thousand dentists and their families. The Cornell form obtains very personal health information including subtle, often overlooked symptoms of illness such as aches, pains, colds, and allergies. The Standard Food Frequency questionnaire obtains information on the quantity and frequency of all foods eaten in a person's diet over a period of time, in addition to data on nutritional supplements regularly used by respondents.

Results Confirm
RDAs Don't Provide Optimal Health

Not surprisingly, the people in the survey with the highest nutrient intake were the healthiest and had the fewest symptoms of illness. Conversely, Dr. Cheraskin found, the less nutrients that were ingested, the more prevalent were the nagging symptoms of ill health. But what was surprising was that the healthiest people were exceeding the government RDAs for vitamins and minerals by five to ten times.

Dr. Cheraskin continued his research, surveying and monitoring his study group of 2,000 dentists and their wives for more than 20 years. He also completed many other supplemental double blind nutritional studies to confirm the initial findings from his original study group. In virtually every study, the healthiest subjects were ingesting five to ten times more of the nutrients than recommended by the RDAs. In a recent telephone conversation, Dr. Cheraskin expressed his strong belief in the influence of dietary factors on personal health. Sure, he said, genetic inheritance is important. But at present, there is not much that can be done about what we inherit. Yet the potential in our genetic inheritance—especially for disease—doesn't have to manifest itself, he went on, because we can modify the influence of our genes by what we do—by what we eat, by how we live. In other words, disease is not predestined. Whether you will be stricken with a disease is often determined by what you do—especially by your diet! You have the power!

Independent Studies Confirm Dr. Cheraskin's Findings

If Dr. Cheraskin's findings were unique from the results of all other such studies, they would be suspect. We really couldn't rely on them. We would have to think that perhaps in some subtle way the physician's passion for optimal nutrition would have prejudiced his results through data interpretation or the study protocols. We would look at them with interest but nothing more simply could be made of them. In Western science, it is only when a study's results can be replicated by another independent research effort that we begin to take notice and give credence to the researcher's findings. In fact, hundreds—perhaps thousands—of studies, many of which are going on at this very moment, have confirmed and will continue to confirm Dr. Cheraskin's pioneering work.

For example:

•In the area of research on the nutritional benefits of optimal ascorbic acid intake, Miller (1977) reports in his investigations for the Eli Lilly company that young, identical twins (aged six to eleven) were given either five times the RDA of vitamin C or received only the vitamin C from the food they consumed. After five months, virtually all twins receiving megadoses of Vitamin C grew more in height—by as much as one inch—than their identical brother or sister.

•Scientists used double blind procedures to test the value of high-dose ascorbic acid supplementation, taking 20 infertile men and giving them a gram of vitamin C daily for 60 days. A second group was given a placebo supplement. At the end of the 60 day period, all wives of the men in the group given megadoses of vitamin C were pregnant; none of the wives had conceived in the placebo group.

•Biochemist Simin Nikbin Meydani "dramatically" increased the immune responses of elderly people by 10 to 70 percent when he gave vitamin E supplements that were 80 to 100 times higher than the RDA (Kotulak 1991).

•In an examination of the role of broad-based nutritional supplements which took place at the Memorial University of Newfoundland in St. John's and was published in 1992 in *Lancet*, Dr. Ranjit Chandra conducted a yearlong double blind study that conclusively demonstrated that those senior citizens who got a daily supplement of vitamins and minerals had a 40 to 50 percent reduction in days of illness.

•Optimal intake of vitamins C and E can help prevent cellular damage to the eye caused by oxygen free radicals which translates in everyday terms to the enhanced prevention of cataract formation (Robertson 1991). Researchers writing in the *American Journal of Clinical Nutrition* report that they have, "Fair to good evidence for causal association between supplementary vitamin C and E consumption and freedom from senile cataracts." Their study, they say, "suggests that the consumption of supplementary vitamins C and E may reduce the risk of senile cataracts by about 50 to 70 percent" (Robertson 1991). This news is especially important in light of the more than 500,000 cataract operations performed annually in the United States.

•Italian researchers reporting in the *Journal of the National Cancer Institute* report that dietary supplementation with vitamins A, C and E seems to be effective in reducing cell proliferation abnormalities in normal-appearing rectal tissue in patients with colorectal cancer (Paganelli 1992). In other words, these researchers reporting in a highly conservative, mainstream medical journal assert that simply put: nutritional supplements seem to have important, life extending anti-cancer effects.

•Various micronutrients may interact *synergistically* in the prevention of cancer. Ramesha (1990) and colleagues, reporting in the *Japanese Journal of Cancer,* found that the combined actions of selenium, magnesium, ascorbic acid and retinyl acetate prevented mammary cancer in experimental animal subjects exposed to the highly carcinogenic chemical 7,12-dimethylbenz[*a*]anthracene.

Do We Meet the RDAs?

Given the wonderful body of knowledge we now have about the benefits we can derive from vitamins, minerals and other nutrients including phytochemicals when they are ingested in optimal amounts often exceeding the RDAs, we must ask whether or not we can make optimal nutrition an everyday part of our lives.

Some physicians and nutrition experts contend that we can get all the nutrients that we need from the average daily diet. But that argument simply doesn't stand up to scientific scrutiny. Dr. Cheraskin estimates that if every adult in the United States answered the Cornell Medical Index and Standard Food Frequency questionnaires only five percent of the respondents would be considered very healthy. Millions of Americans, in fact, wouldn't even be meeting the minimal requirements of the government RDAs, much less the optimal guidelines discovered by Dr. Cheraskin and other researchers. For example:

•Only *one in ten* Americans even eats the recommended minimum of five servings of fruits and vegetables a day.

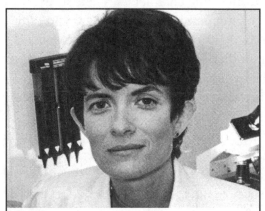

Many fractures in the elderly could be prevented with adequate intake of calcium, says Megan Shields, M.D., a diplomate of the American Board of Family Practice and researcher specializing in the field of chemically related illness. Dr. Shields agrees with other experts who assert that, "It's time to increase our calcium uptake," adding that calcium citrate is the most bioavailable form of calcium to supplement. Dr. Shields also suggests that people begin exercising *now* in order to prevent osteoporosis.

•Even the conservative and sometimes anti-dietary supplement American Medical Association (AMA), which has long maintained that all the nutrients you need can be obtained from a well-balanced diet, has conceded that we may need supplements. Society's overreliance on highly processed foods, between-meal snacks and fast food restaurants results in nutrient-depletion, the AMA has finally acknowledged.

•At the nation's premiere aging research center, the Tufts Human Nutrition Research Center on Aging, Associate Director Dr. Jeffrey B. Blumberg notes that a study of some 1,000 elderly people provided strong evidence that diet alone cannot meet their nutritional needs. The majority of these elderly were consuming at best only 66 percent of the RDAs for minerals and vitamins such as calcium and zinc, and vitamins B-6, B-12, D and folic acid.

•In the Baltimore Longitudinal Study on Aging, nutritionist Judith Hallfrisch was totally surprised by the results of her work which focused on people who were representative of the educated upper middle class and yet who still consumed nutritionally deficient diets lacking proper amounts of iron, magnesium and vitamin E.

One of the interesting nutritional lessons that Dr. Hallfrisch learned is that a common affliction of the elderly, dementia, may be nutritionally related. In fact, she believes that around five

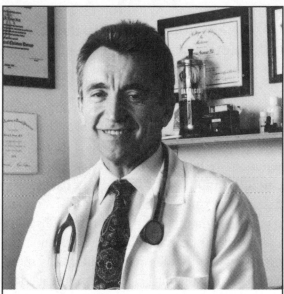

Murray Susser, M.D., past president of the American College of Advancement in Medicine, concurs with other experts that using a daily, broad-based multivitamin, multimineral supplement formulated with nutrients higher than the RDA is a "conservative and very rational thing to do, especially for older people."

percent of people classified as having dementia are probably sickened by suboptimal intake of vitamins in the vitamin B complex. In addition, she warns that the low standards adopted in the RDA for vitamin C aren't enough for optimal immune function.

•Consuming even the minimal amount of calcium would go a long way towards prevention of osteoporosis, says Dr. Bess Dawson-Hughes, chief of the Tufts Calcium and Bone Metabolism Laboratory. Although the RDA for calcium is 800 milligrams daily, the average woman, aged 44 and older, gets less than 500 mg in her daily diet. Each year, Americans suffer some 1.2 million fractures because of thinning bones. Sadly, 20 percent of the 250,00 people who suffer hip fractures annually, die as a result of their injury, and another 20 percent are immobilized for life. And this kind of injury is so preventable through optimal nutrition. Dr. Dawson-Hughes's work demonstrates that calcium supplements help build new bone in women at least six years beyond menopause and reduced their fracture rate (Kotulak 1991). She told reporters, "It's time to increase our calcium intake. No more hedging. No more excuses. No more nothing. Just get the calcium intake up."

•The lesson here is that optimal nutritional habits and the use of dietary supplements (when and where needed) should begin not when people become sick but when they are healthy. Waiting until people are diseased is the wrong time to start being concerned over dietary intake of key nutrients—especially when we're talking osteoporosis. For example, there is strong evidence that calcium supplements should be a part of even the diets of children, based on fascinating studies at the Indiana University School of Medicine in Indianapolis. Experiments with identical twins demonstrated that the siblings who received extra calcium in their diets had nearly three percent more bone than their genetically identical counterparts three years later, reports the *Chicago Tribune* (Kotulak 1991). This increased bone mass early in life may well prevent disabling fractures of the hip and osteoporosis later in life.

It's no wonder with this tremendous body of knowledge that Dr. William Evans, chief of the Tufts University Health Science Center's human physiology laboratory, concludes that, "Many of the biological markers of aging are not valid at all. Rather, they are markers of inactivity and poor nutrition" (Kotulak 1991).

He adds that, "*Taking a broad-based, multivitamin, multimineral supplement formulated at one to two times the RDA is a conservative and very rational thing to do, especially for older people*" (Kotulak 1991).

"Even if you have only minor health problems now, you should still be vitally concerned about your daily nutrient intake. Those minor symptoms are sometimes indicators of potentially much more devastating illnesses," Dr. Cheraskin asserts, adding that, "Many people believe one suddenly contracts disease as though one has suddenly gotten a virus or bacterial infection. But many diseases are progressive. Diabetics may begin as five percent diabetic but because they ignore initially minor subclinical symptoms the disease becomes progressively more devastating."

One of nutritional science's most valuable discoveries is the honest realization that people truly cannot obtain optimal amounts of nutrients from the ordinary foods and beverages that are consumed in the typical diet. Sometimes this dietary deficiency results from nutrient loss during processing, cooking, shipping or storage. At other times, fresh fruits and vegetables are unavailable or prohibitively expensive. Finally, our fast-paced modern lifestyles do not always afford us the opportunity to eat for optimal nutrition. Of course, that doesn't mean that because we recognize the difficulty inherent in obtaining optimal nutrition from our daily diets that we have *carte blanche* to give up on the idea of a good diet and that we can all go on junk food binges, and simply start popping megadoses of vitamin pills. No way! You still must do your best to achieve an optimal daily diet in the foods that you select to fuel your body. The nutrients and fiber you obtain from wholesome everyday foods like fresh fruits, vegetables, grains, meats, dairy, seafood, nuts and seeds are crucial to your health. All we're saying is that if people honestly and objectively examine their nutritional habits, they will find that their everyday diet alone probably isn't enough to achieve optimal dietary standards.

The Total Formula

Because realistically an optimal nutritional intake is truly difficult to achieve from a daily diet alone, many physicians and nutritional experts assert that most people need nutritional supplements for optimal health. The question, of course, is what vitamins, minerals and phytochemicals are the best and most essential for protection against major killing diseases and even minor illnesses. Many experts believe that a good place to start is with an integrated, well-balanced and broad-based daily nutritional supplement.

Many experts such as Dr. Cheraskin, Dr. Hans Kugler, Ph.D., President of the National Health Federation, and Dr. Richard Passwater, Ph.D., author of *The New Supernutrition* believe that an effective supplement program should contain a minimum of some 30 different vitamins, minerals, bioflavonoids and enzymes in quantities significantly greater than the federal RDAs, which are just not enough. Indeed, some of the nutrients recommended by Drs. Cheraskin, Kugler and Passwater haven't even made it yet to the RDA list although they are universally considered vital to healthy lives.

Many of the nutrients that are recommended are well known antioxidants like vitamins A, C, and E. Your body needs a generous supply of these vitamins for many facets of health including optimal cardiovascular function and protection against cancer. Vitamin A (in the form of its safe, nontoxic precursor beta carotene) is extremely protective against lung disease caused by cigarette smoke and pollution. Vitamin C can help detoxify toxic chemicals. For example, when you eat preserved and cured meats such as bacon or bologna, you ingest a chemical called nitrite or nitrate which can interact with substances in your body to form carcinogenic nitrosamines which are, in turn, suspected of causing colon cancer. But vitamin C can actually prevent this reaction from occuring. As for vitamin E, its healthy heart benefits, including tissue oxygen saturation, have been well documented for more than half a century. Each of these nutrients also helps prevent the formation of oxygen free radicals.

Also, of extreme importance are the B vitamins in amounts substantially greater than the RDAs. Among the most important for a dietary supplement are vitamins B-1 (thiamin), B-2 (riboflavin), B-6 and B-12 (cyanocobalamin). The B vitamins help release energy from the food we eat by converting carbohydrates into glucose and increase our ability to fight fatigue. Vitamin B-1 is an excellent antistress nutrient. Furthermore, without enough vitamin B-1 we would suffer severe brain disorders similar in effect to senile dementia. The B complex-related nutrients choline and lecithin are two nutrients that the body needs in order to produce acetylcholine, a neurotransmitting chemical that allows us to transmit messages from the brain to other nerve cells. Recently, the U.S. Centers for Disease Control and Prevention has recommended that pregnant women should be sure to supplement their diets with the B complex nutrient folic acid in order to prevent the occurrence of neural tube birth defects.

Additional minerals that should be in a daily formula include calcium and magnesium in a two to one ratio, especially as a preventive for bone loss as people age. Did you know that every single cell in your body contains calcium? Did you know that calcium regulates your heart beat and that diets rich in calcium can help prevent coronary heart disease and hypertension? Calcium may even help prevent cancer by contributing to the orderly reproduction of your cells. Calcium is often used to help the body excrete heavy metals such as lead. A calcium-rich diet will prevent significant lead absorption in people who have an adequate iron intake. Since today, we are bombarded with lead in our food, water and air, this is especially vital. Scientists have noted that calcium-rich diets actually alleviate the symptoms of anxiety, and they speculate that a calcium-deficient diet may result in anxiety disorders with symptoms such as heart palpitation, tremors, nausea, choking sensations, and blurred vision. Yet, as we shall learn, not just any old form of calcium will do; only certain forms of this mineral are readily utilized by the body.

Zinc supplementation, of course, is essential, says Dr. Kugler, noting that the American diet is often deficient in this mineral. Men, especially, he says are prone to deficiencies in zinc which can then lead to sexual impotency and prostate disease.

And as we will learn, manganese and copper are greatly needed by the body to produce one of its key antioxidants, superoxide dismutase. Furthermore copper plays a role in the production of blood hemoglobin. Indeed, some anemia can be cured only when iron is supplemented with copper. Copper also helps the body use vitamin C. Copper is also able to prevent weakening of the walls of blood vessels, most notably the aorta, thus helping in the prevention of aneurysms and ruptures. Copper also helps prevent radiation damage, which may be in part why the pancreas, spleen and even white blood cells—all of which are naturally low in copper—are the organs most susceptible to radiation damage.

Then there is selenium, another absolutely essential micronutrient. Working together with vitamin E, selenium enhances immune function. It has been shown to prevent cancer, slow the aging process and prevent heart and circulatory diseases. According to Michael Weiner, Ph.D., author of the excellent book *Reducing the Risk of Alzheimer's,* selenium together with vitamin E can play an instrumental role in prevention of Alzheimer's disease.

There are many more important substances including bilberry for vision protection, pycnogenols which are extremely potent oxygen free radical scavengers and hesperidin which is a crucial member of the vitamin C complex.

Nobody is guaranteed a long, healthy life, one that is vital and exciting well into the golden years. Give yourself the best chance for a longer, healthier life. By following optimal nutritional guidelines, basing your dietary supplementation on a foundation such as the guidelines listed *above*, you will certainly provide yourself with the best opportunity for an active, healthy life well into your nineties or older. That's what optimal nutrition is all about!

The Aging Process

The signs of aging happen at different rates in different people but invariably they are nature's way of warning us that we are not immortal--at least not yet! Unfortunately, many of the signs of aging occur subtly and are not noticeable right away. Furthermore, they also occur subclinically and are not easily diagnosed by physicians--until it is too late! That's why it is imperative to take a proactive approach to delaying the aging process.

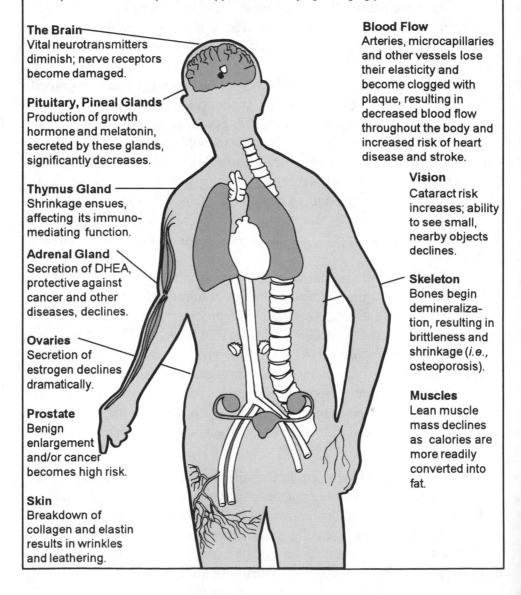

The Brain
Vital neurotransmitters diminish; nerve receptors become damaged.

Pituitary, Pineal Glands
Production of growth hormone and melatonin, secreted by these glands, significantly decreases.

Thymus Gland
Shrinkage ensues, affecting its immuno-mediating function.

Adrenal Gland
Secretion of DHEA, protective against cancer and other diseases, declines.

Ovaries
Secretion of estrogen declines dramatically.

Prostate
Benign enlargement and/or cancer becomes high risk.

Skin
Breakdown of collagen and elastin results in wrinkles and leathering.

Blood Flow
Arteries, microcapillaries and other vessels lose their elasticity and become clogged with plaque, resulting in decreased blood flow throughout the body and increased risk of heart disease and stroke.

Vision
Cataract risk increases; ability to see small, nearby objects declines.

Skeleton
Bones begin demineraliza-tion, resulting in brittleness and shrinkage (*i.e.*, osteoporosis).

Muscles
Lean muscle mass declines as calories are more readily converted into fat.

2. The Free Radical Theory of Aging

Life is a contradiction. Its only consistency is that two truths, totally opposite in effect, often occur simultaneously. The breath of life is oxygen. The kiss of death is oxygen.

Oxygen is our savior. It is ultimately our greatest enemy as well.

When we learn of the mega-importance of oxygen to life and death, we can conceive of our own lives extending in years far greater in number than ever before imagined.

Many millions of years ago all plant and animal life was confined to the sea to escape the destructive and deadly force of ultraviolet radiation from the sun (Harman 1981). Back then at the dawn of life on earth, oxygen was not the life source. Rather, organisms produced energy by breaking down carbohydrates in a process called "glycolysis." Researchers believe that some 500 million years ago atmospheric concentrations of oxygen increased gradually and significantly. Because of this increase, the deadly forces of UV radiation became absorbed before they could destroy life. Life began to emerge from the seas. Evolution accelerated. Sixty-five million years ago primates appeared. Four to five million years ago appeared humans.

In order to stay alive, all cells must have an energy source, and that source is oxygen. But although oxygen enabled life to emerge from the oceans, oxygen also initiates changes that destroy life. In other words, oxygen is destructive. A human breathing pure oxygen could live only two days before his lungs would sustain so much oxygen-related damage that he would die. Fortunately the earth's air supply is composed of only 20 percent oxygen.

The human machine burns oxygen imperfectly and it produces harmful byproducts much like our imperfect harnessing of the atom produces destructive radioactive wastes. No problem. When prehistoric man was busy being chased by saber-toothed tigers and other woolly beasts, he wasn't concerned with a life span of 90 years; he would have settled for living beyond the next 90 seconds! It seems that for most of human kind's existence, Mother Nature didn't really intend for us to live much longer than 30 years—the time required to mature, breed and propogate the species. Men and women back then were breeding machines. Once humans procreated and passed on their genetic structure, it was time to die. Oxygen took care of that! The continual inhalation of oxygen, ultimately, is like a double-edge sword in that it sustains life but also ages the body.

The Free Radical Theory of Aging

An understanding of the dual nature of oxygen in life creation and destruction is essential in order to prolong life.

At least that's what leading experts on aging today like Dr. Denham Harman believe. Dr. Harman is considered the founder of the *free radical theory on aging* which asserts that oxygen-based compounds within our own bodies are the primary cause of human aging. These oxygen compounds, which we shall come to know well throughout the course of this book, are known as *oxygen free radicals.*

The free radical theory of aging, based on Dr. Harman's findings beginning in 1954, is one of the most important theories on life extension developed in the Twentieth Century. The 77-year old University of Nebraska emeritus professor of medicine and biochemistry told reporters recently, "Chances are 99 percent that free radicals are the basis for aging. Aging is the ever increasing accumulation of changes caused or contributed to by free radicals" (Kotulak 1991).

Dr. Earl Stadtman, chief of the laboratory of biochemistry of the National Heart, Lung and Blood Institute in Bethesda, Maryland, agrees that the damage caused by oxygen free radicals is a very important part of the aging process—much more important than medical science was willing to accept in the past. Human life span, says Dr. Stadtman, is dependent on cellular damage caused by oxygen free radicals. The body's cells do resist some oxidation damage but eventually they become so damaged that they can no longer function.

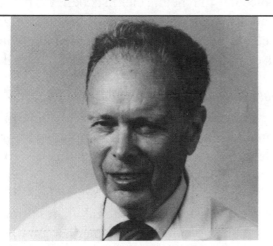

Denham Harman, M.D., Ph.D., is the founder of the Free Radical Theory of Aging, the most important paradigm of the Twentieth Century for understanding the aging process. Through his work, we have come to learn of the value of antioxidant nutrients such as beta carotene, vitamins C and E, in life extension. Dr. Harman, professor emeritus at the University of Nebraska, supplements his diet daily with vitamin E and zinc. He is now 77. Like many of the free radical theorists who have put their findings into practice, Dr. Harman is living proof that aging can be significantly delayed through diet. He is working as hard today as ever; annual meetings of the American Aging Association, under Dr. Harman's leadership, have become the premiere forum for scientists worldwide to present the latest findings in life extension!

Have you ever seen a piece of metal rusting away? Have you ever cut open an apple, and watched it turn brown after a few minutes? Those are two examples of the process called oxidation, caused by oxygen free radicals. The hardened metal and the softened apple both fall victim to oxidation and will eventually wear away. Oil-industry scientists in the 1930s showed that oxygen free radicals could produce spectacular chemical transformations such as the rancidification of fats and oils, says Dr. Roy Walford, M.D., in his book *The 120 Year Diet* (Simon and Schuster 1986). Ultimately, he says, "These discoveries gave birth to the development of the plastics and polymers industry."

What are Free Radicals?

They have been described as "great white sharks in the biochemical sea." They are "cellular renegades: they wreak havoc by damaging DNA, altering biochemical compounds, corroding cell membranes and killing cells outright," says *Time* magazine. "Such molecular mayhem, scientists believe, plays a major role in the development of ailments like cancer, heart or lung disease, and cataracts. The cumulative effects of free radicals also underlie the gradual deterioration that is the hallmark of aging in all individuals, healthy as well as sick."

Looking more closely at oxygen free radicals, we see that they are different from other molecules: their electrons—electrically charged particles found in all atoms and molecules—are unpaired and unbalanced. This is important to note.

Electrons virtually always orbit in pairs—and if electrons could, they'd tell you they'd always like to orbit in pairs. It is in their very nature to exist in pairs.

Now, the chemical reaction for energy creation in the human body is an imperfect process. It strips an electron away from an oxygen atom, resulting in an unpaired electron and very unstable molecule. This is neither good, nor stable.

This forms the notorious oxygen free radical. Because the oxygen free radical is so unstable, it desperately seeks to find a match. But an oxygen free radical can only get an electron from another molecule. This process of searching for a second electron creates cellular mayhem.

The unstable molecule knocks frantically against other molecules in an effort to attract away an electron. The process destablilizes additional molecules within other cells.

Says Dr. Walford, one of the nation's leading anti-aging researchers and founder of the immunological theory on aging, "Once generated, they grab on to everything in reach. And once triggered, free-radical reactions tend to be unstoppable, uncontrollable, and irreversible, almost explosive. Blam! Like Sodom and Gomorrah! Turn you into a pillar of rancid fat!" Incredibly, considering all the damage that they cause, the life span of an oxygen free radical is only a few thousandthsof a second.

Accumulating evidence indicates that aging is largely due to free radical reaction damage. Ultimately, explains Dr. Harman (1981), free radicals damage the coded messages of genes and damage enzymes and other cellular processes that occur in the mitochondria, the energy producing centers of the cells. Dr. Harman says that the damage to cellular mitochondria is especially noteworthy. He points out that mitochdondria—so essential to energy production for our bodies—are like biological time clocks and that death ensues when the function of the mitochondria is impaired below a critical level.

Oxygen free radicals released in our bodies also destroy the proteins that are essential constituents of our body and which regulate our hormones and enzymes and compose our nerves, muscles, skin, and hair. In other words, those wrinkles that we all fear are also the dirty work of oxygen free radicals.

Dr. Walford explains their effects: "Chief sites of attack are against cell membranes, both those inside cells (mitochondrial and nuclear membranes) and those forming the external walls of cells . . . . The radicals may also damage DNA, the hereditary blueprint for life within each cell. Indeed, many of the substances that cause or promote cancer may do so by stimulating cells to produce free radicals which then damage or alter the blueprint until the cell becomes cancerous."

Dr. Harman (1981) notes that studies strongly suggest that free radical reactions play a significant role in the age-related deterioration of the cardiovascular and central nervous systems. Free radical reactions may also be significantly involved in the formation of the neuritic plaques associated with senile dementia of the Alzheimer type, he says. These plaques were much higher in senile people than normal people.

Richard Passwater, Ph.D., (1991) describes free radicals as chemical terrorists and asserts that their reduction in number and protecting the body from their effects is the key to slowing aging and preventing cancer, heart disease and arthritis. One free radical can damage a million or more molecules.

"Free radicals alter cell membranes in such a way as to kill the cell or change it to a cancer cell," he says in his excellent book *The New Supernutrition* (Pocket Books 1991). "Free radicals can also bind compounds together in such a way as to alter their function or the physical characteristics of the entire tissue. As an example, young, babylike skin can be made as tough as leather by the actions of free radicals produced by sunlight."

Furthermore, according to Dr. Passwater, free radicals damage the body in a handful of ways by causing:

•Damage to fatty compounds causing them to turn rancid which causes the release of more free radicals.

•Undesirable cross linking between DNA and protein which prevents DNA from carrying out its replicative duties and instead produces cellular garbage.

•Loss of the optimal functioning of cellular membranes which disrupts nutrient absorption and waste disposal ultimately causing the death of the cell.

•Destruction of the lysosomal membrane allowing the spill over of lysosomes, which are strong cellular digestive enzymes, into the general areas of the cell and causing damage to other cell functions.

•Formation of lipofuscin, also known as age pigment, which accumulates in cells until it interferes with vital processes.

Over time, free radical damage accumulates especially in our cellular genetic materials. Dr. Bruce Ames, director of the National Institute of Environmental Health Sciences at the University of California at Berkeley, estimates that the genetic materials in each cell are hit 10,000 times a day by free radicals. The cells that are damaged ultimately repair themselves. But the repair process is only 99.9 percent perfect. Thus, everytime a cell is struck by an oxygen free radical, the damage becomes a little more devastating and the repair process a little less perfect; the damage to the cell is said to be *cumulative*. For example, one such free radical, called hydroxyl, damages the DNA in human breasts, and when enough damage accumulates to the genetic materials, cancer may follow, according to research performed by Dr. Donald Malins, a cancer researcher at the Pacific Northwest Research Foundation in Seattle and published in the journal *Cancer Research*.

Even as you're reading this passage, oxygen free radicals are being produced in your body at an enormous rate, they're streaming through your body's cells, creating molecular mayhem. Considering their destructive impact and the fact that the genetic materials of each cell are hit by oxygen free radicals some 10,000 times daily, our resilience is indeed miraculous!

Free radicals live only a millionth of a second and that has prevented researchers from studying them as thoroughly as they would like. Nevertheless, the body of research that has been built leads many experts to believe that oxygen free radicals are responsible for a plethora of maladies:

•Atherosclerosis

•Alzheimer's disease
•Cancer
•High blood pressure
•Schizophrenia
•Parkinson's
•Down's syndrome
•Stroke
•Paralysis
•Cataracts
•Arthritis
•Emphysema
•Hang-over
•Dandruff
•Wrinkling
•Memory loss
•A rapidly increasing list of other diseases of both major and minor significance.

Is It Possible That We Can Stop Oxygen Free Radical-Related Damage?

It seems that Mother Nature intended for us to reach our peak physical health in our third decade of life—primarily for the purpose of reproduction. Once we procreated and continued on the genetic transference of the species our lives-our individual lives—weren't all that important—at least in an evolutionary sense. *You're born, you mate, you die.*

Sound bleak? All of this probably sounds so ominously destructive and deadly that you are probably left wondering how anybody makes it past age 30.

But there is hope that we can be more than simply nature's reproductive machines.

The scientific quest to extend the human life span has led medical science to discover that despite our evolutionary programming to begin the self-destruction process after age 25 or 30—we can counter this process.

Free radicals would completely destroy our health, tremendously reducing our life span, if it weren't for *two evolutionary adaptations—cellular compart-*

The Cell Under Attack!

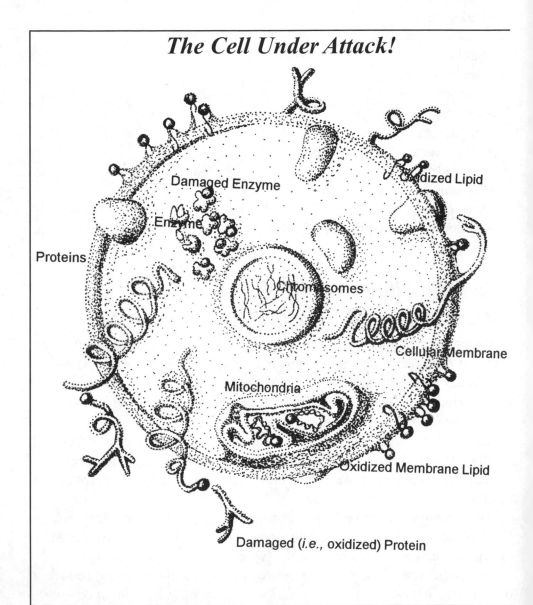

But there is hope that we can be more than simply nature's reproductive machines.

The scientific quest to extend the human life span has led medical science to discover that despite our evolutionary programming to begin the self-

Chromosomes
When damaged by oxygen free radicals, DNA no longer accurately produces the proteins that are involved in producing hormones and enzymes.

Enzymes
Enzymes are protein catalysts secreted by cells. They are responsible for many activities including scavenging oxygen free radicals. But when damaged by oxygen free radicals, enzymes can become deactivated, leading to cellular damage.

Mitochondrial DNA
The energy centers of the human cell, when damaged by oxygen free radicals, mitochondria can be destroyed, literally starving the cell. In addition, the mitochondria produce oxygen free radicals during the course of energy production. But when the mitochondrial membrane is damaged, oxygen free radicals spil into the cell, creating additional damage.

Cell Membrane
The membrane is responsible for selectively allowing nutrients in the cell and keeping out harmful substances. When the lipids (*i.e.,* fats) that make-up the membrane are damaged, it no longer protects the cell, resulting in damage to enzymes.

Protein
Proteins make-up 75 percent of dry cell matter and are involved in various structures including hormones and enzymes. When they are oxidized and damaged, the production of other protein-dependent structures is also hindered.

DNA Under Attack!

DNA is the repository of inheritance, responsible for the orderly reproduction of cells. If a single strand of DNA is damaged by oxygen free radicals, reproduction of the cell may be adversely effected.

In the developing fetus, damaged DNA may result in birth defects. In adults and children, damaged DNA may result in cancer and other diseases as well as diminished reproduction of proteins that constitute essential elements of both enzymes and hormones.

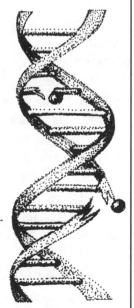

Base damaged by oxygen free radical (*i.e.,* oxidized)

Oxygen free radical-damaged strand of DNA

mentalization and antioxidants, both of which prevent free radical damage. Through the ages, nature evolved compartmentalization within the cell, says Dr. Walford. The mitochondria, where energy is produced and many free radicals are generated, are separated from the rest of the cell by their own unique membranes. Still, the burning of oxygen is imperfect. There is spill-over into the rest of the cell, and the mitrochondria could be mortally damaged by their exposure to oxygen free radical molecules. That is why antioxidants are produced by our bodies from the nutrients available in our diets "Nature developed, within each cell, the ability to manufacture protective free-radical neutralizers—'scavengers,' or to use the more popular term, 'antioxidants,'" says Dr. Walford.

Dr. Harman, who postulated the free radical theory of aging more than 30 years ago, remains one of the nation's leading scholars in this area of medicine. He points out that the free radical theory of aging assumes that there is a single basic cause of aging, modified by genetic and environmental factors. He says that if there is one basic cause of aging then it follows that if you control damage caused by oxygen free radicals you can control aging.

His research demonstrates that in animal subjects, their life spans are correlated with their ability to repair free-radical damage. Indeed, the good news is that our bodies have the ability to strongly control free radicals before they inflict too much damage. Dr. Harman recommended in 1981 that future diets should contain "increased amounts of substances capable of decreasing free radical reaction damage, such as a-tocopherol (vitamin E), ascorbic acid, selenium or one or more synthetic antixodants." In fact, says Dr. Harman, when substances are added to the diets of experimental animals that are designed to counter the effects of free radicals, average and maximum life span increases do occur.

We now know of many antioxidant nutrients. Many of these will be discussed in later chapters in this book.

Present Research

So important is research into the prevention of free radical-related damage to the human body that the National Institutes of Health has begun a five-year, $17 million study with more than 40,000 women to determine the role of free radical-fighting nutrients such as vitamin E and beta carotene to prevent cancer and heart disease.

The research being conducted currently provides important insights on how we can best use dietary supplements for the prevention of damaging oxygen free radical processes:

•Kenneth Munkres and Raj Rana at the University of Wisconsin's Laboratories of Molecular Biology and Genetics reported in *Mechanisms of Aging and Development* that free radical activity and lipid oxidation are the major cause of cellular deterioration resulting in the aging of the human body. The best preventives are antioxidants, they said, pointing out that their own research demonstrated that antioxidants prolong life by 14 percent.

•Einstein and Gershon, of the Biology Laboratories of the Israel Institute of Technology, concur in *Mechanisms of Aging and Development* that antioxidants can considerably prolong average life span.

•Researchers Robert Bolla and Nathan Brot, at the Roche Institute of Molecular Biology in New Jersey, report in the medical journal *Archives of Biochemistry* that the antioxidant *a*-tocopherol quinone increased life span by approximately 19 percent in experimental animal subjects.

•Comfort and Gore at the University College, London, demonstrated a 22 percent increase in life span with the use of antioxidants.

•Dr. Harman at the University of Nebraska College of Medicine reported in the *Journal of Medical Sciences* that animal subjects in a double blind study who were given antioxidants had virtually no tumors when they died compared to the control subjects who had *many*. Dr. Harman notes that studies with antioxidants such as ethoxyquin, a chemical feed additive, and 2-mercaptoethylamine (first developed by the Atomic Energy Commission to protect against radiation exposure), have both increased life span of experimental animals by 20 to 50 percent depending on the dose.

•Brugarolas and Gosalvez found the antioxidant TCA clearly had an antitumor effect.

•Jaime Miguel and A. C. Economos, at the National Aeronautics and Space Administration's Ames Research Center, found that TCA increased life spans by eight to fourteen percent.

•Brugarolas and Gosalvez report that when aged, experimental animal subjects are given antioxidants, they mate more frequently and act younger.

•Independent studies by Miguel and Economos confirmed findings of increased vitality and improved sex drive in aged animals.

•Clapp reports in the *Journal of Gerontology* that not only do antioxidants increase life span in animals, they have thicker, more lustrous coats and fur.

•In research, performed by Robert Floyd, a molecular toxicologist at the Oklahoma Medical Research Foundation and John Garney of the University of Kentucky, the industrial antioxidant PBN has been used with profound results. Essentially, the researchers showed that memory can be restored in aged animals with optimal nutrition. The scientific researchers used aged gerbils in their study and treated them for two weeks with PBN which first stopped free-radical related damaging processes and then increased the amount of other chemicals in their brains, allowing their nerve cells to communicate more efficiently and clean out proteins damaged by free radicals. The gerbils were placed in physically confusing enclosures and forced to learn their way through them by using their memory. Amazingly, the PBN-treated subjects performed on a level equal to that of their younger counterparts. Unfortunately when the PBN was withdrawn, the old gerbils began once again showing their age. By now, the researchers knew that memory loss was related to free radical damage. So impressed was the NIH's Dr. Stadtman that he was moved to announce that age-related memory loss could finally be overcome by reversing oxygen free radical-related cellular damage.

•Dr. John P. Richie Jr., of the University of Louisville School of Medicine, used antioxidants to increase the life span of rats by 42 to 64 percent. Still other scientists have shown that antioxidants might be able to hold back diseases like Parkinson's, stroke, heart disease, cataract and some cancers.

•Research for the World Health Organization discovered that men in 16 European cities with the lowest levels of vitamin E in their blood were more likely to suffer fatal heart attacks than those with the highest levels. So strong was the link that researchers ruled out cholesterol levels as a contributing reason for this startling difference between those with the lowest and highest amounts of the antioxidant in their bodies. Not surprisingly, the researchers also recommend that people use nutritional supplements. Dr. Daniel Steinberg of the University of California at San Diego says that there's "a reasonable amount of evidence"antioxidant supplements like vitamin E may help prevent arterial disease.

•Even alcohol-induced birth defects may be nutritionally related, at least to some extent. So says Harvard Medical School researcher Dr. Paul Gallop who was able to isolate a substance called PPQ. Dr. Gallop believes that when PPQ is missing or at low levels in pregnant female alcoholics, their babies will suffer the worst retardation.

The Future Direction of Antioxidant Research

As medical scientists learn more about oxygen free radicals and how to limit the cellular damage which they can cause, people will enjoy longer, healthier lives.

Biochemist Bruce Ames of the University of California is optimistic that people eventually will be living *a lot longer.*

"Conservatively speaking, antioxidant therapy has been estimated to slow the aging process at a mean rate of 15 to 20 percent," says Dr. Richard D. Lippman (1980).

"We all can't live to be a hundred years old, but we can live much longer than we would if we didn't protect ourselves from premature aging with supplements and life-style changes," says Dr. Passwater (1991). "The most important benefit will be in the quality of our lives."

We now know that many common nutrients work as antioxidants—vitamins C and E, beta carotene (a precursor of vitamin A) and selenium are able to limit oxygen free radical-related damage. But many other antioxidants that are less well known also are becoming available. Many more are yet to be discovered and many more, about which we know little, certainly demand a much more thorough investigation of their disease-fighting benefits.

That's why the federal Government has asked scientists at 21 U.S. research centers to search out these chemicals in the rain forest, in the oceans and even in space.

Many of the most important of these yet-to-be-discovered substances very likely will be oxygen free radical fighting antioxidants, says cell biologist Michael Wargovich of the University of Texas' M.D. Anderson Cancer Center in Houston.

Dr. Harman and other like-minded anti-aging experts such as Hans Kugler, Ph.D., say that researchers have three tasks today that must dictate future

research and be achieved *as soon as possible*:
   •Find the optimal level of naturally occurring antioxidants.
   •Develop new and more powerful antioxidants.
   •Determine the best combination of antioxidants that will provide people with the opportunity to live strong and healthy lives and extend their maximum human life span.

   "My research in slowing the aging process involves more than preventing damage by slowing free-radical reactions," Dr. Passwater adds. "The damage caused by free radicals can continue to age the body by tying up needed components such as DNA. Also, body compounds that are misproduced can cause immunological reactions that hasten aging. The damage that has occurred from free-radical reactions must be *undone* if appreciable life extension is to occur. The body has repair enzymes such as macroxyproteinase and phospholipases that can undo part of the damage."

   But we don't need to wait for the final outcome of all this research. Indeed, we can start living vital healthy lives today with nature's own miracle antioxidants which are available to us to supplement our diet.
   By taking advantage of the already numerous nutritional breakthroughs in antioxidant therapy, you can extend the best years of your life by *several decades*.
   Some of the most helpful, known antioxidant and related nutrients which you can begin using *today* for life extension include:

   Beta Carotene
   Vitamin B-6
   Vitamin C
   Pantothenic Acid
   Selenium
   Zinc
   Glutathione
   Methionine
   Arginine
   Cysteine

Lysine
Ornithine
Superoxide Dismutase
Coenzyme Q-10
Pycnogenols
Ginkgo biloba

Each of these nutrients and many more, representing exciting discoveries in the field of human nutrition and longevity, will be discussed in the following chapters of this book.

Your adventure is about to begin!

3. Superoxide Dismutase

In the Bible, Methuselah lived more than 900 years. Someday, through the combination of genetic engineering and optimal nutrition, we may be as long lived as Methuselah.

In America today, the *average* life span for men and women is somewhere between 70 and 80. A closer look, however, at increases in productive life span during this century provides evidence of a great need for new approaches in fighting aging.

Between 1900 and 1955, average life span increases were rapid and even dramatic, increasing from about 49.5 years in 1900 to 68.5 years some 50 years later (Kinsella 1992).

Yet despite the post-World War II boom in medical and pharmaceutical technology, recorded increases in life span since the early to mid 1950s have been minimal. Although in the first 50 years of the century the gain was nearly 20 years, in the 40 years since 1950 we have gained only about seven years (Kinsella 1992).

Today, average life span for the U.S. male is 72.1 years and 79 years for the average female. These are indeed small advances. They raise the important issue of the distinction between *average* life span and *maximum* life span.

The reason for the early dramatic jump in life expectancy can be attributed to increases in *average* life span, due largely to the "expansion of public health services and facilities combined with disease eradication programs greatly reduced death rates, particularly among infants and children" (Kinsella 1992). The decrease in infant mortality has led to an increased life span for the *average* U.S. male and female.

As for *maximum* life span, we've not done as well in its extension. Joe Weissman, M.D., author of the important book *Choose to Live* (Grove Press 1988) notes that we're not much better off today in the last decade of the Twentieth Century than the average man or woman in the mid-Nineteenth Century. Dr. Weissman points out that although in the mid 1850s one's youth was filled with many potentially deadly health catastrophes—particularly infectious disease—if a man or woman of that era were fortunate enough to make it to his forties, there was an excellent chance that he or she could be as long lived as men and women of today.

We have, in other words, done a good job in eradicating infectious diseases. But our efforts at halting other sorts of "modern" disease like cancer, stroke, Alzheimer's and atherosclerosis have been minimal.

More recently in the 1980s, only "very slight" gains have been noted in most developed countries (Kinsella 1992).

Because of this plateauing of increases in life expectancy, the free radical theorists such as Drs. Denham Harman, Emanuel Cheraskin and Linus Pauling are now advancing their theories as the key to increasing life expectancy. Even eliminating cancer would add only about two years to present life expectancy, asserts Dr. Harman (1981). "At best," he says, "complete elimination of overt causes of death would increase life expectancy to about 85 years."

Now that we've discussed average life expectancy, we also need to consider *maximum* life span which is generally thought to be about 115 years with the ultimate healthy lifestyle alone—meaning that as a nation most of us are now falling about 35 to 45 years short of living out the full potential of our lives. *But just think—if only we could unlock the secrets of longevity scripted in the genetic structures within our own bodies, 40 more years of healthy living could be ours—enough time to embark upon second careers, live out our creative fantasies, travel the world and, in a very real sense, enjoy the opportunity of living two distinctly different lives.* It is time to move into the brave new world of research examining new methods for alleviating the damage caused by oxygen free radicals, say longevity scientists.

"The free radical theory of aging predicts that the healthy life span can be increased by minimizing deleterious free radical reactions while not significantly interfering with those essential to the economy of the cells and tissues," Dr. Harman asserts. "The data now available indicates that this can be done by keeping body weight down, at a level compatible with a sense of well-being, while ingesting diets adequate in essential nutrients but designed to minimize random free radical reactions in the body."

Such diets would contain minimal amounts of components prone to enhance free radical reactions such as polyunsaturated fats found in many kinds of vegetable oils; synthetic toxins such as highly toxic pesticide residues and even natural toxins such as excessive iron which can form harmful oxygen free radicals.

Optimal diets should also include increased amounts of substances capable of decreasing free radical reaction damage such as:
  •Ascorbic acid (vitamin C) found in citrus
  •*A* tocopherol (vitamin E) found in oils and nuts
  •Beta carotene (a precursor of vitamin A) found in foods such as carrots and collard greens
  •Selenium found in unrefined grains grown in vital soils
  •One or more synthetic antioxidants such as PBN, produced by the Monsanto Corporation and presently used in animal feed.

Dr. Harman asserts that, "It is reasonable to expect this approach will decrease the morbidity and mortality due to degenerative diseases and nonspecific age changes . . ."

Superoxide Dismutase

In this chapter, we will discuss the recent rapid advances in free radical research and antioxidant substances, such as superoxide dismustase, which is known to fight damage done by these cellular renegades.

Both the oxygen free radical called superoxide and its beneficial nemesis superoxide dismutase (SOD) were discovered by Duke University biochemist

Irwin Fridovich and colleagues in 1968 (Kotulak 1991). In fact, the discovery of SOD ranks among one of the first breakthroughs in longevity research that demonstrated that the body not only produces free radicals but that in its infinite wisdom also produces substances which offer important protection.

How excited is the research world over the discovery of SOD? When you realize that one in three Americans is struck with cancer and that approximately 22 percent of the population will die from this disease, you can get a pretty fair idea of the excitement over a substance that may play a pivotal role in halting or preventing the onset of this disease in individuals. "Cancer is a disease that has resisted man's efforts at understanding since the beginning of its study," says Dr. Larry Oberley, one of the nation's leading SOD researchers. "This lack of understanding is obviously because a vital link in the biochemistry of the cancer cell has been missing. Many groups around the world are now examining whether superoxide dismutase (SOD) is that missing link."

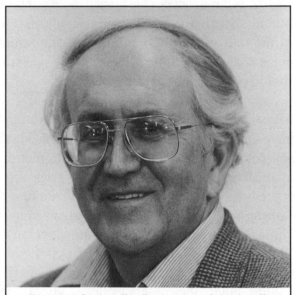

Richard Cutler, Ph.D., is one of the leading researchers and proponents of the oxygen free radical theory of aging. His research has focused on oxidative stress and aging. Dr. Cutler has helped demonstrate that free radicals are an important part of the aging process. The life spans of some one dozen species of animals have been correlated with the abundance of SOD and other antioxidants in their bodies, says Dr. Cutler. His own supplement program consists of 800 IU vitamin E (half morning/evening), 300 millgrams of pure beta carotene, 500 mg vitamin C, plus a multivitamin *without iron*.

Since its discovery, SOD has been ceaselessly investigated for its life extending properties. The life spans of some one dozen mammalian species have been positively correlated with the amounts of SOD found in their bodies, says Dr. Richard Cutler, of the Gerontology Research Center of the National

Institutes of Health in Baltimore.

Study after study of SOD activity in cancerous cells has shown that the levels are highly diminished at the time of malignancy, Oberley says, adding that these findings have led researchers to conclude that, "If oxygen radicals are the cause of normal cell damage and if low antioxidant levels in target tissue are potentiating factors, then these facts suggest that adding back antioxidants should prevent normal tissue damage."

Additional research has shown that SOD may well possess characteristics with direct implications for the protection of human health from the ever increasing belt of radiation contaminating our atmosphere as a result of natural sources such as sunlight coupled with depletion of the protective ozone layer; increasing pollution from past above-ground nuclear testing; nuclear reactors; nuclear waste; and other humanmade sources of nuclear radiation. SOD has been shown to be highly effective against environmental radiation effects in clinical trials, says Dr. Richard Passwater, author of *The New Supernutrition* (Pocket Books 1990). In this regard, Dr. Oberley points out that, "SOD has also been used to protect against normal tissue damage by ionizing radiation." Double-blind, placebo-controlled studies of people undergoing high energy radiation therapy for bladder tumors have shown that SOD has a very strong protective effect against ionizing radiation.

There are many startling examples of SOD's power to protect the body from oxygen free radical damage:

•One example of how SOD works comes to us from Duke University's Department of Medicine and Biochemistry. Researchers there, using *in vitro* techniques (meaning studies occuring outside the living body—usually in a test tube) exposed one set of white blood cells to SOD and left the other group unprotected. Free radicals were introduced to both groups of white blood cells. The SOD-protected cells remained alive; those without SOD died.

•At the Institute of Biology, Physics and Chemistry in Paris, researchers performed a similar experiment using samples of ribonuclease, an enzyme located in the lysosomes of cells that splits RNA at specific places in the molecule. Both samples were exposed to free radicals. But only that sample which had the protective insurance of SOD survived and flourished, remaining largely unaffected by free radicals.

•In yet another *in vitro* study, researchers added SOD to one cell culture and left the other without protection. To both were added known carcinogens. The SOD-protected culture remained healthy. The unprotected culture became cancerous.

•Experimental animals with induced head trauma recovered in half the normal time when treated with SOD (Michelson 1988).

•Nuclear radiation creates free radicals and it would be difficult for us to conceive of any living organism being able to exist within nuclear reactors. Yet the bacterium *radiourans* is able to survive within the core of nuclear reactors. Not surprisingly, no living organism on earth has more SOD within its system per gram of body weight than *radiourans*.

Thus far the study results appear promising. Some scientists believe SOD's anti-inflammatory properties ultimately will be harnessed to relieve rheumatoid arthritis and Duchenne muscular dystrophy, as well as oxygen-induced lung

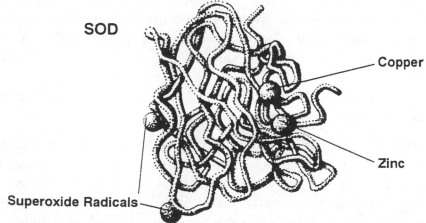

This is Superoxide Dismutase!

In this drawing, demonstrating how SOD works in the human body, the SOD molecule is guiding superoxide free radicals towards copper and zinc atoms that participate in destroying harmful oxidants.

SOD

Copper

Zinc

Superoxide Radicals

"Superoxide dismutase is now used to reduce inflammation and is under study for other applications, potentially including amelioration of degenerative diseases that become common late in life," reports *Scientific American* in its December 1992 issue.

damage in premature infants. SOD may well even find a role in the prevention of heart attacks.

High SOD Level Means Increased Life Span

One area of important research into human longevity is in developing the ability of medical professionals to intervene in limiting the cellular damage caused by the body's production of oxygen free radicals.

Geneticists have uncovered certain genes in the human body which, when manipulated and turned *on* or *off*, possess the potential to one day dramatically increase the maximum human life span. Researchers, who are intimately involved in longevity-related genetic engineering—and are aware of its tremendous potential—believe that some day people will routinely live to 200 years or more. These fascinating, anti-aging genetic structures within our bodies are known as *Methuselah* genes and they are responsible for the production of SOD (Maugh 1992).

An enzyme produced by one of these so-called Methuselah genes is capable of destroying oxygen free radicals and researchers believe that by studying the Methusaleh genes, they are actually studying a "blueprint" for the production of the SOD enzyme which destroys free radicals. When more of this enzyme is produced, the body more effectively prevents harm caused by the production of oxygen free radicals. And, so the theory goes, if we can halt free radical damage, we can live considerably longer lives.

Two studies shed light on the potential of using genetic engineering techniques for increasing maximum life span:

•University of California biologist Michael R. Rose found that delaying reproduction in experimental animals ultimately prolonged the life span of future generations by as much as 80 percent (Maugh 1992). *The researcher believes his long-lived subjects had an advantage in that his selective breeding techniques produced strains which possessed unusually high amounts of superoxide dismutase in their systems.*

•Using genetic engineering techniques, molecular biologist James Fleming of the Linus Pauling Institute of Science & Medicine, in Palo Alto, California, demonstrated the power of SOD by taking a different research tact. In his work, Fleming "inserted" extra copies of the Methusaleh gene for SOD into experimental fruit fly embryos. Those which underwent the genetic engineering lived as long as those that were bred in Rose's multi-generational experiment.

But for the time being, widespread practical applications of genetic engineering have been relegated to the animal and agricultural laboratories. Although genetic engineering is being used for the palliation of diseases, the ethical debate surrounding human genetic engineering as it applies to life extension for healthy individuals must be resolved before we are likely to see its widespread and direct human benefits in prolonging life.

So where does that leave you and me? Sure, we'd love to live longer, healthier lives. But we can't sit around waiting for the genetic engineering techniques of tomorrow. They may not become reality until it's too late for us! What can we do now?

There's a lot we can do, and we're learning more all the time about how to induce production of SOD in our own bodies.

Although it is true that the human body manufactures SOD, the raw materials required for optimal production—especially zinc, copper and manganese—are not always present in ideal quantities in the foods people consume. For example, Dr. Passwater (1991) reports on a study conducted at Pennsylvania State University that found the recommended portions of the basic four food groups do not ensure adequate amounts of essential nutrients including zinc—which is needed by the body for synthesizing SOD.

A deficiency in one of the building blocks of SOD can mean significant decreases in body tissue levels. We know this to be true from studies such as those performed by researchers at the Department of Internal Medicine at the University of Utah College of Medicine in Salt Lake City. Researchers there found that deficiencies in copper in the diets of experimental animals decreased SOD activity in body tissues (Williams 1975). Other researchers report that depriving experimental animals of dietary manganese—also needed by the body for the production of SOD—significantly diminished the amount of SOD in their tissues including their liver and brain.

On the other hand, SOD levels were increased by manganese supplements, according to a report in the *American Journal of Clinical Nutrition*. The research was done at the University of Wisconsin and examined 47 women who ingested either a placebo, 60 milligrams of iron, 15 milligrams of manganese or both mineral supplements for 124 days. Only the groups ingesting manganese had increased blood levels of SOD.

The human health consequences of SOD depletion are noteworthy. Although researchers are not completely certain at this time, they speculate that as a result of being deprived of the nutrients necessary for producing SOD, our cells may survive for shorter periods and that their membranes may become weakened (Williams 1975). For you and me, this translates into a greater amount of damage done to our cells by free radicals. And this is a theory worth noting, since most of the research correlates diminished SOD activity with diminished cellular health and increased oxygen free radical activity, according to Dr. Oberley. Compounding the damage is the fact that your body's ability to synthesize SOD decreases as you age. Yet, at the same time, pollution of all kinds, disease, other environmental factors, stress and the aging process itself lead to increased amounts of free radical stress on your body.

Induce SOD Production in Your Body

That's why a supplement designed for stimulating your body's production of SOD has enormous potential.

If you want to obtain your *maximum* life span, not the *average*—your body needs help in fighting cellular damage caused by free radicals. Dietary supplements designed to induce SOD synthesis have the potential to help.

As parents and concerned adults we often find ourselves insisting that our children or that we ourselves take vitamins everyday. And that's commendable. But let's not stop there with the job only half done. Now you will find it equally rewarding to take SOD-inducing supplements everyday.

This brings up the quandry that we presently face. Oral administration of SOD is ordinarily not a successful way of stimulating increased SOD activity within the body. That is because SOD is an enzyme quickly broken down by the body upon ingestion. Although upon oral ingestion a small increase in blood SOD activity was noted in one research report, the elevation was not considered significant and the researchers concluded that oral supplementation with SOD does not affect tissue SOD activity. But they added one interesting and important caveat: "Oral supplementation of SOD did not have any effect on the SOD activity of the tissues analyzed *when the animals were consuming a nutritionally adequate diet.*" In order for us to accept these study results as indisputable, we would need to see the effects of oral administration of SOD on animals whose diets are nutritionally deficient. Such a study would also bear more relevance to many Americans whose diets are also nutritionally deficient— especially in zinc.

The Raw Materials of SOD

But let's put aside this issue on scientific study protocols for a moment and return to the really only essential point: how can concerned health-conscious individuals, who wish to take advantage of modern breakthroughs in medical research, increase SOD activity in their body? The answer probably lies in ensuring that the body recieves the raw materials necessary for the synthesis of SOD. These nutrients include copper, manganese and zinc.

Since studies have demonstrated conclusively that diets deficient in these nutrients result in diminished SOD activity in experimental animals (Williams 1975), the inference that we can draw is that by supplying our bodies with enough of the raw materials for SOD production we can ensure that we have enabled the body to naturally produce SOD.

So what nutrients should you be using to ensure your body has the necessary raw ingredients for synthesizing SOD? There appear to be three key nutrients that your body requires for synthesizing SOD, and each of these can be ingested in optimal amounts with exceptional eating habits or with the more practical and predictable aid of dietary supplements. By ingesting them, there is every probability that you will be helping your body defend against the effects of damaging oxygen free radicals.

Dr. Passwater personally recommends the following forms of nutrients—(all of which are attached to amino acids for easier assimilation):

SOD-Inducing Micronutrients And Recommended Daily Amounts

Zinc (Glycine, histidine dipeptide chelate)	5 mg
Copper (Lysine dipeptide chelate)	500 mcg
Manganese (Glycine dipeptide chelate)	2 mg

By ingesting these nutrients in the proper amounts, you can stimulate your body to produce optimal amounts of SOD. This will promote further antioxidant activity in your body. You will not feel any different, at least not in the short run. But as you age you will find that you retain your youthful vigor, vitality and energy longer than the people around you who have neglected to nourish their bodies.

Over time, the cellular damage caused by pollution, disease and other inducers of oxygen free radicals will be minimized and you will enjoy a longer extension of life span accompanied by perfect health!

Where to Find the Formula

Editor's Note: An excellent antioxidant formula is available that you should know about. It is called SOD Complex and combines the building blocks of superoxide dismutase—copper, manganese, and zinc in chelated form—together with the entire superoxide dismutase molecule. It could be an important breakthrough supplement because of its ingredients' proven abilities to stimulate the body's own SOD production. Order by calling (800) 825-8482.

4. ACF 223: The Patented Antioxidant Formulation

Free radical damage not only causes diseases such as cancer and heart disease but hardening of the skin and wrinkling as well. Beauty, as we are about to learn, starts from within with a healthy body and circulatory system. One particular antioxidant formula not only has demonstrated potential to help prevent cancer, it can help keep your skin smooth and wrinkle-free.

One strong piece of evidence that the free radical theory of aging has become accepted as an important working paradigm for health professionals in the area of the prevention of aging and age-related disease is that the U.S. Patent and Trademark Office awarded on Sept. 22, 1987 an actual patent to an anti-aging supplement formulated with several synergistic, pharmaceutically acceptable antioxidants.

Perhaps most unique about this patented antioxidant formula is that the support documentation clearly asserts that when we take measures to prevent the oxygen toxicity caused by free radicals not only do the benefits appear internally as in the halting or slowing of the onset of atherosclerosis, stroke and cancer—additional benefits also include the postponement of wrinkling and hardening of the skin. This is an important insight for people concerned about their outward appearance. *It's crucial to remember that taking of care of your appearance starts from within. The cellular havoc wreaked upon our bodies through the inefficient processes of oxygen metabolism and those cellular sharks known as free radicals becomes evident in the wrinkling and hardening of the skin.*

"Free radical pathology mechanisms seem to be involved at key points in the etiology and pathogenesis of cancer, occlusive atherosclerosis and *wrinkling*," notes the U.S. patent.

Indeed, by controlling the same processes that cause hardening of the arteries and heart disease we can also control age-related hardening and wrinkling of the skin.

Both skin and arteries consist of supportive material called *collagen* and *elastin*. *Collagen* is the major protein of the white fibers of the connective tissue, cartilage and bone. *Elastin*, or elastic tissue, is the major connective tissue protein of elastic structures such as the large blood vessels and the skin and it enables these structures to stretch, and then resume their original size and shape.

Both collagen and elastin contain fibers internally linked together by chemical bonds called an *imide* bond. It is theorized that aging involves the oxidation of these imide bonds to *amide* bonds. In both the skin and arterial collagen and elastin, as more and more amide bonds are formed, the collagen and elastin fibers become increasingly less elastic and flexible. In man it is known that these fibers harden at a rate of approximately seven percent per decade after the age of maturity (approximately in the mid-twenties). This means that arterial-vascular system currently has a theoretical life span of approximately 140 years before becoming 100 percent rigid. Obviously, nobody has yet lived long enough to die of old age—largely as a result of the damage done to collagen and elastin fibers through oxygen free radical action. Yet through the use of antioxidants, this conversion process can be delayed, says the patent, noting specifically that the compounds in ACF 223 "are useful in retarding the aging phenomena of skin wrinkling."

The Swedish inventors of ACF 223 first learned about the free radical theory of aging as undergraduate students in Sweden; they were intrigued by this area of research, particularly in explanations of why the body's cells age. The research team began doing graduate research work in the area of cell biology in the mid-1970s in Sweden at the University of Uppsala's Department of Medical Cell Biology. The researchers had access to some of the most sophisticated technology available worldwide for measuring microscopic cellular functions and changes that occurred as a result of disease and aging.

They learned that one of the major problems with aging is that cells lose their integrity. The cell walls become weaker, the genetic materials become damaged, the enzymes inside cells become damaged. Now some cells, like those of the skin, can be completely replaced but other cells like those of the heart, brain and central nervous system, once damaged, remain damaged for the rest of one's life. In other words, they are damaged forever.

For example, the human brain can decrease from an average weight of 1,500 grams in a young human adult to 1,000 grams or less in a human of advanced age. A brain that has decreased in size is highly forgetful, unable to memorize new information and cannot react quickly to external stimuli. Shrinkage with age is also found in other organs such as the heart, liver, kidneys, lymph nodes, skeletal muscles and vertebrae. Such shrinkage often corresponds with the accumulation of peroxidized, free radical products seen as brown-yellow age pigment and brown age spots (known technically as *lipofuscin*).

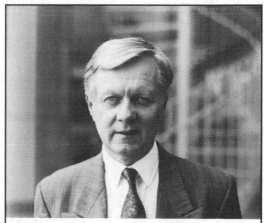

Who uses ACF 223? The patients of Dr. Kaj Alvestrand do—along with thousands of the most knowledgeable longevity seekers in Sweden, Italy, the United States, and Canada. The Stockholm, Sweden, nutritionist heads his own anti-aging clinic and is editor of *Anti-Aging Breakthroughs*. He regularly prescribes ACF 223 to his clients because of its dynamic synergistic complement of anti-aging nutrients, found in no other product available in the U.S.

Other corresponding changes associated with aging are wrinkled skin, depleted fat deposits, fewer dermal melanocytes, brittle bones, low infection resistance, poor exercise tolerance and lack of reproductive ability.

The researchers were able to do an enormous number of tests and document that ACF 223 really did offer something concrete to combat the effects of aging.

In their research the inventors administered ACF 223 to volunteers who allowed researchers to perform highly detailed tests that would document clinical changes in the function of their bodies' vital organs. They found that the ACF formula truly is beneficial. They found that especially middle-aged and older people were benefiting from using ACF; their liver function was like that of teenagers. Often people experience reduced liver function as they age, especially if they have abused their bodies with heavy consumption of alcohol and fatty foods. The mechanism that increased their liver protection was ACF's ability to offer protection from different oxidants (oxygen free radicals) in the body.

The ACF formula has been approved for use by regulatory agencies in both Sweden and Italy and patented in the U.S. and Canada.

So what exactly does ACF 223 have that other supplements don't?

Nordihydroguairetic acid (NDGA)

The ACF research team had done a great deal of research on the effects of nuclear radiation fall-out, especially at test sites in the American southwest. They learned that radiation exposure induces releases of huge amounts of oxygen free radicals and that it is their abundance following the initial exposure which produces the severe damage to the human body. Yet despite the enormous damage that high energy radiation can cause to living organisms, there were certain plants at Ground Zero at the Nevada test sites that grew back within nine months following testing. The ACT research team made the decision to travel to America and during the course of their research they visited Death Valley in Eastern California. This desolate yet beautiful national landmark has the highest temperatures on the planet and is one of the driest spots as well. To give you an idea of how dry Death Valley is: the humidity on an airliner is about nine percent and that's pretty dry. The humidity in Death Valley is one or two percent and that's *very* dry.

Yet despite these extreme conditions, the research team noticed that there was an abundance of wildlife in Death Valley. With the aid of infra-red binoculars enhancing their vision at night when the fauna of the valley came to life, they observed that virtually all the animals had one thing in common: they consumed a certain brush, known as chaparral, or creosote.

The researchers began asking questions. They wanted to know why they were eating only this cactus. "Could this be related to the reason why they

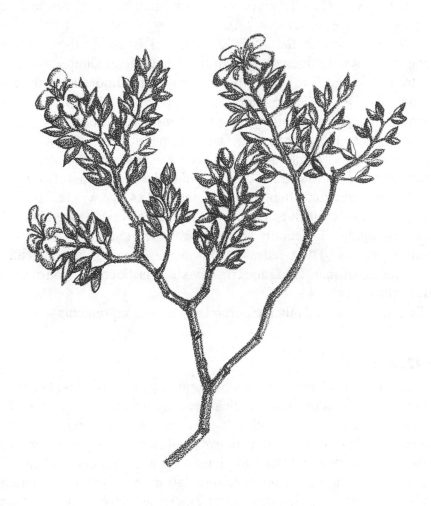

Creosote (Chaparral)

survive and even thrive in this inhospitable environment?" they asked.

The scientists gathered a small amount of this bush for testing. In the ensuing laboratory analysis, they learned that this particular cactus contained the radiation-protective substance we now know as nordihydroguairetic acid (NDGA). It is this compound which enables the animals that consume it to withstand extreme ultraviolet radiation from the sun. Ultimately, they found a source of this substance in the low lying, remote desert regions of northern Arizona. The ACT team received legal permission for its harvest and began extracting the active substances.

Yet there is more to the ACF 223 story. Discussing the outcome of experimental animal studies, the patent notes that in one example, two groups of experimental mice were fed standard lab chow. In addition, one of the groups was also fed NDGA. The mice that were given the additional nutritional support, says the patent report, "were visually more youthful and healthy at 26 months of age than the control mice. The last remaining control mouse showed significant hair loss, pigmentation loss, poor eyesight and difficulty in movement as compared with the four NDGA-fed mice that were also still living at this stage of the experiment." In other words, the NDGA that was fed to the mice not only extended their lives but prevented their physical appearance from prematurely aging. Especially apparent was the greater skin wrinkling in control mice versus NDGA-fed mice. This increased wrinkling is indicative of collagen and elastin hardening and cross-linking via the conversion of imide to amide bonds.

ACF contains several other important antioxidant ingredients.

Vitamin E

Although vitamin E is one of the most commonly found antioxidants it is not to be underestimated in its free radical scavenging ability. Harman (1981) asserts that, "the declining death rate from gastric carcinoma in the United States may be related to the introduction of breakfast cereals, particularly wheat cereals, rich in tocopherol (such as vitamin E) and other antioxidants." The value of ACF 223 lays in its ability to stimulate the synergistic interactions of a number of protective antioxidants so their increased activity is greater than the sum of their effects if they were used separately. Vitamin E, for example, can be combined with other antioxidants to have highly acceptable values of antioxidant effect through the phenomena of synergism.

Butylated Hydroxytoluene (BHT)

There are many other equally important antioxidants. For instance, buty-lated hydroxytoluene, known as BHT, is one of the most common food preservatives used today, because of its ability to prevent oxidation. All you need to do to see how common BHT is today is pick up a box of cereal or a candy bar. You will see that BHT (or its relative BHA) is frequently listed on the label. Its application in human health in the form of a supplement also holds promise. BHT was widely used during World War II to preserve the foods of soldiers out in the field. Researchers noticed a side effect of the use of BHT was that the incidence of stomach cancer was half of what it was among soldiers in the 1930s. In experimental studies, BHT has also protected against acute lethality of X-rays and prevented cancer-causing chemicals from causing tumors. Research shows that the free radical scavenging effects of vitamin E are "enhanced" by the addition of BHT to the formulation.

2-Mercaptoethylamine (MEA)

Another free radical scavenger gaining importance as a supplement is 2-mercaptoethylamine (MEA). Dr. Denham Harman (1981) notes that the addition of MEA to the diets of experimental mice "increased the life span by 30 percent; this increase is equivalent to raising the human life span from 73 to 95 years."

MEA has another unique function: preventing the damage caused by iron-based oxygen free radical compounds. As *U.S. News & World Report* noted in its September 21, 1992 issue, a "provocative study by Finnish researchers, published... in the American Heart Association's scientific journal *Circulation*, concluded that the amount of iron stored in the body *ranks second only to smoking as the strongest risk factor for heart disease and heart attacks.*"

In fact, experts cited by *U.S. News & World Report* place iron ahead of high cholesterol, high blood pressure, and diabetes as a leading cause of heart attacks.

What does iron do once in the body? As Dr. Hans Kugler, Ph.D., explains,

"Your body produces hydrogen peroxide as a byproduct of metabolism—the burning of oxygen.

"Scientists believe that iron combines with hydrogen peroxide in the body to cause a cascade of cellular-damaging oxygen free radicals which can damage heart muscle as well as the nerves and fatty acids of the heart. Damage of these nerves may mean that you will need a pacemaker in your later years to renew electrical nerve impulses to the heart that can no longer be efficiently transmitted from your brain. Furthermore, oxygen free radical damage of your heart's circulatory tissues can mean that they will plug up with plaques or fatty acid streaks. This could mean that you may need heart surgery—if a heart attack doesn't strike first!"

Taking an aggressive and proactive approach to your health means making sure the iron in your body doesn't lead to the formation of cell-damaging, iron-based oxygen free radicals. ACF 223 is one of the few supplements medically tested to safely scavenge free iron. In their research at the Department of Medical Cell Biology at the University of Uppsala in Sweden, investigators actually tested their formula for its potential to scavenge free iron in the presence of heart muscle before it forms harmful oxygen free radicals. In addition, ACF 223 was extensively clinically tested to determine the proper dosage so that people won't develop anemia.

So for protection against iron-related heart disease, cut down on rich sources of iron such as red meat and organ foods, and use a dietary supplement like ACF 223.

Catalase

Catalase is another important enzyme in the body's total defense mechanism against free radical-related aging. Activities of catalase have been found to be diminished in tumor cells in many studies.

Synergy

Few supplements today contain the proper amounts of these particular antioxidants, and only ACF 223 contains a combination of BHT combined with catalase, MEA and NDGA and vitamin E in a patented formulation. Remember, when all these anti-aging substances are combined, the end result is greater than taking only one of them. Many aging processes are promoted by free radical reactions. Selective mixtures of antioxidants and other related geroprotectors should guard against these processes.

5. *Pycnogenol*

Along the southern coast of France a tree grows that could save your life. It is able to withstand the brisk, salty Atlantic winds and withering intense summer heat. Its active ingredients saved the lives of the men who discovered Canada.

Many of the most well known and widely used vitamins like C and E and minerals such as selenium are recognized today by the medical community for their powers as antioxidants. Individuals with even the most rudimentary knowledge of nutrition tend to use vitamins such as C and E. That's a good practice with which we have no quarrel.

But many lesser known substances are also being recognized for their antioxidant powers and are available as supplements in your quest for optimal nutrition. You may not have heard much about them. But if you desire the opportunity for a long-lived, healthy life you should know about them. That way you will be able to take advantage of being on the cutting edge of optimal nutrition's influence on longevity.

For many years now and many more years to come, scientists have been, and will continue, studying a group of approximately 500 known varieties of botanical substances known as flavonoids which are commonly found in photosynthesizing cells of the plant kingdom; flavonoids are the pigments that lend color to plants (Havsteen 1983).

In addition to their free radical scavenging activity, flavonoids have demonstrated many other excellent anti-aging properties including resistance to viral infection. For example Havsteen (1983) reports that viral infections in your body remain completely harmless until the protein coat surrounding the nucleic acid has been removed by lysosomal digestion. The removal of the protein coat surrounding the nucleic acid apparently requires the fusion of the virus with the lysosomal membrane. This fusion happens with the help of a proton known as ATPase and possibly an enzyme known as phospholipase A2. "Both of these enzymes," says Havsteen, "are inhibited by flavonoids and similar compounds."

In other areas of health, the flavonoids appear to play helpful roles. For example, in the case of diabetes mellitus which can cause narrowing of the blood vessels and micro-bleeding; both can be stopped by flavonoids. These plant substances have also demonstrated anti-cancer properties in experimental animal studies, says Havsteen (1983).

It isn't enough, of course, that a substance show antioxidant or other anti-aging, health promoting properties for it to become part of your optimal nutrition program. There are conditions for membership into this exclusive health promoting longevity fraternity.

Criteria for Determining Useful Herbs & Botanicals

Dietary supplement ingredients must conform to several pharmaceutical standards which include:

•*Bioavailability when ingested.* Some free radical scavengers are enzymes which means that in many cases much of their bioavailability when taken orally is limited since they will be hydrolyzed into their constituents within the digestive system. One such example is superoxide dismutase when taken orally; although a small amount may make its way into the bloodstream, for the most part SOD is broken down into other compounds.

•*Low toxicity in both short-term and long-term use. In vitro,* for example, some agents have shown tremendous capacity for free radical absorption. The flavonoid quercetin is a fantastic free radical scavenger but has demonstrated potential mutagenic (gene-altering) properties and is in fact one of the most potent mutagens in the *Salmonella* tester strains (Middleton 1984). The *Salmonella* tester strains are used by toxicologists to determine whether a chemical is potentially cancer-causing. Very often chemicals that cause mutations in the *Salmonella* test are considered to be potentially cancer-causing. Yet even here it isn't always easy to tell friend from foe. Havsteen (1983) asserts that when discussing so-called gene-damaging qualities exhibited by quercetin and other plant substances known as flavonoids—the possibility must be discussed that the standard procedure for testing, the Ames *Salmonella* test, is unable to distinguish between depression of normally inactive genes and true mutagenesis. In the case of the flavonoids, says Havsteen (1983), the observation which prompted the positive results was only the appearance of new traits, which may have many consequences other than causing cancer in animals; indeed, quercetin is widely used by many people who believe that its so-called mutagenicitiy is a bad rap. In fact, no serious side effects have been observed with the use of flavonoids, including quercetin, at moderate doses.

  •*Therapeutic action with results that are not only statistically significant but also capable of being replicated in double blind tests using standardized protocols.* A substance must prove itself effective in several studies before it can be said to be helpful—at least by the standards of Western medical science.

Despite these strict requirements that truly are difficult to meet, there are those times in nutritional history when a nutrient is discovered that seems to hold great promise without any of the drawbacks—when it seems to meet all the qualifications in terms of bioavailability, safety and therapeutic effect. When this happens, nutritionists become very excited.

Ironically, as so often happens in medicine, the lay and nutritional community herald the appearance of such substances as though they've only been recently discovered.

In the case of the antioxidants we're about to discuss—the pycnogenols—it's really a matter of their being rediscovered.

Proanthocyanidins

One substance that seems to hold great promise for fighting the effects of aging is Pycnogenol, which is the registered trademark name for a specially developed antioxidant product. This brand of antioxidant is made from substances that are a sub-family of a more general grouping known as the plant *proanthocyanidins*, which are a highly specialized and narrow group of plant flavonoids characterized by bioavailability through the oral route and their lack of toxicity including lack of mutagenic, teratogenic and allergenic effects (Masquelier 1987).

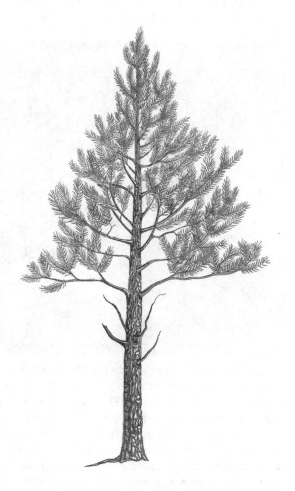

The powerful product called Pycnogenol that we're going to discuss is made from substances that are derived from the bark of the maritime pine, *Pinus maritima*, growing

The Bordeaux pine of France is able to withstand the harsh winds of winter and brilliant sun of summer. Its special antioxidant properties have now been harnessed so that you too can withstand the harsh elements of the environment and enjoy greater antioxidant protection.

along the coast in the pine woods of southern France from Bordeaux to the Spanish border. These pines have a very thick bark that protects them from the salty winds of the Atlantic Ocean and from the intense summer heat.

Although many treelike plants contain this water-soluble flavonoid, not all kinds are good sources and suitable for the production of this natural remedy. The best source is the pines that grow outside Bordeaux.

The bark contains the largest amounts of the active ingredients contained in Pycnogenol, says Dr. Jack Masquelier, who is generally credited with the rediscovery of these healing, life-promoting nutrients.

"Interestingly," he adds, laughing, "[the active ingredients found in] Pycnogenol [are] also found in the Bordeaux red wines."

In towns like Dax, in the south of France, wood processing plants extract the active ingredients that eventually go into the brand product known as Pycnogenol. The process of gathering the active ingredients from the pines produces a yellowish powder that is very valuable: 500 kilograms of pine bark is required to gain one kilogram of the

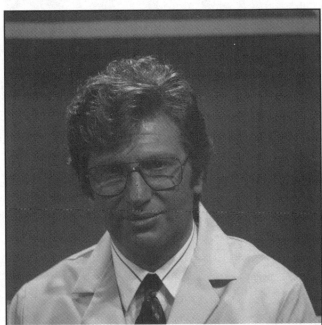

Dr. Benjamin Friedrich, geriatrics specialist of the Geriatric Institute of Romania, studied under professors educated by Ana Aslan, M.D., one of the pioneers of longevity therapy with the advent of Gerovital H3 (*see Chapter 30*). Dr. Friedrich notes that he frequently suggests longevity seekers stay up with the latest findings in nutritional science and use powerful, new and safe antioxidant supplements such as pycnogenols in order to prolong the best years of their life. He has found that pycnogenols not only prevent free radical damage to internal organs but also help prevent skin wrinkling. He is particularly enthusiastic about the multiple benefits that stem from the use of pycnogenols, especially for older patients in helping improve circulation.

powder which sells for at least $1,000.

Pycnogenol is 50 times more potent than vitamin E and 20 times more potent than vitamin C as antioxidants. Some researchers, in fact, strongly believe Pycnogenol is the most powerful naturally occurring free radical scavengers yet discovered. If not *the* most powerful free radical scavengers, it is certainly near the top of the list.

Cartier Discovered More Than Canada

It's strange how we so often lack historical perspectives on medical advancements. In the U.S. many health professionals are hailing Pycnogenol as a brilliant new discovery. Yet, their powers have been known for at least four centuries.

It all started with French explorer Jacques Cartier and his crew of 110 men who in 1534 were unexpectedly blocked by ice on the St. Lawrence River in an area of what is now known as Quebec.

The men had only salted meat and biscuits to eat—no fruits or vegetables. Disease set in. Soon, 25 died of scurvy and 50 others lay near death. Those who did survive were so weak that they were unable to dig graves for their companions. They simply buried the bodies in the snow (Masquelier 1980).

Desperate, Cartier persuaded a Quebec Indian medicine man to help them. The native healer made a drink and a poultice from the needles and bark of a large pine tree which he called *Anneda*. Fearful and mistrustful of the native healer's presumed remedy, Cartier allowed just two of his men to be treated. They became well within days. Quickly, Cartier allowed the same treatment for all of his men. They were all saved.

Little did Cartier know that he had stumbled upon what would become known as one of the most powerful anti-aging nutrients of the Twentieth Century—the flavonoid family known as proanthocyanidin.

Vitamin C Alone Doesn't Cure Scurvy

Modern scientists have been fascinated by the proanthocyanidin family for more than 50 years. Their interest was first sparked when they found that pure vitamin C did not repair the bleeding gums and peeling skin caused by scurvy, yet lemon juice did. Evidently, they concluded, some undiscovered factor remained in the lemon rind or its pulp that also was present in juice.

In 1968, French scientist Professor Jack Masquelier of the University of Bordeaux identified the substance that potentiated the effects of vitamin C as a receptor on cell membranes for ascorbic acid. Masquelier had been working at Quebec University when he began a study of flavonoids in nutshells. Ultimately, he discovered that the active, cell-wall protecting compound that prevents scurvy is one of the hundreds of natural compounds contained in the bark of most trees and woody shrubs (Masquelier 1980). Today we know those compounds are proanthocyanidins.

Ironically, not even Masquelier knew the historic background of the active ingredients that make-up Pycnogenol. It was only after the announcement of his scientific discovery that Masquelier learned of Cartier's voyages to the New World which led to the discovery of Canada and of the pine that comprised the tea administered to the seaman's dying crew which restored their health.

Multiple Powers

Yet, Pycnogenol is much more than a tool to be used with vitamin C. Their other demonstrated powers include:

•*Blocking Cholesterol.* Dr. David White of the University of Nottingham in England put it very simply at a scientific symposium in France on Oct. 6, 1990, when he called Pycnogenol "a powerful, nontoxic anti-oxidant that may block the accumulation of cholesterol" (Passwater 1991).

•*Preventing Cancer.* Dr. Stewart Brown, yet another researcher at the University of Nottingham, asserts that Pycnogenol prevents build-up of a cancer-related chemical that is present when cells become malignant.

•*Improving Circulation.* Pycnogenol has been demonstrated to have effects that may help prevent heart disease by improving circulation and strengthening the body's veins and arteries. It has proven particularly effective in patients suffering from circulatory disorders and eye disease related to poor circulation. One researcher reports that the oral use of Pycnogenol for four weeks resulted in an overall satisfactory improvement in 70.3 percent of the symptoms associated with patients suffering odemea including varicose veins and blood clotting. In the area of diabetic-related eye disease, Pycnogenol appears to hold a special place for treatment of symptoms, says Maynard (1970).

•*Relieving Arthritis.* Pycnogenol can also help relieve arthritis and improve joint flexibility by fighting inflammation; help prevent cataracts; and, in the area of youthful appearance, this substance can even improve skin smoothness and elasticity (Passwater 1991).

•*Improving Skin Texture and Preventing Wrinkling.* Researchers report that Pycnogenol appears to exert a protective effect on collagen, the protein underlying the skin, responsible for skin texture and elasticity. When taken soon enough, Pycnogenol may even aid in prevention of early facial wrinkling (Passwater 1991).

•*Protecting From Oxygen Free Radical Damage.* Pycnogenol is one of the few dietary anti-oxidants that readily cross the blood/brain barrier to directly protect brain cells from free radicals' damaging effects. In experimental animal studies that examined their effects on circulatory function, rats—bred to be genetically prone to early death from stroke—lived much longer than expected when Pycnogenol was added to their diet.

Dozens of studies have been done on the safety of Pycnogenol. Dr. Peter Rohdewald, of the Pharmacology Institute of the University of Munster in Germany, asserts that when used in recommended dosages there is no danger of toxicity. Pycnogenol is neither mutagenic nor do they cause reproductive damage or birth defects. Other studies on its bioavailability when taken orally indicate that it is well absorbed.

Since Pycnogenol has been proven effective for so many health maladies— from heart disease prevention to diabetic-related eye disease, we have detailed its five major benefits:

•Strengthens connective tissue by cross linking collagen
•Reduces inflammation by blocking histamine formation
•Scavenges free radicals
•Carries vitamin C to various body tissues
•Protects vitamin C from free radical oxidation

There are 18 areas of use for Pycnogenol where its efficacy has been verified in double-blind, controlled studies or appears to hold promise. These include:

Arthritis
Asthma
Athletic Injury

Capillary Fragility
Cataract
Detoxification
Diabetes Mellitus
Inflammatory Bowel Disease
Inflammatory Joint Disease
Inhalant Allergies
Interstitial Cystitis
Multiple Sclerosis
Oedemia (Tissue Swelling)
Peptic Ulcer
Poor Vision
Retinal Degeneration
Stroke
Vascular Disease

More than 400 years ago, Cartier stumbled upon the power of substances contained in the bark of a pine tree native to Canada and a tea made from it saved the lives of his men. Cartier waited until his men were deathly sick and some had died before taking advantage of this miracle natural substance. If only he had known about the proanthocyanadins within the bark *before* his men became ill!

Some nutritionists will tell you about this *newly discovered* substance called Pycnogenol. You now know better.

6. *Chromium Picolinate and Life Extension*

You could feel the excitement bursting through the auditorium.

These were the most distinguished longevity scientists in the world. They were men and women of prestigious universities, research centers, and think tanks from throughout the world. Yet the presentation being made that October afternoon in San Francisco, Calif., based on research conducted at a little known university in the state of Minnesota, was about to herald a new era in longevity research, for finally one of the keys to life extension—one that would impact 90 percent of all Americans—had been discovered. Now suddenly everything fit together, and advances in life extension would proceed on two essential fronts. There were reporters covering the scientific meeting from the nation's leading daily newspapers including the Los Angeles Times, Washington Post, and New York Times. Longevity magazine had sent a special correspondent. Everybody wanted the story—even though all too few Americans would come to understand the significance of the story that was unfolding and which had become the centerpeice of the conference.

Calorie Restriction Myth Exploded

For years, mainstream scientists have maintained that the only way to obtain significant advances in life extension is to cut calories. Sixty years ago researchers noted that rats fed diets containing only 60 percent to 65 percent of their normal calorie daily intake lived 50 percent longer. Additional species, ranging from one-cell protozoa to fish and even primates have also enjoyed significant life extension with caloric restriction. One of the world's leading experts on life extension, Dr. Roy L. Walford, a pathologist at the University of California at Los Angeles, has even begun to consume a low-calorie diet.

And for sixty years that was where science was firmly entrenched. Reduce calories and increase life span. And what a hellish dictate for most people. Let's face it: Most people like to eat. They like to eat a lot, they like to eat frequently, and the last thing they want is to live a life of restriction. There must be an easier way. *There is—with chromium picolinate.*

Federal Scientists' Findings

Researchers with the U.S. Department of Agriculture (USDA) have developed and patented a form of chromium, called chromium picolinate, which can be more easily absorbed by the body.

One of the primary researchers into this new form of chromium is Dr. Gary W. Evans of Bemidji State University in Minnesota. Dr. Evans had conducted previous studies with Dr. Jack Geller and Dr. Raymond I. Press at Mercy Hospital and Medical Center in San Diego that demonstrated chromium picolinate can reduce levels of low-density lipoproteins (LDLs, i.e., the "bad cholesterol") in humans while increasing their high-density lipoproteins (HDLs, i.e., the "good cholesterol").

These studies pointed up the fact that chromium picolinate can reduce incidence of atherosclerotic plaques, which encrust the arteries and cause heart attacks.

But there is more, Dr. Evans discovered. Studies in animals had shown that chromium picolinate increased lean muscle mass and reduced body fat.

So Dr. Evans began providing members of the Bemidji football team 200 micrograms daily during the season while they were engaged in weight lifting on a regular basis.

Those players who were given the chromium picolinate enjoyed a 22 percent drop in total body fat compared to only 1 percent for those who did not receive the supplement. The men receiving chromium picolinate also enjoyed a 42% greater increase in lean muscle mass.

Wonder Pill, Say Scientists

Many scientists now call chromium picolinate a wonder pill. "It is certainly something most everybody could benefit from by having more of it," notes Richard Anderson of the USDA in Beltsville, MD.

But the real excitement came at the 22nd annual meeting of the American Aging Association in San Francisco last fall when Dr. Evans announced the dramatic effects of chromium picolinate on life extension when tested on experimental animals.

Dr. Evans took three groups of rats. One group received chromium chloride, another chromium dinicotinate, and the third chromium picolinate. Their diets began quickly after weaning and continued throughout the life span of the animals. They were allowed to eat as much and as frequently as they wished (*ad libitum* feeding).

The rats receiving chromium picolinate lived an average of one year longer than the others. After nearly four years, when all of the rats in the first two groups were dead, 80% were alive in the group receiving chromium picolinate. Their life spans had been increased by 33%. Considering that all other benefits of chromium picolinate that are found in animals also apply to humans, many researchers now believe the life extension properties of chromium picolinate will also benefit people.

Dr. Caleb Finch of the University of Southern California is one of the nation's leading experts on life extension. Dr. Finch, commenting on the findings, notes that Dr. Evans's work represents "a new and unexpected potential variable in life span that deserves serious consideration in long lived species."

Now we return to the caloric-restriction theory and its connection with chromium picolinate.

The reason that calorie restriction seems to work so well is that it reduces the amount of sugar (glucose) circulating in the animals' blood streams. When glucose is found at high levels in the human body, it almost always causes a process called glycation which damages the body's veins and arteries, causing an accumulation of damaged proteins which is thought to be one of the primary causes of aging.

Dr. Evans, however, found that blood sugar and glycated hemoglobin levels were consistently and markedly lower in the rats receiving chromium picolinate and were, in fact, 60% lower than in the other groups.

So now we know that there are many roads to a longer, healthier life, and that both supplementation with chromium picolinate and caloric restriction work. One, however, means a life of restriction. On the other hand, Dr. Evans notes, chromium picolinate has such a profound effect on insulin function and lowering blood sugar levels that its benefits are comparable to calorie restriction. Yet you can eat all you want!

"This could be a potentially major finding," notes Anderson of the USDA. He adds that more than 90% of U.S. adults have a dietary deficiency of chromium, however, because it is poorly absorbed and because plants do not require chromium for growth and may be grown in chromium-depleted soils.

Indeed, this fact is underscored by a recent study published in the *Journal of Applied Nutrition* which found that conventionally grown foods had far less mineral content than organically grown foods. I am truly a believer that we need to supplement this important mineral, and the best form to use is chromium picolinate.

In fact, chromium picolinate has so many benefits that Dr. Evans states, "I would very definitely suggest that people take chromium picolinate on a regular basis."

7. The Immune System

"In a world of disease, a good immune system is your best self-defense," says Dr. Hans Kugler, president of both the National Health Federation and International Academy of Preventive Health & Medicine in California. "If you had no choice but to live in a hostile environment, what would be your first concern? Naturally, to protect yourself with every possible means. In respect to your health you have no choice. You do live in a hostile environment that threatens you with cancer-causing substances, factors that age you prematurely, and with microorganisms like the AIDS virus. If we would interview cancer-researchers, gerontologists and virologists, and ask them—What is the single most important factor in protecting yourself against disease and aging?—most would agree on one answer: having a good immune system."

It's saddening to realize that it has taken a massive tragedy like the AIDS crisis in America to focus our nation's attention on the purpose and well functioning of the body's immune system. Perhaps this is because scientists and health care professionals alike are intrigued by the fact that, while some 100,000

Americans have died or are in the throes of dying from full-fledged AIDS, many millions more of our nation's men, women and children have been exposed to the HIV virus, yet they remain relatively healthy. Current research suggests that the answer lies in the strength of their immune systems. A strong immune system is more capable of defending the body's cells from the deadly effects of HIV. A weak immune system is not. But what makes one person's immune system so much stronger than someone else's? Of course, part of the answer is genetic. Some people seem to have been born with very strong immune systems while others are cursed with systems which are relatively weak and inefficient. Interestingly, there is evidence to support the idea that we can use our knowledge of optimal nutrition to strengthen our body's immunity to outside toxins including viruses, bacteria, radiation, pesticides, industrial chemicals and other compounds that threaten our health. Based on future studies, new RDAs for newly recognized immune-related nutrients will need to be formulated and applied widely in medical and public health practices and public education.

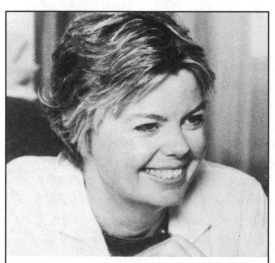

Joan Priestley, M.D., is a strong believer in the power of the immune system to ward off disease. In her practice, she specializes in immune system enhancement for prevention, palliation and cure of HIV/AIDS, candida sensitivity, Epstein-Barr, chronic fatigue syndrome, PMS and degenerative diseases. Among the most helpful immune boosters is quercetin which seems to also promote the activity of vitamin C, she says.

In light of the immense environmental pollution and biological toxins burdening our body's immune systems, the information we are acquiring about optimal immune function is of paramount importance. Beisel (1990) comments on the role of micronutrients for enhancing immune function and reports that the future is bright in the field of nutrients and immunity. Recent advances in technology will permit the design of many new research studies, and an increased application of the findings to clinical and public health practices, the researcher says. More researchers will need to be trained in the fundamentals of both nutritional and immunological sciences. Yet although additional basic knowledge is desperately needed in both fields, the scientific and clinical value of merging these two fields is already well established. Dr. Kugler says that, along with the free radical theory, the immunologic theory on aging is extraordinarily important. "By eliminating factors that impair immune functions, like smoking cigarettes and environmental toxins, and by improving the immune system with super nutrition and vitamin and mineral supplements, very impressive life span increases were achieved on cancer-prone animals," he says adding that he believes the same impressive results can be shown to be true for people as well.

Does the typical American need a supplement for improved immune function? Many health experts would answer this question with a resounding and affirmative *Yes!* With pervasive environmental pollution, increased cancer incidence striking Americans at the rate of one in three and with predictions that the percentage may well be one in two within a few decades— the need for optimal immune function is absolute.

Other less progressive thinkers—plagued with the anachronistic belief that nothing new happens under the sun—would tell you that all you need is to consume an "average" diet. But such views are rather outdated in light of the many recent breakthroughs in nutrition.

Note these examples:
•Researchers reporting in *The American Journal of Clinical Nutrition* looked at 32 healthy women and men greater than the age of 60 who were placed in a double-blind, placebo-controlled trial of vitamin E supplementation at 800 IU daily for 30 days or placebo. In the vitamin E-supplemented group, there was an increased antigenic response to the delayed-hypersensitivity skin test and increased production of the important immune agent interleukin II. There was a decrease in prostaglandin E2 synthesis and plasma lipid peroxides (Meydani 1990). This study demonstrated for the first time, in a double-blind, placebo-controlled trial, that vitamin E enhances immune function in healthy elderly individuals and suggests that elderly individuals might benefit from supplementary intake of vitamin E. This is a very significant finding that a single nutrient may be immunoenhancing in healthy adults consuming the recommended daily

allowances from their diets. Dietary intervention is also the most practical modality for delaying or reversing the rate of decline of immune function.

•Another team of researchers reporting in *The American Journal of Clinical Nutrition* gave modest doses of beta carotene to 10 healthy men and 10 healthy women who were an average of 56 years of age. With dosages of 30 mg/d or greater for two months, there was an increase in the percentage of lymphoid cells with surface markers for T-helper, natural killer cells and cells with interleukin II. This relationship was dose-dependent (Watson 1991). In the elderly subjects the singular elevation of T-helper cells without affecting suppressor cells is significant. This is an area of immune deterioration in adults which may increase their incidence of cancer development. This study suggests that beta-carotene has immunostimulating capabilities in humans.

•*The Lancet* reports that healthy male volunteers between the ages of 21 and 34 years of age ingested 30 grams of arginine per day in divided doses for three days. There was a mean increase over the pretreatment natural killer cell cytotoxicity by 91 percent. The increase was greatest in those who had the lowest baseline activities. The enhancement of natural killer cells and lympho-kine-activated-killer cells by large doses of arginine may prove beneficial in immunosuppressive states such as AIDS and malignant diseases.

•Researchers reporting in the *Canadian Medical Association Journal* state that enteral diet supplements to enhance immune function are becoming increasingly available, and they're working. Certain amino acids, omega-3, omega-6 and short chain fatty acids can all have a pharmacological effect on immune function. Arginine enhances immune function by stimulating lympho-cyte reactivity. Supplementation with an "immuno-nutrition" product con-taining arginine, RNA and omega-3 fatty acid for seven days after surgery resulted in fewer infections and significant reduction in hospital stay compared to the standard enteral diet.

•Selenium supplementation among elderly residents of a nursing home, suffering from osteoarthritis, hypertension, residual stroke and other age-related diseases, enhanced lymphocyte response, report researchers from the Department of Rheumatology and Physical Medicine, Saint-Pierre Hospital, Brussels, Belgium (Peretz 1990).

•In the journal *Age and Ageing*, researchers found that modest supplemen-tation of vitamins A, C and E among 30 elderly individuals resulted in an increase in most of the indices of immune function but not in the placebo-controlled group (Penn 1990). These results suggest that supplementation with vitamins A,C and E in combination can improve cell-mediated immunity and may prevent premature mortality.

•Castillo-Duran and colleagues reported in the *American Journal of Clinical Nutrition* in 1987, that zinc supplementation has significant effects on weight gain and host defense mechanisms in infants—*despite normal plasma levels for these nutrients.*

•Not surprisingly, given the above studies and many others, researchers at the Nutritional Immunology and Toxicology Laboratory of the U.S. Department of Agriculture Nutrition Research Center on Aging, at Tufts University in Boston, assert: "Dietary manipulation of the immune system has been proposed as a practical approach to intervening in its age-related functional decline."

Don't Wait Until You're Sick

You might question the wisdom of those who say that you don't need nutrients to stimulate your immune system. Essentially they're telling you to wait until you get sick with a viral infection or cancer before you start strengthening your immune system. It would seem that, by then, the proverbial horse (saddled with disease) is out of the barn. Those health professionals who favor strengthening the immune system through dietary supplements believe strongly that an active, assertive approach to personal health is a wiser choice—one that will help prevent or ameliorate most serious and mild illness before it destroys your health. In other words, why wait to scamper for a cure after you become ill when you can take a pro-active role in your own health care by taking advantage of the preventive measures available to you beforehand? Part of the answer must lay in ignorance. Many people simply do not know how to take care of themselves. Optimal nutrition nutrition should be required at every stage of a student's education.

We must teach our children that sickness is not the normal state of life. Many sicknesses probably can be avoided altogether or at least delayed through optimal nutrition and good health practices.

We know ultimately that prevention is the most important concept in medicine. This belief is extraordinarily important when we discuss the health of the human immune system. There is no longer any doubt among many health professionals that people need nutritional boosters to fortify their body's immunity. This is the underlying principle behind many cancer and AIDS therapies.

Nobody is Safe

But again what about the average person who is not overtly suffering from any diseases? Is the average person's immune system in need of help? Before you can answer that question, you need to determine who the *average* person is. *Whose immune system isn't being assaulted?*

Is a woman who lives in Wisconsin's potato-growing region average? How about residents of small farm towns in the upper San Joaquin Valley of California? Are residents of New York City the average American? How about an office worker in downtown Dayton, Ohio? A wheat farmer in Kansas? What about a young girl living in New Jersey? An elderly couple in Los Angeles? Is any one simply *average*?

In other words, each of us is so vastly different from everybody around us that there may not be an average person anywhere in this nation. Furthermore, nobody is protected from pollution, viral agents and bacterial disease; our exposure to environmental and biological pollution may be having the insidious effect of burdening our immune systems and wearing down our cells by causing toxic oxygen free radical reactions within our bodies. This kind of environmental pollution is serious in major urban areas of the country where the greatest concentrations of the population are located.

But moving to the rural areas of America may not prove to be much safer when it comes to environmental pollution.

Recently a study was done of women in Wisconsin's potato growing region where a pesticide called aldicarb has been used extensively on the crop. This pesticide is so toxic that even a drop can kill a full grown man. In 1985, this same pesticide poisoned more than 1,000 people in the Western U.S. who ate watermelons grown in the Kern County area of California that were contaminated with illegal residues of this deadly substance. California state health officials say that this incidence was the largest food borne poisoning outbreak

How The Immune System Protects Your Health

The human body has many ways of defending itself against toxins including bacteria, viruses, and pollutants. Two ways the immune system works are via the *innate* and *adaptive* immune systems.

The Innate Immune System

Your body contains many kinds of defenses that are often taken for granted, such as your skin, nose hairs, and even the digestive juices released by your stomach. Many of these physical and chemical defenses are considered to be part of the innate immune system.

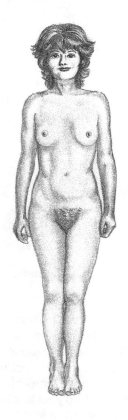

You might not know that the tears of your **eyes** contain an anti-bacterial enzyme which protects your body from bacterium that might otherwise be able to enter via the openings of your ocular cavity.

Your **skin** does more than hold in your skeletal system and make you look youthful or aged. Your skin, when unbroken by cuts and abrasions, screens out many bacteria and viruses (including the AIDS virus). Your skin also contains sebaceous glands which secrete anti-bacterial chemicals.

Your **nose hairs** may not seem to be the most aesthetic part of your face, but their usefulness, in preventing microscopic bits of dust and organisms riding on dust from entering your respiratory tract, cannot be denied. Your nose hairs have probably saved your lungs and respiratory tract many times over from both physical and bacterial toxins that would otherwise have destroyed your health.

When you eat you salivate. Contained in your **saliva** are anti-bacterial enzymes called lysozymes which protect your body from the many varieties of bacteria contaminating the food which you ingest.

How many times has your **stomach** saved you from food poisoning? Many contaminants, including potentially deadly bacteria such as salmonella and listeria, may be found in food which you swallow. However, the stomach secretes a powerful acid to which most bacteria succumb. Those that do survive the power of your stomach acid encounter another defensive system: your intestinal lining contains many beneficial bacteria which compete with harmful bacteria and help control their population.

The **respiratory tract** of humans contains mucus, which are able to detain bacteria and hold them in place while phagocytes, which are a form of white blood cells, destroy them. Alternately, the cells of the respiratory tract have tiny hairs, called **cilia**, which can expel bacteria, for example, when you cough.

A woman's **vagina** and **urethra** contain both beneficial bacteria and mucus which help prevent bacterial illness. In men, semen contains a substance called spermine which may have anti-bacterial properties.

The Innate Immune System in Action

But what happens when your body's protective barriers are broken through and bacteria, a virus or toxin enters the bloodstream, threatening your health? Let's take as an example what happens when you accidentally step on a tack, which penetrates the skin barrier.

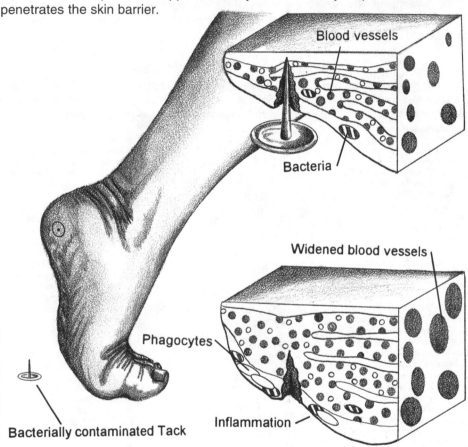

Blood vessels

Bacteria

Widened blood vessels

Phagocytes

Inflammation

Bacterially contaminated Tack

The first thing that will happen is that the body's blood vessels will widen and weaken, while blood will flow from them into the damaged tissues. At the same time, inflammation will set in, and the body will release chemicals such as histamine. Thanks to the leakage from the vessels to the site of infection, the body's phagocytes can travel to the site of infection where they are able to engulf and digest potentially poisonous bacteria and viruses. So when your foot becomes inflamed with pain and swelling, as painful as this might seem, it is your body's way of dealing with a potentially dangerous situation.

Phagocytes—Part of Your Body's Innate Immune System

Phagocytes are white blood cells that literally surround and gobble up harmful bacteria with the help of powerful lysosomes.

Phagocytes work in three steps:

1. Recognition of the bacteria or microbe as being a threat to the body is the first step. The phagocyte is helped by the body's release of chemicals during inflammation. In the first stage, the phagocytes attaches itself to the microbe.

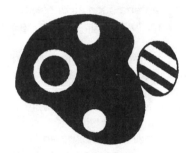

2. In the second stage, the phagocyte surrounds the microbe while its powerful lysosomes ready themselves to destroy the invading bacterium.

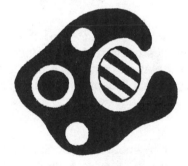

3. In the third and final stage, the lysosomes release their enzymes which destroy the microbe. Once the microbe is digested, the phagocyte rids itself of remaining debris.

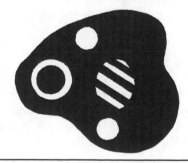

The Adapative Immune System

The Adaptive Immune System consists of cells called lymphocytes which are produced in the bone marrow and then develop into two groups: B lymphocytes and T lymphocytes. The B lymphocytes belong to the Humoral Immune system. The T lymphocytes belong to the Cellular Immune System.

The Humoral Immune System

The Humoral Immune System is especially effective against viruses such as measles, bacteria such as cholera, and parasites such as *Crypto sporidium.*

There are four basic steps in the activities of the humoral immune system.

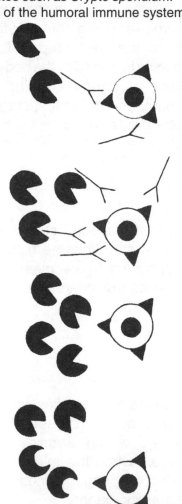

1.   The first step begins when a foreign substance or organism enters the body, say for example a bacterial microbe. This foreign microbe will have on its surface an antigen, a protein which is not part of the body and which the B-lymphocytes recognize as being foreign to the body.

2.   In the second step, the B-lymphocytes begin rapid reproduction and form plasma cells which produce antibodies that "adapt" to the specific organism and attack.

3.   When enough antibodies have been produced, they migrate towards the bacterium with the foreign antigen, attaching themselves to the antigen.

4. Fortunately, some of the B-lymphocytes involved in this process have memory imprints and become memory cells, remaining in the body. If the same antigen enters the body, antibodies are produced rapidly.

Cellular Immunity

Cellular immunity is particularly important for the prevention of viral diseases and cancer. In the cellular immune system, T-lymphocytes are released. Actually, the history of your body's T-lymphocytes begins before birth in the thymus gland which "educates" them. Although the thymus gland eventually shrinks in size and virtually disappears as a person ages, the lymph nodes continue to process and "educate" T-lymphocytes.

There are a number of different kinds of T-lymphocytes: Helper cells help the B lymphocytes from the Humoral Immune system to produce more antibodies. Suppressor cells notify the B cells when to turn off. Killer cells destroy foreign tissues and bacteria. These T-lymphocytes produce a family of chemicals known as lymphokines.

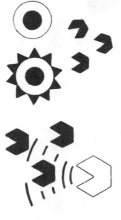

Celluar immunity proceeds in four steps.

1. First, a T-lymphocyte recognizes an antigen (foreign protein) on the outside of an abnormal cell. Upon recognition, additional T-lymphocytes are mobilized.

2. Helper cells aid killer T-lymphocytes to multiply as the body readies itself to vanquish the foreign cell.

3. When enough killer T-lymphocytes have been produced, they intercept the rogue cancer cell, attaching themselves, and killing it. Killer T-lymphocytes may continue to killer any other similar cells.

4. The killer T-lymphocyte cells that remain behind develop a memory for the antigen. If infection reoccurs, the killer T-lymphocyte cells quickly attack and destroy it.

Types of Lymphocytes

What are lymphocytes? Lymphocytes are one of the most important parts of the adaptive immune system and are responsible for subduing invading bacteria, viruses, cancer cells and even, though ineffectively in many cases, the AIDS virus. Lymphocytes make-up some one-third of the white cells in the blood stream. Though all lymphocytes originate in the bone marrow, two kinds of lymphocytes have evolved in the human body.

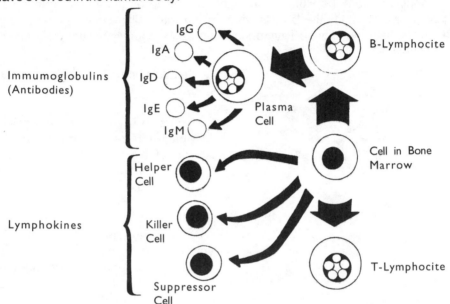

B-Lymphocytes

The B-lymphocytes are part of the humoral branch of the immune system. B-lymphocytes produce plasma cells which then produce many kinds of antibodies, also known as immunoglobulins, as in IgG, IgA, IgD, IgE, and IgM. The B-lymphocytes are most adept at defending the body against viruses, bacteria, and some parasites.

T-Lymphocytes

The T-lymphocytes make-up the cellular branch of the immune system. They are made and educated in the thymus gland early on in a person's life and later in the lymph glands. T-lymphocytes produce chemicals call lymphokines which have many individual protective functions. Among the various kinds of T-lymphocytes are helper cells which assist the B-Lymphocytes in producing antibodies to fight bacteria, viruses, and parasites. Suppressor T-lymphocyte cells help the B lymphocytes to know when to stop producing antibodies. Killer T-lymphocytes destroy foreign tissues and infectious agents. T-lymphocytes are more adept at destroying viruses, bacteria, fungi, and tumor cells.

The Disappearing Thymus Gland

The thymus gland is the major programmer of the immune system. The thymus gland contains T-lymphocytes, and when you are young, the thymus gland teaches lymphocytes to recognize self from "non-self," so that the body's immune system does not attack and destroy itself. Interestingly, medical science has learned that some 95 percent of the T-lymphocytes produced in the thymus gland are actually destroyed, because they have the potential to turn against the body.

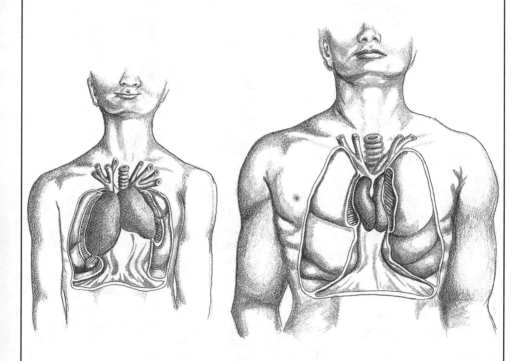

As a child, your thymus gland is as large it will ever be. But as you mature, your thymus gland decreases significantly in size. This shrinkage is testimony to the thymus gland's importance in educating immune cells. Many rejuvenation therapies are built upon the premise of restimulating the thymus gland and improving the body's overall immunity. (*See Chapter 31.*)

in U. S. history. Aldicarb residues have even contaminated the potatoes which you bring home from the supermarket.

Despite the accumulating evidence that aldicarb is a deadly, acute poison that also presents long-term health risks, it is now being found in the drinking water supplies of communities located in Wisconsin, New York and at least 15 other states. Researcher Dr. Michael Fiore used laboratory techniques to examine the immune system function of a group of Wisconsin women who were regularly drinking water from such tainted supplies, and what he found is unsettling. Even at levels as low as one to ten parts per billion, significant clinical abnormalities in immune system function were noted, especially in the women's T8/T4 ratios. Even the researchers who made the findings are unsure of the significance of these clinical abnormalities. But how would you react if you were told that a pesticide in your drinking water had caused changes in your body's immune system and that nobody was sure what it meant?

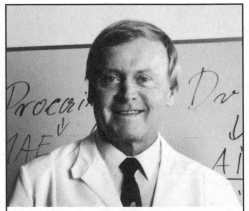

Hans Kugler, Ph.D., president of the National Health Federation, a former researcher at Roosevelt University and author of four best selling books on longevity, says that a strong immune system is a person's best defense in a polluted world. Dr. Kugler uses many of the immune boosters described in this book, especially Phycotene and DMG (*see Chapter 8*).

What is even more unsettling about the Wisconsin study is that this is not an isolated case of immune system alteration. In fact, the drinking water supplies of millions of Americans are tainted with cancer causing pesticides and other questionably safe chemical compounds such as trichloroethylene, perchloroethylene, toluene, benzene, chloroform, alachlor, ethylene dibromide, atrazine, di-bromo-chloropropane—chemicals which have been documented to harm the central nervous system, cause cancer and potentially even cause reproductive problems such as sterility or birth defects. It is an unfortunate fact that the toxicological studies of these same chemicals' effects on the human immune system are sadly lacking, and medical science really doesn't know all that much about what high level cumulative residues of these chemicals are doing to our bodies, especially our immune function.

It's clear to many health professionals that our concern must be focused not only upon the acutely toxic effects of chemical pollution but on their long-term, cumulative effects at high levels. Yet we need not go searching remote areas like the Wisconsin potato growing region for immune devastating pollutants. We need go no further than our kitchen shelves. We all know that our foods are contaminated with pesticides. Some foods like pork/beef frankfurters and peanut butter are highly contaminated with cancer causing pesticides (Steinman 1992). We have discussed that cellular repair mechanisms are at best 99.99 percent perfect. But when each of our cells' genetic materials is known to be hit 10,000 times daily by free radicals which are created when our body fights antigens such as pollutants, bacteria and viruses, we can begin to understand the meaning of *cumulative* damage and the gradual wearing of the cells. Our enemy is omnipresent. The result of neglecting the health of our immune system is that its cells ultimately do not perform their functions as well. Dr. Pauling (1986) asserts that the immune system has the difficult task of distinguishing foe from friend by first recognizing nonself (the invading vectors of disease, such as bacteria or malignant cells) as distinct from self (the normal cells). Dr. Pauling says that such recognition depends on the evaluation of differences in molecular structure between friendly molecules and those which threaten harm. Fortunately, unfriendly viruses and bacteria have striking differences from those that are beneficial and for which distinctions are easily made by our immune system. *But cancer cells have only slight differences from healthy cells and the immune mechanisms must be highly competent in order to be effective. Unfortunately as we age, immune function decreases.* Lesourd (1990) says quite explicitly that aging leads to decrease of immune function and notes that all functions of cell mediated immunity are decreased in the elderly, and that especially our immune cells are less mature and suffer decreased functioning.

Yet nutritional support improves the immune defects in aged ill patients *and many health experts believe dietary supplements are of value in improving this deficiency in immune function even when administered to aged healthy subjects.*

Thus health seekers face a dual challenge: On the one hand, as they age, their immune function naturally decreases. At the same time, achieving an optimal diet through meals alone may be difficult for many people. The challenge is to maintain optimal immune function through optimal nutrition.

Unfortunately, many of the initial symptoms of an altered, damaged or weakened immune system are subclinical, which means that under ordinary circumstances they will not be detected by physicians. But quite probably millions of Americans are suffering from cumulative subclinical symptoms of low level poisoning from both synthetic and natural toxins and environmental stresses. Their immune function may also be hampered by such exposures.

Fortunately an increasing number of responsible health professionals question the wisdom of allowing people to become sick and only then instituting measures to bolster an individual's immunity. Rather, these health professionals assert preventive measures should be implemented in a health-promoting regimen long before there are clinical signs of illness. It is this proposition that must be put forward before the medical community and embraced with the passion with which it has embraced vaccination, low fat diets and eating fresh fruits and vegetables.

The wisest health professionals in the future and even today will combine nutritional therapy with advancements in technology because both are equally important in a health-oriented program and both are where disease prevention is headed.

We need technology. We need it to help us more closely examine the bountiful supplies of potentially helpful substances available in our natural pharmacy. Science is perhaps best defined as the capacity to *see*—to view nature at its most essential levels, to strip it bare in order to see its inner workings. We need look no further, for example, than the creation of the compound microscope. When scientists began to see microbial clusters through the lens of the first primitive microscopes, a whole new world became visible. With the coming of the electron microscope, once again science was given the power to view a natural world which had been previously invisible to the naked eye. And with the power of chromatography we are now able to identify isolates in plant and animal materials that are the potent chemicals from which so many of our most powerful therapeutic drugs have been derived. In a very real sense, nutritional advancements are so much the result of technological advancement.

Once again we stress that our concern is that the substance employed not only improves cellular mediated immune responses but that it be without potentially harmful side effects. The first immuno-modulating agents were bacteria and bacterial products but they had several undesirable side effects. For example, during Benjamin Franklin's era, the first smallpox vaccinations were created based on the finding that milk maids who were exposed to small amounts of small pox did not come down with the disease. One of the problems was that researchers were not able to determine how much was enough and how much was too much to inject into subjects. The result was that many people died. In fact, the Franklin family vehemently opposed small pox vaccinations!

Yet although recent work has demonstrated that undernourished individuals have impaired immune responses, don't think for a moment that we are speaking only in terms of the nutritional habits of Third World peoples. Because in fact, single nutrient deficiencies among otherwise healthy people living in highly industrialized and wealthy nations can have profoundly adverse effects on immune function.

Chandra (1987) notes that it is now established that deficiencies of single nutrients also impair immune responses and that the best studied are zinc, iron, vitamin B-6, vitamin A, copper and selenium. Daly and colleagues (1978) note dietary protein and individual amino acids have a profound effect on immune function. The researchers observed that in a series of experiments with normal animals that arginine was demonstrated to enhance cellular immune mechanisms, in particular T-cell function. Thompson (1987) once again points up the fact that aging in experimental animals and in humans is associated with a significant "defect" of helper/inducer T lymphocytes. For the aged ill and even the aged healthy, there is oftentimes a deficit in protein and zinc.

Some phytotherapeutic nutrients, vitamins and minerals are widely recognized as immune stimulators. The rush is on to discover the most potent immune stimulators by searching our vast natural botanical and wildlife resources worldwide, identifying the most bioactive immune strengtheners and harvesting or synthesizing them in the laboratory.

In preparing a supplement program for patients or people who would like to prepare their own, a number of important nutrients are available that either stimulate the immune system or aid the body in producing its own antiviral, antibacterial, and anti-toxin substances.

One of the most interesting aspects about these potent nutrients is that, like the free radical scavengers, they often perform a number of tasks. Perhaps today's deadliest diseases can someday be controlled by using solutions from the past. Or perhaps we'll find the answer from technology. More than likely, we'll be combining both—looking back and towards the future—taking full advantage of our historic pharmaceuticals, while at the same time using technology to develop and isolate startling new immune strengtheners.

8. *Immuno-Stimulators*

Why do sharks never contract cancer? What native American flower, now proposed for the endangered species list, protects users from viral infections? And more to the point: what dietary supplements can you incorporate into your daily health program to stimulate your immune system into a state of super immunity?

The following nutrients have been proven in experimental studies to improve immune function and they are available *now*:

Alkylglycerols

The story is told of Dr. Astrid Brohult, a Swedish doctor who in 1952 conceived of the idea that children suffering from leukemia could be helped by being given the marrow from the bones of freshly slaughtered calves. In fact, although the results were at first uneven, the calf bone marrow in many cases strongly stimulated white blood cell counts in children. Her husband, biochemist Sven Brohult, analyzed the active substance in the bones that appeared to have stimulated increases in the white blood cell counts and found that the chemicals were alkylglycerols, a group of three natural substances first discovered in 1922 by Japanese researchers and were first synthesized by Nobel prize laureate Sir Robert Robinson. Ultimately, the Brohults' work with bone marrow extracts paid off when their published reports demonstrated more than a decade later that patients with cancer of the uterine or cervix who received alkylglycerols before their primary radiation treatment had a significantly better survival rate than patients not given alkylglycerols (Brohult 1977).

One of the reasons that physicians are so adamant infants be breast fed is that immune stimulating nutrients such as alkylglycerols are found naturally in mother's milk at levels 10 times greater than in cow's milk. Other rich sources of alkylglycerols include spleen tissue and bone marrow; alkylglycerols are also produced by healthy individuals in their liver as well.

A Swedish pharmaceutical manufacturer discovered that the liver oil of the Greenland shark is one of the best sources of natural alkylglycerols. Ultimately, a purification process was developed that was able to remove nonessential substances such as cholesterol, squalene, vitamins A and D, and other fatty acids as well as pollutants such as polychlorinated biphenyls (PCBs) and pesticides while retaining the alkylglycerols. It has been only since 1986 that purified shark liver oil containing alkylglycerols has become publicly available.

The immuno-stimulating effects of alkylglycerols are gaining wide recognition for their benefits in the medical and scientific communities. Yet once again we find that other cultures in other lands have beaten us to the punch—in this case it's the immune stimulating "punch" of shark liver oil. For more than 2,000 years, medicinal shops in China have made available the oil from shark livers to treat burns and cuts, heal stomach ulcers, and increase fertility. Likewise, fishermen around the world—from Norway to Argentina—swear by the healing properties of this unique substance.

Alkylglycerols are involved in the production of white blood cells. In fact, some scientists believe that their presence in the human body is as important to white blood cells as iron is to red blood cells.

Technically known as leukocytes, white blood cells are responsible for the production of antibodies, special kinds of blood proteins which circulate in the plasma and attack antigens that are toxins harmful to the body.

The human body can produce some one million types of antibodies. Each is a rather large protein molecule, consisting of about fifteen-thousand to twenty-five thousand atoms. Each kind is able to recognize a particular group of atoms (Pauling 1986) and vanquish this antigen before it does us in.

Modern health researchers, wondering why shark oil is such a potent immuno-stimulator, were stunned to discover that shark liver oil contains an incredible concentration of alkylglycerols. When researchers discovered that liver oil from the Greenland Shark (*Somniosus Miccephalus*) contained approximately 30 percent alkylglycerols and that other species such as *Chiamera Monstruosa* contained up to 90 percent alkylglycerols—scientists suddenly had an adequate supply source; a new era of human immuno-defense research began.

Studies show that alkylglycerols:

•Cause an increase in the white blood cell and platelet count when given to AIDS patients.

•Alleviate the two most common side effects of radiation therapy—leukopenia (white blood cell reduction) and thromboctopenia (blood platelet reduction).

•Reduce the drop in the white blood cell count accompanying chemotherapy especially if their use is begun before the onset of treatment.

•Possess the ability to promote the production of all types of white blood cells including T-cells as well as the large white blood cells known as macrophages which consume yeast and viruses (Boeryd 1980).

•Can be used as general immune stimulators in conditions where elevation of immunity is required as in chronic yeast and viral infections.

•Arrest or limit the growth of tumor cells in *in-vitro* tests.

Dimethylglycine

In 1981, researchers studying the human immune defense system found that dimethylglycine (DMG) was a successful immunomodulator which had the ability to increase immune defense functions by causing certain elements to move more quickly through the blood. Graber (1981) notes in *The Journal of Infectious Diseases* that DMG enhances immune responses in humans.

Reap and colleagues (1990) conclude that their results "show that DMG given orally can potentiate the immune response in a whole animal model" and that although the mechanisms by which DMG enhances the immune response are unknown, it is of considerable importance to examine new nontoxic immunoenhancers. "Immunologic aberrations are well-known consequences of aging," the researchers said, "in which both cellular and humoral branches of the immune system are altered. Immune function in these various states might profit by treatment with a nontoxic immunomodulator, such as DMG."

Phycotene

Phycotene is an extract made from both spirulina and dunaliella algae which together contain at least 17 beta carotenes, vitamin E and two immune-enhancing substances. Phycotene has been shown to increase tumor necrosis factor (TNF) by 600 percent more than beta carotene, reports Dr. Hans Kugler. Furthermore, Harvard University researchers found that in experimental studies where cancers were induced in the oral pouches of hamsters, 30 percent of the animals treated with Phycotene experienced total tumor regression and 70 percent showed partial tumor regression, says Dr. Kugler.

The Viral-Aging Cycle

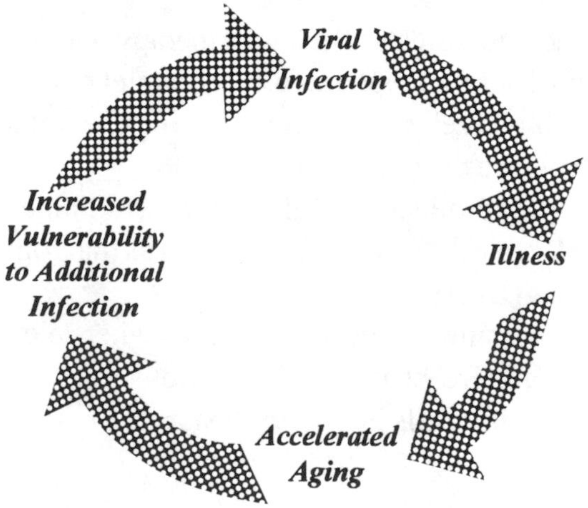

Viral Infection

Illness

Accelerated Aging

Increased Vulnerability to Additional Infection

Viruses play an important role in many diseases including influenza, chronic fatigue syndrome, leukemia, cervical cancer, uterine cancer, liver cancer, lymphoma, meningitis, herpes and encephalitis. Each time a person is ill, it takes a toll on their overall health with the release of free radicals and ensuing immune system damage. To break this cycle, protect yourself with immunostimulators, say doctors. In the above illustration, the viral cycle of aging and its circular nature is shown. A strong immune system, however, can break the circle of viral aging, say experts such as as Dr. Hans Kugler.

Another Harvard University study found that animals exposed to the carcinogen DMBA and who received Phyco-tene at the same time failed to form tumors even after seven months of constant exposure to DMBA, says Dr. Kugler. In yet another study, reported in 1988 in *Nutrition and Cancer*, experimental animals were treated with DMBA. One group received Phycotene, another beta carotene and another canthaxanthin which also stimulates TNF. Only the Phycotene-treated animals developed no tumors; however, both the beta carotene- and canthaxanthin-treated animals also had lower than normal numbers of tumors.

Dr. Kugler explains, "Dr. Joel Schwartz of Harvard University, trying to identify the anti-cancer mechanism of phycotene, found that phycocyanin-C (found in the Phycotene mixture), seems to alter the environment around a tumor and makes it more difficult for the tumor to grow. However, the most important finding was that Phycotene greatly stimulates TNF formation." Kugler points out that research into immune function has shown that TNF is an extremely potent immune system activator. But there's more to this story than simply activating TNF, Kugler explains. Another immune activator is Interferon. When both TNF and Interferon production are stimulated, the effect is greater than additive—it's synergistic. An important activator of Interferon is DMG which has been shown to stimulate production by more than 500 percent. So when DMG is combined with Phycotene, it's a fantastic immune stimulator. Furthermore, studies published in *Medication and New Drugs* in 1966 indicate that two to three grams daily of spirulina will slow loss of white blood cells.

Echinacea

One of the primary healing nutrients in the 19th Century, *Echinacea* is another immune booster, fighting infections by destroying germs as well as increasing the body's white blood cell count. It is an important part of daily optimal nutritional programs, meant to stimulate the immune system. In addition to a substantial body of German research which documents this herb's ability to stimulate the immune system, particularly the production of disease-fighting T-cells, Mowrey (1986) explains that: "In recent years, research has discovered the mechanisms by which *Echinacea* may work to prevent infection. One of the primary defense mechanisms of the body is known as the hyaluronidase system. Hyaluronic acid (HA) is the [material] that occurs in the tissues between cells to 'cement' them together. It forms a very effective barrier against infection. There is an enzyme that attacks HA in a way not fully understood. When it does, the HA quickly loses viscosity, like jello turning to water. This is the weak link in the system. If the enzyme is allowed to destroy the integrity of the HA barrier, pathogenic bacteria such as staph and strep penetrate the tissues and make you sick. A similar mechanism is thought to be involved in rheumatism and tumor formation and at the beginnings of malignancy." *Echinacea*, says Mowrey, has been shown to prevent the enzyme from dissolving HA. "It's that simple," he says. "The herb acts to effectively close down one of the major routes of bug-invasion."

Unfortunately *Echinacea* is in trouble. One of nine North American species of *Echinacea* has been proposed for federal listing as an endangered species, reports *HerbalGram*. There are many species of this plant and *Echinacea laevigata* is the rarest. But other species are also disappearing.

Echinacea—the purple cone flower—is certainly one of the most important herbal medicines of the American continent.

Echinacea laevigata grows in the Appalachian region. Only 6,000 individuals of this form of *Echinacea* are known from only 19 natural populations. The largest cluster of plants is on a site recently under consideration for a proposed Environmental Protection Agency regional toxic waste incinerator. A Bush administration moratorium on new government regulations prevented immediate listing of the species in 1992. Furthermore, the listing of this species, that would offer its protection, must also be be justified on economic grounds. "It is an excellent example of a species from an important medicinal plant group that has far greater economic potential if maintained extant, compared to any intrinsic economic value derived from allowing it to become extinct," comments *Herbal Gram*.

Arginine

The amino acid arginine has been shown to stimulate pituitary gland production of human growth hormone whose levels decline as we age. In studies, lowered levels of human growth hormone have been associated with increased incidence of major killing diseases such as cancer, stroke and heart disease. In addition, human growth hormone stimulates the thymus gland which plays an integral role in human immune function.

Hormones are carried in the blood throughout the body and they have an effect on almost every tissue. If their activity is decreasing with age and then enhanced with dietary supplements, their rejuvenating influences will be felt on many other organ systems. Without adequate production of hormones, the body is like a large and complex army without any battle commands and therefore no chance of winning a war, say experts. Hormones trigger responses from target cells, either locally or far from their point of origin in an endocrine gland. They are transported around the body in the bloodstream. Their overall responsibility is to maintain the metabolic equilibrium of the body.

For example, we know that maintaining the immune system is essential as we age in order to prevent virtually all diseases from cancer to bacterial and viral infections. Perhaps no organ is more essential to the immune system than the thymus gland. But in order for the thymus gland to function optimally, many small hormones known as peptides are essential. In particular, thymus peptide hormones are required for optimal immune efficiency. But once again as we age, one of the best known thymus peptides, thymulin, decreases. That leads to diminished immune function and more days of illness.

Arginine + Lysine = Immune Power!

Fortunately, researchers are truly excited about the use of two amino acids for reversing the aging process. Indeed, Italian researchers report that the all important thymus gland can be rejuvenated through nutritional intervention. *The bottom line is that age-related decline of thymic hormonal activity is reversible, say these researchers.* Through nutritional intervention with amino acids, the neuroendocrine network can be reactivated and the production of thymic hormones stimulated.

"An amino acid combination of lysine and arginine is able to increase the synthesis and/or release of thymulin to values comparable to those recorded in young subjects," report researchers from the Italian National Research Centres on Aging in Ancona, Italy.

Melatonin

Though pineal function and the production of its hormone remained a mystery through much of medical history, clinical research on melatonin during the last ten years has begun to unravel its biochemical secrets.

Melatonin is the main secretion produced by the pineal body, an endocrine gland located in the mid-brain area, and is produced in darkness during a circadian or 24-hour schedule. Production of this pineal hormone is curtailed by light.

As people age, pineal gland function begins to shut down, producing less and less mela-

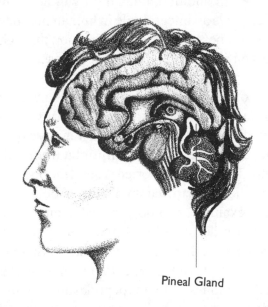

Pineal Gland

For years, medical science knew virtually nothing of the function or purpose of the pineal gland. Now, however, scientists have learned that this tiny member of the endocrine system secretes a hormone—melatonin—that is one of the keys to life extension.

tonin each year. Once again, dietary supplements can rejuvenate the pineal gland. For example the life span of mice was doubled with melatonin supplementation in a test environment. This has led biochemists to believe that one of the secrets to staying young is tied up with melatonin production.

Other studies suggest melatonin may protect people from the damaging effects of oxygen free radicals entering the body from smog, rancid food oils, or other environmental pollutants.

For women, supplementation with melatonin may hold strong potential for the prevention of breast cancer:

•A study published this year suggests electrical power together with electro-magnetic force fields shuts down pineal gland production of melatonin in women working on computers and thus, may increase their risk of developing breast cancer.

•Human breast cancer cells treated with melatonin were inhibited in growth.

•Melatonin specifically blocked estrogen-induced tumor cell proliferation in breast cancer cells.

Coenzyme Q10

Experts call CoQ10 a significant immunologic stimulant. Coenzyme Q10 is a lipoidal vitamin-like substance similar in structure to vitamin K. Also known as CoQ10 or ubiquinone, it was first isolated in its pure form in 1957, according to the American Institute for Biosocial Research and it is an essential substance in cell respiration, electron transfer, and the control of oxidation reaction.

Dr. Richard Passwater, director of research for Solgar Nutritional Research, reports that CoQ10 doubled the immune system's ability to clear invading organisms from the blood and has been demonstrated to double antibody levels as well as offer protection and resistance to viral infection. It is an experimental life extender. Dr. Passwater also reports, "Animal studies have shown that the mean life span can be increased significantly by CoQ10 supplementation, with a significant number of the animals having life spans well beyond the acknowl-edged maximum life span for that species. But, more importantly, the longer-living animals were younger appearing and younger acting."

No significant side effects have been noted with extended use. Dr. Passwater (1987) reports that a study of more than 5,000 persons taking 30 milligrams of

CoQ10 daily as a food supplement found fewer than one percent had gastric discomfort, nausea or diarrhea. He calls it a "significant" nutrient for the nineties.

Anti-Nutrients

We need to limit our intake of anti-nutrients such as pesticides and industrial toxins and bacteria which put additional stress on the immune system. It would also be wised to limit consumption of polyunsaturated fatty acids such as vegetable oils because they also negatively affect immune system function. Many homemakers today cook with polyunsaturated vegetable oils—a big mistake. Dr. J.E. Kinsella, professor of lipid biochemistry at the Institute of Food Science at Cornell University in Ithaca New York, notes that dietary polyunsaturated fats exert significant damaging and pervasive effects on several facets of the immune system. He goes on to say that linoleic acid found in polyunsaturated vegetable oils suppresses the immune response and that, in general, diets high in omega-6 fatty acids "suppress" immune competence in experimental animals.

We must also make sure that we provide our bodies with optimal amounts of pro-nutrients including:
•Alkylglycerols
•Arginine
•Lysine
•Melatonin
•CoQ10
•DMG
•*Echinacea*
•Phycotene

If we could derive adequate nutrients from our daily diet, it would be great and we could forget about the need for these proven immuno-stimulators. But the fact is that most of us don't. Supplements are helpers in both maintaining health and curing illness. They can stimulate your immune system and may well extend the healthiest years of your life.

9. *The Healthy Heart*

*The heart in itself is not the beginning of life;
but it is a vessel formed of thick muscle,
vivified and nourished by the artery and vein
as are the other muscles.*

*Leonardo da Vinci (1452-1519)
The Notebooks of Leonardo*

*From 1964 to 1985, the age-corrected death rate
from coronary heart disease dropped by more than 42
percent resulting in 350,000 fewer deaths in 1986 than
would otherwise have occurred, reported the U.S. Surgeon
General in his 1988 Report on Nutrition and Health. Was it
better medical intervention and lifestyle changes that caused
this precipitous and most welcome decline in heart disease?
Or was it the use of nutritional supplements? You might be
surprised to know that the use of dietary supplements may
well have played an important role in the decline in heart
disease deaths in the U.S. Despite this decline, however,
heart disease still accounts for more deaths annually than*

any other disease or group of diseases; more than 1.25
million heart attacks occur each year, two-thirds of them in
men; more than 500,000 people die as a result.

The number of persons afflicted with cardiovascular disease in the U.S. is truly astounding. But then when you think about the nutritionally inadequate diets so many people consume—including highly fatty foods, laced with pesticides and salt, their lack of exercise and stress—perhaps the numbers shouldn't be astounding. For example, in his 1988 report to the American people, the surgeon general estimated that 57.7 million people have hypertension (one of the underlying causes of heart attack and stroke), 6.7 million already have developed full blown coronary heart disease, 2.7 million have cerebrovascular disease and another 2.9 million suffer from rheumatic fever and cardiac arrhythmias.

Many people in the lay community believe that the number one enemy of cardiovascular health is high blood pressure; still others will tell you the culprit is cholesterol.

Every expert has a theory on the causes of heart disease. But that's the beauty of honest science—experts are always arguing, learning, growing and striving for greater perception and understanding of underlying causes.

Some experts' views, unfortunately, are so hardened that they cannot accept new theories. This is the case with many physicians and health care professionals who have denigrated the idea of supplements having any potential whatsoever to prevent heart disease. It is unfortunate that all too many health professionals appear to be willing to accept only the most publicized causes of heart disease as being legitimate.

But another way of looking at heart disease is that it is a killer whose causes we are only in the infancy of understanding. It shouldn't be the mission of health professionals to prove one theory right and another wrong but rather to examine to what extent each theory explains the causes of a disease that is responsible for nearly 50 percent of all deaths annually in the U.S. The prudent popular message of making necessary lifestyle changes is undeniably important. But what about combining these changes with nutritional molecular breakthroughs?

The key to understanding heart disease is that it involves a series of chemical changes in the body. Fats alone are not the culprit. It's the changes they trigger that are so detrimental. The conclusion we can draw is that we must act to influence these chemical changes.

Certainly cutting down on fat intake is prudent. Fat contains many harmful natural and synthetic substances that spark production of free radicals which may cause atherosclerosis, cancer, and central nervous system, liver and kidney damage.

In addition to decreasing fat intake, some physician-prescribed drugs such as cholestryamine may not be very effective in prevention of heart disease and may even result in increased risk of gastrointestinal cancer (Passwater 1991). Indeed, in discussing claims made by pharmaceutical firms for their cholesterol-lowering drugs, the *New England Journal of Medicine* reports the results of studies were inaccurately interpreted to misleadingly magnify the positive benefits derived from such drugs and the advertising accompanying choles-terol-lowering drugs "stretches the truth to the limits."

Furthermore, "the implications of long-term drug therapy for millions of Americans are unknown," according to *The Surgeon General's Report on Nutrition and Health.* "There are documented side effects of the anti-hypertensive drugs. Thiazide diuretics, for example, can induce short-term increases in serum cholesterol, low density lipoproteins (LDL), and triglyceride levels in some persons."

Some studies suggest these effects decrease or disappear with long-term therapy, although some clinical trials have shown persistence of the adverse effects (JNC IV 1988). Beta blockers tend to lower high density lipoprotein (HDL) levels.

These and other risks of drug therapy call attention to the potential benefits of non-pharmaceutical treatment of high blood pressure (Kaplan 1985).

But our understanding of heart disease has broadened in recent years to include a multitidue of causes which can work together to bring on the onset of disease. Our approach in prevention of heart disease is called the *multifactorial* approach.

The following topics discuss risk factors that are among the major influences on heart disease. Pay attention to them and eliminate those that you know are part of your lifestyle.

Hypertension

Hypertension—also known as high blood pressure—is responsible for a major portion of cardiovascular disease, according to *The Surgeon General's Report on Nutrition and Health* (1988). Hypertension affects 20 to 30 percent of the adult population, approximately one in four people—or roughly 40 million Americans. High blood pressure can cause heart failure and stroke.

Blood Pressure Self Test

It is impossible to make a correct diagnosis of high blood pressure in a doctor's office with a single reading, report James F. Balch, M.D., and Phyllis A. Balch, C.N.C., authors of *Prescription for Nutritional Healing* (Avery Publishing 1990).

"The test needs to be repeated throughout the day to be accurate," they report. "Home testing is best because it enables the person to periodically monitor the condition. To take your blood pressure at home, purchase a sphygmomanometer—a device with an inflatable bladder inside a hollow sleeve that fits around the arm and is pumped up. There are electronic models that are very easy to use."

The authors note these key points to keep in mind when doing a blood pressure self-test:

•The arm must be relaxed, supported, and held at chest level. (The reading will be excessively high if the arm is too low.)

•Do not speak while pressure is being measured.

•Slip the cuff on the upper arm and tighten. Pump up the bulb.

The sphygmomanometer measures the distance that mercury would move given the amount of pressure that the blood is exerting on it. A normal blood pressure reading is 120 mm Hg systolic over 80 mm Hg diastolic (120/80). It can vary from a normal of 110/70 to 140/90. Borderline hypertension reads 140/90 to 160/90 or 160/95. Any pressure over 180/115 is severely elevated.

High blood pressure is associated with coronary heart disease and atherosclerosis, in addition to kidney disorders, obesity, diabetes, hyperthyroidism and adrenal tumors.

Public health efforts have increased public awareness and knowledge of the risks and appropriate treatment of this condition. Today, almost the entire adult U.S. population has had at least one blood pressure measurement and 73 percent of all Americans have had their blood pressure checked within the previous six months, according to *The Surgeon General's Report on Nutrition and Health* (1988).

Where do you fit in this picture?

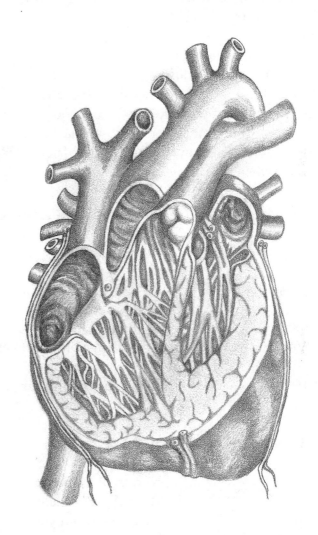

The health of your heart depends upon keeping your arteries free from plaque and other deposits which inhibit blood flow and can be a cause of hypertension.

Understanding Your Blood Pressure Reading

We have used the surgeon general's report to classify blood pressure in adults 18 years or older. You can compare your blood pressure reading to the following figure.

Remember, blood pressure ratio is expressed as systolic/diastolic. A classification of borderline isolated systolic hypertension (SBP 140 to 159 mm/ Hg) or isolated systolic hypertension (SBP 160 mm Hg) takes precedence over high normal blood pressure (diastolic blood pressure 85 to 89 mm Hg) when both occur in the same person. High normal blood pressure (DBP 85 to 89 mm Hg) takes precedence over classification of normal blood pressure (SBP < 140 mm Hg) when both occur in the same person.

Classification of Blood Pressure in Adults 18 Years or Older

Range, mm HG   *Category*

Diastolic

Range, mm HG	Category
<85	Normal blood pressure
85-89	Normal high blood pressure
90-104	Mild hypertension
105-114	Moderate hypertension
>115	Severe hypertension

Systolic

Range, mm HG	Category
<140	Normal blood pressure
140-159	Borderline isolated systolic hypertension
>160	Isolated sytolic hypertension

Hypertension is often asymptomatic and has been called the silent killer because there remain so many people with high blood pressure who don't even know they have the disease; another one-fourth know, yet do nothing!

Advanced warning signs of hypertension include:

•Headache
•Sweating
•Rapid pulse
•Shortness of breath
•Dizziness
•Vision disturbances

Atherosclerosis is a common precursor of hypertension and it involves a thickening, hardening and loss of elasticity of the walls of arteries; they become obstructed with cholesterol plaque and circulation of blood through the vessels becomes difficult. When the arteries harden and constrict in this way, the blood is forced through a narrower passageway and as a result blood pressure becomes elevated. Eventually the vessels can become completely blocked, causing heart attack or stroke.

Dietary causes of high blood pressure and heart disease include:

•Excessive intake of saturated fats, protein and salt (Meneely 1976)
•Alcohol
•Coffee (Lang 1983)
•Sugar (Hodges 1983)
•Too little fiber

Non-dietary causes include:

•Excess weight (Hvalik 1983)
•Smoking (Kershbaum 1968)
•Lack of exercise
•Stress
•Medications (especially antihistamines)
•Heavy metals (Beattie 1976)

Cholesterol

Heart disease is also thought to be a result of free radical-related damage brought on by excessive "bad" cholesterol in the body. The best illustration of the good cholesterol/bad cholesterol concept is the story of Helen Boley. She is a scientific superstar.

A resident of Kansas City, Missouri, the 61-year-old retired State Department worker's blood is drawn once a week and rushed to the National Heart, Lung and Blood Institute in Bethesda, MD. There, her blood is studied by scientific experts whose quest is to learn how her body handles high- and low-fat diets (Kotulak 1991).

Boley is unique because the level of high density lipoprotein in her body is the highest ever recorded in medical history (Kotulak 1991). Known as the "good" cholesterol, the level of HDL in Boley's body is nearly five times higher than normal. The *Chicago Tribune* reports that researchers have learned that HDL has the unique, "ability to halt the damage to cells caused by free

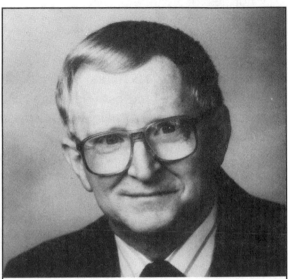

One of the nation's most trusted nutritional advisors and respected innovators, Richard Passwater, Ph.D., says that heart health is as much a matter of what is missing from the diet as what is present. He strongly urges people to use a special supplement program containing many of the nutrients discussed in this chapter including CoQ10 and vitamins B-6 and C. Also important, says Dr. Passwater: chromium picolinate and beta sistosterol. His best seller *The New Supernutrition* is the ultimate guide to a healthy heart.

radicals, the 'sparks' thrown off by the oxidation process that produces energy in our cells. *Free radicals can damage arterial walls, thus leading to the dangerous buildup of fatty plaques and eventual heart attacks or strokes*" (Kotulak 1991). HDL normally takes excessive blood cholesterol from the blood circulation to the liver where it can be metabolized out of the body. Whereas LDLs take cholesterol from the liver and put it into the circulation when the body needs it. Too much LDL means having too much cholesterol in the bloodstream and greater oxygen free radical damage to the walls of the arteries.

Boley's physician Dr. William Harris, head of the lipid laboratory at the University of Kansas Medical Center, told reporters: "She's preventing oxidation damage like crazy. Her arteries are probably squeaky clean."

Boley is a genetic anomaly in that she appears to have inherited a double dose of one of the body's Methuselah genes—those that presumably can extend life for virtually hundreds of years. In this case, this particular Methuselah gene regulates body HDL. Boley is naturally endowed with the genetic structures that produce very high HDL levels. Not surprisingly, her relatives are all long-lived, and experts expect that Boley will be no exception in coming close to reaching a second century of healthy living.

Scientists are busily learning more about the powers of HDL to halt free radical-related damage and increase longevity—and even how the genetic structure of this particular Methuselah gene can be engineered to provide all of us with increased amounts of body HDL.

But these genetic engineering breakthroughs are likely to be years and even decades away. The question for the average person is what we can do until these breakthroughs are available. Your body may not have a double dose of the HDL-regulating Methuselah gene like Helen Boley's body. But nutritional supplements certainly will help you improve your HDL level.

Overweight

Early studies on the association between body weight and blood pressure have been confirmed in epidemiologic studies of primitive as well as developed populations where body weight does not increase with age and neither does blood pressure (Surgeon General 1988). The Hypertension Detection and Follow-Up Program (1977) reports that 60 percent of the participants with hypertension were more than 20 percent overweight. It has been suggested that control of obesity would eliminate hypertension in 48 percent of whites and 28 percent of blacks (Tyroler 1975). According to the surgeon general (1988),

"Even when weight loss does not reduce blood pressure to normal, health risks may be reduced, and smaller doses of anti-hypertensive medication may be needed as a result."

Weight loss also elevates levels of HDL, says Dr. Hans Kugler, one of the primary investigators in a study that demonstrated that specific nutritional supplements can perform the dual function of stimulating weight loss and improving the body's ratio of HDL to LDL, the dangerous low density lipoproteins that are associated with increased heart disease risk. In a controlled study, Dr. Kugler discovered that those subjects who experienced significant weight reduction also enjoyed decreased LDLs and increased HDLs.

Weight loss is a safe, effective way of lowering blood pressure. For many people, even a limited weight loss program can produce completely normal blood pressure. The best way to lose weight is through a proper high-fiber diet and exercise or physical activity.

Weight loss is helpful. But in keeping with our multifactorial theory of optimal heart health people with high blood pressure or other symptoms of heart disease can do more than just controlling their weight.

Excess Sodium Intake

The role of a high sodium/low potassium intake in the development of hypertension has been considered extensively and conclusively (Meneely 1976, Khaw, 1984). Excessive consumption of dietary sodium chloride (salt), coupled with diminished dietary potassium, induces an increase in fluid volume and an impairment of blood pressure regulating mechanisms which results in hypertension in susceptible individuals.

The normal amount of salt needed daily is about 300 mg. Most people consume over 10,000 mg a day. It is important to note that sodium restriction alone does not improve blood pressure control but must be accompanied by a high potassium intake (Skrabal 1981). Some food additives that are high in salt include soy sauce, baking soda, canned vegetables, meat tenderizers, softened waters.

Excess Alcohol Intake

Along with sodium consumption, chronic alcohol consumption is one of the strongest predictors of hypertension (Gruchow 1985), along with excessive alcohol intake. Even moderate amounts of alcohol produce acute hypertension in some individuals as a result of increased adrenaline secretion (Formann 1983, Potter 1984).

High Sugar Intake

Common table sugar, also known as sucrose, can elevate blood pressure. It may cause increased sodium retention by elevating adrenaline secretion (Hodges 1983). It appears that increased adrenaline production may be the primary cause of increased blood vessel constriction and increased sodium retention. Sugar also causes hypertension because it is converted into fat which in turn is changed into cholesterol and triglycerides.

Smoking

Another substantial heart-risk factor is smoking. The hypertensive response to nicotine is due to its adrenal stimulation which results in increased adrenaline secretion (Kershbaum 1968). Smoking can contribute to hypertension because it constricts blood vessels. One cigarette can constrict blood vessels for as long as two-thirds of an hour. Cigarette smokers also tend to have higher concentrations of lead and cadmium in their bodies and lower concentrations of ascorbic acid than non-smokers (Pelletier 1968)—all of which are causes of heart disease.

Lack of Exercise

Lack of physical exercise contributes to heart disease because the body does not take in as much oxygen as it should. People who don't do at least 20 to 30 minutes of exercise daily—such as walking, bicycling, or swimming—have 16 times less oxygen in their system. As a result, body cells die. In other words, body tissues do not live as long, organs do not live as long and the individual ultimately doesn't either.

Stress

Stress is one of the primary contributors to hypertension because it causes the blood vessels to constrict. However, do not construe stress to be the sole cause of hypertension.

Heavy Metals

Chronic exposure to lead from environmental sources, including drinking water, is associated with increased cardiovascular mortality. Elevated lead levels have been found in a significant number of hypertensive individuals (Beattie 1976, Pierkle 1985). Areas with soft water (*i.e.,* lacking minerals such as calcium and magnesium) have increased lead concentrations in the public drinking supply due to the acidity of the water, and people living in these areas may suffer greater accumulation of lead and subsequent increased risk of hypertension. Soft water also is low in calcium and magnesium which have a beneficial effect in fighting hypertension. Cadmium has also been shown to cause hypertension. Untreated hypertensive individuals have blood cadmium levels that are three to four times higher than those in matched people with normal blood pressure (Glauser 1976).

Dietary Fat Intake

Diet can play a pivotal role in the prevention of heart disease. Eliminating fats from your diet and making them no more than 10 percent of your total caloric intake is an important breakthrough for people who must take special steps to prevent heart disease. It is also important to read labels. Be absolutely certain to cut down on your use of partially hydrogenated oils and fats, eliminate fried foods and polyunsaturated cooking oils. Some of the most commonly consumed foods that can contain excessive fat include cheeses, lunch meats, sausages, hot dogs, and many packaged foods.

Low Fiber Intake

The high fiber diet is effective in preventing and treating many forms of heart disease. If a person is on a low-fiber diet and is constipated, there is no way for the cholesterol to get out of the body. Bowel movements are essential for expelling cholesterol from the body. An extra advantage to a high fiber diet is that cholesterol binds to the fiber and is carried out of the system by fiber. The types of dietary fiber that are of the greatest benefit are the water soluble gel-forming fibers such as oat bran, apple pectin, psyllium seed husks, guar gum and gum karaya. The type of grains that are most helpful are the natural whole grains in whole food form—like brown rice, millet, oats, barley, wheat, rye and buckwheat. The more fiber in the diet the better. When you eat a lot of whole grain foods you produce more bulk in your body and fat is moved through your system much more quickly.

The Role of Optimal Nutrition

Research appears to be pointing in the direction of the multitude of additional benefits to be gained through nutritional manipulation of the body to prevent those chemical reactions that cause heart disease. It's true that a low-fat diet together with high-fiber meals and exercise and no smoking are all important components of a healthy heart program. But they are far from being the only components, and if people go no further than this for their healthy heart program, they will be doing only half of what they could to ensure their best chance at extending the healthiest years of their lives.

We know:

•Vitamin E is absolutely essential to a healthy heart and a handful of studies have shown that it can halt the onset of atherosclerosis. It is an antioxidant and improves the ability of tissues to absorb oxygen.

Heart Disease Incidence Among People Taking 1,200 IU or more of Vitamin E for Four or More Years

Age Group	Number in Group	Expected Number with Heart Disease (National Rate from HEW Figures)	Actual Reported Number with Heart Disease (Possible Undetected Cases in Parentheses)	Percentage of Expected Number with Heart Disease
90–98	1	0	0 (0)	—
80–89	64	28	0 (0)	0
70–79	284	114	2 (2)	1.8
60–69	356	114	4 (3)	3.5
50–59	333	67	1 (2)	1.5
	1,038	323	7 (7)	2.2

1200 IU or more of vitamin E taken for 4 years or more is strongly associated with reducing the incidence of heart disease prior to 80 years of age from 32 per 100 people to 10 per 100 people.

Source: *The New Supernutrition*

•Deficiency in vitamin B-6 causes increases in heart disease incidence. As long ago as 1951 scientists learned that experimental animals on high cholesterol diets failed to develop arterial plaques when they were given generous amounts of vitamin B-6. These studies have been confirmed in additional research and many experts believe that this theory is more solid than the present theories on cholesterol reduction, *leading some researchers to conclude that levels of vitamin B-6 substantially higher than the RDA may be required for the prevention of heart disease* (Passwater 1991). Furthermore, a large number of persons over age 65 are deficient in vitamin B-6. We also know that the average annual imports of synthetic vitamin B-6 increased by 5,400 percent from the mid-1960s to the mid-1980s and have continued to increase, according to the U.S. Department of Commerce. *Could it be that our increased supplementation of vitamin B-6 is, in part, responsible for our nation's welcomed declining rate of death from heart disease?*

•Men and women with the highest vitamin C intakes and who took regular vitamin C supplements had 25 and 45 percent lower coronary mortality rates, respectively, than subjects with a low vitamin C intake, according to the National Health and Nutrition Examination Survey. Vitamin C helps regulate the conversion of cholesterol to bile acids and, in cases of high cholesterol, may help lower it. Vitamin C also protects against free radical oxidation of cholesterol in the water soluble environment and has been found to prevent free radicals from damaging lipids. Vitamin C stimulates prostacyclin, which is a prostaglandin that keeps blood cells from sticking together and causes dilation of arteries. As little as two to three grams of vitamin C daily can reduce platelet stickiness. According to *Clinical Pearls News*: "Vitamin C levels are reduced in disease states or conditions such as diabetes mellitus, smoking, hypertension, elderly and male subjects, that are associated with an increased risk of coronary artery disease.

•Some 20 percent of deaths from heart attacks are caused by coronary artery spasms which are in turn caused by deficiencies in magnesium and tryptophan.

•Coenzyme Q-10 may improve tissue strength of the heart muscle, preventing congestive heart failure.

How important is optimal nutrition in maintaining cardiovascular health? At best, high cholesterol and a sedentary lifestyle explain only half of the potential causes of heart disease. Dr. Passwater (1991) says: "If eating rich, fatty foods, smoking, and lack of exercise were the only causes of heart disease, then prudent dieting, abstinence from smoking, and exercise would wipe heart disease off the map. Yet, in those groups making the prudent changes, heart disease incidence hasn't been cut by anywhere near half." Dr. Pauling (1986) asserts that the death rate from heart disease "could be decreased greatly, probably cut in half" through the use of vitamins and other nutrients.

In a certain sense, says Dr. Passwater (1991), "the dietary component of heart disease is not so much what you eat as what you don't eat. *The vitamins and minerals that are missing from most diets are more important than the excess fats."*

If you're seriously interested in optimal health, you should combine improvements in lifestyle together with an optimal nutrition program that goes to the heart of the problem, directly influencing body chemistry.

There are a number of nutrients which can certainly be used for both prevention of heart disease and healing the body of cardiovascular disease.

Chromium Picolinate

Chromium can help prevent and lower high blood pressure, says Dr. Earl Mindell, author of the *Vitamin Bible.* Its deficiency is a "suspected factor in arteriosclerosis and diabetes." This is especially important to know because as we age we "retain less chromium" in our bodies, according to Dr. Mindell. Dr. Kugler explains that people with adequate chromium levels have little evidence of arterial plaque when compared with people whose blood levels show little chromium. And Jeffrey A. Fisher, M.D., (1990) reports that, "There have been several tests in which elevated cholesterol, elevated triglycerides, and reduced HDL ('good') cholesterol in non-diabetics have improved following chromium supplementation. Subjects who had the highest insulin levels . . . tended to improve the most. Dr. Evans and his colleagues, before demonstrating the muscle-building effect of chromium, tested the ability of chromium picolinate to lower cholesterol. His were the best and most consistent results obtained: a seven percent decrease in total cholesterol and an eleven percent reduction in LDL cholesterol after only six weeks on 200 micrograms per day of chromium." The form of chromium you choose is important. Many chromium supplements contain the trivalent form of chromium—chromium chloride—which is very poorly absorbed (Fisher 1990). The most bioavailable form is chromium picolinate (Fisher 1990).

The U.S. Department of Agriculture reports that 90 percent of Americans take in less chromium than is needed for normal health in part because by the time food manufacturers have processed their products, especially grains, more than 80 percent of the natural chromium has been removed. Furthermore eating simple sugars causes the body to excrete large amounts of chromium.

Allium sativum

Allium sativum has been shown in studies to reduce cholesterol and its daily intake also is associated with improved HDL/LDL ratios. *Allium sativum* lowered serum cholesterol levels in normal human

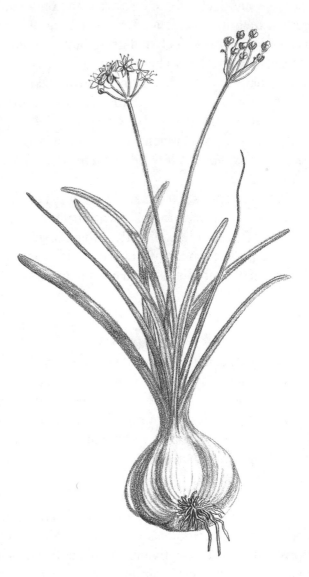

Nature's cholesterol buster, Allium sativum should be the first alternative to prescription drugs for reducing blood pressure and cholesterol, say many medical experts.

volunteers, and Kamanna (1982) reports that *Allium sativum* "caused a marked reduction" in the serum cholesterol levels in experimental animals. Its important properties include potential protection from atherosclerosis as Bordia (1973) discusses in *The Lancet*.

Beta-sistosterol

One of the more interesting qualities of vegetarian diets is that although they tend to be very low in cholesterol, they're exceptionally high in common plant compounds known as phytosterols. One such phytosterol is beta-sistosterol, which is similar to cholesterol although its functions are different. Because it is carried in the blood by the same system that transports cholesterol, its presence in high quantities in the diet blocks the accumulation of cholesterol. The best time for taking beta-sistosterol is immediately prior to eating so it has the best opportunity for blocking cholesterol absorption.

For those people who find changing their diets impossible, beta sistosterol is the perfect supplement. Matson (1982) reports that beta-sistosterol lowered cholesterol in people whose diets otherwise remained the same.

Charcoal

Activated charcoal is like a filter. It adsorbs cholesterol as well as many other potentially toxic chemicals. Although charcoal may also adsorb nutrients, its effectiveness is tremendous. One study from Finland found that seven grams of activated charcoal daily for a month lowered LDL cholesterol by 41 percent (Passwater 1991).

CoEnzyme Q10

If you're one of millions of Americans who is at risk for cardiovascular disease or if you've already had a heart attack you need to know about the powers of CoQ10.

CoQ10 is an essential component of the metabolic processes involved in energy production. Individuals with cardiovascular disease often are deficient in CoQ10 and require increased tissue levels of this nutrient. Clinical studies demonstrate that CoQ10 is of considerable benefit in the treatment of hypertension and other cardiovascular diseases, lowering blood pressure and improving heart function (Folkers 1977, 1984).

For anyone determined to achieve the best possible health and a longer, richer life, CoQ10 is mandatory.

A biochemical compound and nutrient, CoQ10 has intrigued scientists around the world (Passwater 1987, Hunt 1987). Indeed, its function is both unique and critical, for it contributes to the production of energy cells, and, in particular, to the production of energy in heart cells (Passwater 1987). In fact, says Dr. Passwater, a number of heart attacks, induced by coronary spasms, may be the result of a deficiency in CoQ10.

Although the human body manufactures CoQ10, its output often drops because of the aging process. And though CoQ10 is present in much of what people eat, it can't survive food processing and storage (Passwater 1987). Result: Millions of people worldwide take CoQ10 in the form of nutritional supplements (which produce no significant side effects) to counter heart disease, high blood pressure, aging and weakened immunity, along with many other conditions (Passwater 1987).

In Japan alone, more than 12 million people "take daily doses of CoQ10, prescribed by their physicians as the medication of choice for preventing and treating heart and circulatory diseases" (Hunt 1987).

Researchers in 1957 first isolated CoQ10 in its pure form and subsequently discovered that the nutrient was critical to cell respiration, electron transfer and oxidation-reaction control. Over the following years, CoQ10 was found to be of clinical value for cardiovascular disease, angina, heart failure, hypertension and other serious disorders.

Researchers also found correlations between CoQ10 deficiencies and the incidence of diabetes, periodontal disease and muscular dystrophy. What's more, a six-year study by scientists at the University of Texas showed that congestive heart-failure patients who took CoQ10 in addition to conventional therapy had a 75 percent chance of surviving three years—in contrast to a 25 percent survival rate for patients taking standard treatment only (Hunt 1987).

A related study, by the University of Texas and the Center for Adult Diseases in Japan, revealed CoQ10 could lower high blood pressure without medication or diet changes (Hunt 1987*).*

And in the course of examining CoQ10's effect on angina and heart-attack patients, Japanese researchers discovered that it cut by 50 percent both the rate of angina attacks and the need for nitroglycerine (Passwater 1987).

Chondroitin Sulphate A (CSA)

An important dietary supplement, which is gaining in importance these days, is chondroitin sulphate A (CSA)—also known simply as chondroitin sulfate.

In addition to making sure your body is getting optimum antioxidant protection, CSA can play an integral role in cardiovascular health. But we must warn you that your learning curve will be so greatly accelerated by this report that your knowledge on the subject of CSA may put you ahead of even your physician's present knowledge.

The arteries are the biggest of the blood vessels and when their walls become clogged with plaque deposits they lose their elasticity and become hard. This is why arteriosclerosis is commonly referred to as "hardening of the arteries."

CSA is a mucopolysaccharide, which is a hormone-like nutrient as important as vitamins, minerals, and amino acids. Naturally occurring in cartilage, bone and connective tissue of arterial walls, CSA is essential to maintaining the elasticity of blood vessels to keep our arteries structurally sound.

CSA is found in large proportions in the arterial "intima," the inner layer of the artery wall and the first part of the body subject to the effects of degenerative disease. In healthy individuals, this inner layer is elastic in structure and protects vessels from interference by outside factors, defending them against cholesterol-containing plaque deposits.

Blood clots are fatal. One of the most important things that you should know if you are at risk for heart disease is that CSA has anti-thrombogenic properties. Thromboses are blood clots. They can clog the walls of arteries. But when they dislodge from the arterial wall, they can often have fatal consequences. CSA helps dissolve blood clots.

"That's why doctors at the forefront of preventative medicine use mucopolysaccharides routinely to help prevent the degenerative diseases that lead to arteriosclerosis, heart attack, and stroke," reports Dr. Earl Mindell, Ph.D., R.Ph., author of the *Vitamin Bible.*

Dr. Mindell goes on to explain, "As we age, the natural circulating level of CSA decreases and begins to break down our arterial defense system. Persons suffering from coronary heart disease also experience a decrease in arterial wall CSA. The rationale for oral supplementation of CSA is to supply these deficiencies in the arteries to help reduce the incidence of heart disease and lower serum cholesterol levels. Research data confirms that oral supplementation of CSA is effective toward this end."

That's why experts such Dr. Mindell make sure to supplement with CSA daily.

Coronary heart disease has now reached epidemic proportions throughout the world. In the United States, it is responsible for 55 percent of all adult deaths. Yet, more than one million heart attacks a year might be prevented in the U.S. with oral supplementation of CSA, reports Dr. Lester Morrison, professor and director of the Institute for Arteriosclerosis Research at Loma Linda University School of Medicine in California.

Dr. Morrison conducted a six-year study that proves his assertion of the amazing power of CSA to prevent heart attacks and other cardiovascular-related diseases. In his study, 60 randomly selected patients with histories of heart disease were given supplements of CSA in addition to their conventional therapy. The progress of this group was then compared to a control group of 60 patients treated by conventional medications only. Overall, the number of "coronary incidents" during the six-year period in the CSA-treated patients was about one-sixth the number of incidents reported for the control group. Further, sixteen fatal heart attacks occurred in the drug-treated group, while only four fatalities were reported in the CSA-treated group.

CSA has many more documented benefits to your health. In addition to its anti-coagulating and anti-atherogenic functions, CSA has anti-inflammatory, anti-allergic and anti-stress properties. It aids in wound healing and recovery from bone fractures. It stimulates cellular metabolism and increases growth, size and quantity of certain cells. CSA also increases RNA and DNA synthesis in the body.

"In the area of deficiency diseases, many conditions are associated with changes in the mucopolysaccharide content of the tissues involved," explains Dr. Mindell. "Among these conditions are atherosclerosis, rheumatoid arthritis, asthma, and emphysema. Mucopolysaccharides are also related to the degenerative changes associated with aging."

During the six-year study conducted by Dr. Morrison, no adverse side effects were observed from CSA use. In fact, no reports of CSA toxicity have ever been recorded in the medical literature.

Dimethylglycine (DMG)

An amino acid which we discussed earlier for its potential to boost immunity and prevent cancer, DMG can also lower cholesterol. One study found that after nine months of administration DMG caused a 41 point drop in cholesterol levels with improvements in HDL (Passwater 1991). Thus, we learn that one nutrient plays many roles in promoting optimal health!

Fish Oils

Studies show that the American diet is unusually low in omega 3 oils. A deficiency of this oil can cause abnormalities involving heartbeat, kidney malfunction, fatty degeneration of the kidneys and liver, brain damage, elevated cholesterol and triglycerides, and high blood pressure. Adding one or two tablespoonfuls of an oil rich in omega 3 is an important part of a healthy diet. A particularly excellent source of omega 3 oil is eicosapentaenoic acid. Also known as EPA, it's a very important supplement for reduction of blood pressure. EPA is an omega 3 fatty acid and comes from cold-water marine fish in its most generous amounts; eating for your heart means consuming halibut, salmon, mackerel and albacore tuna. EPA has been shown to favorably change the ratio of HDLs to LDLs. When people take EPA the net result is that they have a higher HDL to LDL ratio and much lower blood cholesterol and triglycerides. Fish oils may also be of benefit because of their ability to reduce inflammatory substances on the arterial wall, keeping blood cells from sticking together, reducing triglycerides. In the *Journal of Cardiopulmonary Rehabilitation,* Dattilo (1992) recommends the inclusion of such fish in the diet. The studies are generally ovewhelmingly positive, even dramatic, in demonstrating the potential of this oil to lower cholesterol and improve the HDL/LDL ratio.

Oil of Evening Primrose

Oil of Evening Primrose assists in balancing blood cholesterol with triglyceride levels and is rich in the essential fatty acid linolenic acid.

Flax Oil

Flax oil (linseed oil) is the only oil rich in both omega 3 and omega 6 fatty acids that can be used on salads, making it invaluable as an everyday healthy heart food.

A healthy heart begins with a healthy diet. Sure, it would be pleasant to think that you're going to be one of the few Americans who gets everything needed for a strong heart from your everyday diet. But if not, then your heart could benefit from a well-designed program of dietary supplements.

Where to Find the Formula

Editor's Note: There are several important heart formulas that readers should be aware of combining many of the herbs and nutrients discussed in this report. Each of these formulas provides different assistance to the heart assistance. One formula Cardia-Forté provides direct assistance to the heart muscle for regularity and a powerful beat, as well as helping keep the arterial passages unblocked with plaque. Hyperbalance combines herbs that have been shown to reduce blood pressure. Complex CL-3 provides fiber, niacin, and plant sterols which all have been shown to reduce cholesterol. Each of these formulas can be ordered by calling Gero Vita International at (800) 825-8482.

10. Cancer Prevention

Cancer accounted for 22 percent of all deaths in the United States in 1984. It has been estimated that 965,000 new cases of cancer were diagnosed and 483,000 people died of cancer in the United States in 1987. Cancer may arise in any organ in the body, but tumors of the lung, colon and rectum, breast, skin, and prostate occur most frequently. Cancers of 10 sites—lung, colon-rectum, breast, prostate, pancreas, leukemias, stomach, ovary, bladder and liver-biliary cancers—account for more than 73 percent of all cancer deaths in the United States. Although the exact proportion is unknown, several researchers have attempted to provide quantitative estimates of the percentage of cancer in the United States attributable at least in part to diet. One group estimated the proportion of cancer deaths attributed to diet to be 40 percent in men and 60 percent in women and another estimated it to be 35 percent overall, with a range of 10 to 70 percent.

More than $1 billion annually is being spent on cancer research, yet the progress we are making is little and tenuous at best. "Despite the great amount of money and effort expended in the study of cancer, progress during the last twenty-five years has been slow," says Dr. Pauling. "Significant increase in survival time after diagnosis was achieved about thirty years ago, largely through improvements in the techniques of surgery and anesthesia. During the last twenty-five years some improvement in treatment of certain kinds of cancer has been achieved, mainly through the use of high-energy radiation and chemotherapy, but for most kinds of cancer there has been essentially no decrease in either incidence or length of time of survival after diagnosis, and it has become evident that some new ideas are needed, if greater control over this scourge is to be achieved."

According to the National Cancer Institute, between 1950 and 1985 in the United States:

•Cancer incidence among children under 12 (who provide an early warning system that will afflict the overall population as it ages) increased 32 percent.

•Urinary bladder cancer incidence increased 51 percent.

•Testicular cancer incidence increased 81 percent.

•Kidney and renal pelvis cancer incidence increased 82 percent; mortality increased by 23 percent.

•Reported incidents of non-Hodgkin's lymphoma rose by 123 percent with 26,500 new cases in 1985.

•Between 1973 and 1985 breast cancer incidence increased 14 percent.

It is widely accepted by scientists today that at least 50 percent of human cancers can be attributed to specific causes, including tobacco smoke, ionizing radiation, occupational exposures to toxic chemicals such as asbestos and benzene, and viral and hereditary influences. The extent to which the remaining 50 percent of cancer incidence is due to pesticides and industrial chemicals in our food, water and air is a subject of great debate. Naturally occurring carcinogens in food may cause some. The National Cancer Institute supports the theory that the high fat content of the American diet promotes cancer. And chlorinated tap water is associated with higher rates of breast cancer in virtually every study conducted for the agency where it has been specifically looked for, according to Dr. William Marcus, Ph.D., of the Environmental Protection Agency.

Michael A. Evans, Ph.D., associate professor at the University of Illinois College of Medicine at Chicago, states that 70 to 90 percent of human cancer incidence is the result of exposure to environmental factors, including cigarette smoke, synthetic chemicals, food additives, agricultural chemicals, and other factors such as sunlight and dietary components. Dr. Evans further notes that "additionally, most of the environmental factors that contribute to the overall cancer burden are not complete carcinogens in themselves but probably act together or in combination with other environmental and genetic factors to produce their carcinogenic effect.'

For all the argumentation, scientists simply do not know an exact percentage of cancers caused by our exposure to toxic chemicals in our food, water and air. But what scientists do know is that cancer can be prevented or delayed through optimal dietary supplementation! There are more than 500 naturally occurring carotenoids alone which are potent antioxidants and immune stimulants that can help prevent cancer, reports *Hematology/Oncology Clinics of North America* (1991).

Consider that ordinarily cancer can be induced in 85 to 90 percent of experimental mice fed the cancer-causing chemical dimethylbenzanthracene (DMBA). That number can be reduced to five to 15 percent with antioxidant nutrients, reports Dr. Richard Passwater in *The New Supernutrition*.

Indeed, there is a certain synergy that antioxidants create when they are supplemented in combination.

"When I used strains of laboratory mice that inherently had high cancer rates without having to add cancer-causing chemicals to their diets, the results were the same," reports Dr. Passwater. "When only one antioxidant nutrient was used at high levels, sometimes the induced cancer would not show up where expected but would be found in another organ. The combination of antioxidants totally prevented the induced cancers."

In another study vitamin B-12 and vitamin C together prevented the growth of transplanted mouse tumors and produced a 100 percent survival rate; however, neither vitamin alone at the same dosage had any effect on prevention of tumor growth, according to a report in *Experimental Cell Biology* (Poydock 1979).

How Antioxidants Protect from Cancer
•They destroy free radicals.
•They promote optimal liver health.
•They promote the integrity of cellular membranes so that cancer-causing

chemicals can't enter the cell.

So important is antioxidant research that the National Cancer Institute has funded more than two dozen studies currently to look at the role that such nutrients play in the prevention of cancer. Among nutrients currently being tested are vitamin A, beta carotene, vitamins C, E, B-6, B-12, folic acid and selenium.

Although we won't have conclusive results from these studies until the mid- to late-1990s, many medical experts believe that the average person should not wait until those results are available but rather should start a prevention program *now* that is based on dietary supplementation with key immune boosters and antioxidants such as beta carotene, vitamins C and E, dimethylglycine and selenium. In addition, non-vitamins are important—phytochemicals such as indoles, glycosinates, glucarates and ellagic acid. All of these plant substances should be part of your diet both through optimal eating habits and supplementation. Diets rich in raw vegetables are associated with reduced risk of several kinds of cancers—possibly through antioxidant action.

Selenium

Studies have shown that persons with the lowest levels of selenium have twice the incidence of cancer of those persons with exceptionally high selenium

---

Relationship of Selenium Intake and Breast Cancer Mortalities

In this chart, the role of selenium in breast cancer prevention is clearly presented. As you can see, in nations such as the Netherlands, U.K., Canada and U.S., where adequate selenium ingestion is particularly deficient, breast cancer rates are highest. In countries such as Taiwan, Japan, Yugoslavia and Bulgaria, where selenium intake is optimal, breast cancer incidence is at its lowest. The message is clear. If you are at risk for certain cancers, such as that of the breast, optimal selenium intake is essential for prevention.

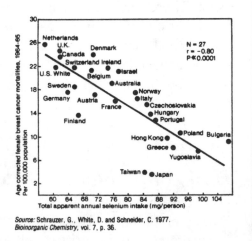

Source: Schrauzer, G., White, D. and Schneider, C. 1977. Bioinorganic Chemistry, vol. 7, p. 36.

levels. Dr. Passwater asserts that both selenium and vitamin E must be present in the body at ample levels in order to prevent cancer, and he cites numerous studies that attest to the significant synergistic action of these two nutrients in prevention. In addition, selenium is one of those nutrients that can also cause cancer regression, asserts Dr. Passwater.

Dr. Passwater also reports that selenium is seemingly essential for prevention of breast cancer. "In 1976, Dr. Christine Wilson, a nutritionist at the University of California at San Francisco, reported her study showing that high-selenium diets protected against breast cancer. After comparing the nutrient content of an average non-Western diet supplying 2,500 calories to that of a typical American diet providing the same number of calories, Dr. Wilson determined that the Western diets contained about a fourth of the selenium of the Asian diets. Also significant was the presence of less 'easily oxidizable' polyunsaturated fat (7.5 to 8.7 grams a day) than in the Western diets (10 to 30 grams).

"The combination of high selenium and low polyunsaturated fats may be protecting Asian women against breast cancer," concludes Dr. Passwater.

Beta Carotene

You might be surprised to know that nonsmokers eating little beta-carotene had a slightly higher incidence of cancer than those people who had been smoking for more than 30 years but were getting adequate beta carotene! In other words, says Dr. Passwater, "Beta carotene is a better protector against cancer than not smoking!" Many studies have demonstrated the need for optimal beta carotene intake for lung protection.

Vitamin C

Vitamin C strengthens the immune system and has antiviral properties. "Large doses of vitamin C may be used to both prevent cancer and to treat it," says Dr. Pauling.

"In 1951, it was reported that patients with cancer have usually a very small concentration of vitamin C in the blood plasma and in the leukocytes of the blood, often only about half the value for other people," reports Dr. Pauling. "This observation has been verified many times during the last thirty years. In

1979, Cameron, Pauling, and Brian Leibovitz listed thirteen studies, all showing large decreases in both plasma and leucocyte concentrations. The level of ascorbic acid in the leucocytes of cancer patients is usually so low that the leucocytes of cancer patients are not able to carry out their important function of phagocytosis, of engulfing and digesting bacteria and other foreign cells, including malignant cells, in the body. A reasonable explanation of the low level of vitamin C in the blood of cancer patients is that their bodies are using up the vitamin in an effort to control the disease. The low level suggests that they should be given a large amount of the vitamin in order to keep their bodily defenses as effective as possible."

Vitamin C also offers protection against toxic chemicals. Cured and pickled foods such as luncheon meats, ham and bacon contain nitrites and nitrates which react with amino acids in the stomach to form highly carcinogenic chemicals called nitrosamines. "A good intake of vitamin C destroys the nitrites and nitrates and prevents stomach cancer."

Vitamin C's powers to prevent colon cancer have been demonstrated in human studies. In one study, four grams of vitamin C plus 400 IU of vitamin E daily, along with a high-fiber diet, produced a greater decline in polyps than a high-fiber diet without the added vitamins, reports Dr. Passwater.

Vitamin E

Vitamin E may reduce the level of mutagenic substances in the stool. In one experimental 1980 study vitamin E supplements reduced stool mutagen levels by as much as 79 percent, according to the *American Journal of Clinical Nutrition*. Furthermore vitamin E, like vitamin C, can prevent formation of cancer-causing nitrosamines in the human body. Vitamin E at 400 IU was effective in blocking the formation of nitrosamines in 10 students fed nitrate and proline, according to a 1985 study in *Cancer Research*.

In an observational study of more than 6,000 people, low vitamin E and lipid levels were correlated with mortality from bowel cancer, according to a 1984 study in the *Journal of the National Cancer Institute*.

As for breast cancer, in an observational study, the level of vitamin E in 5,004 women was significantly lower than in control subjects who had been matched for age, menopausal status, parity and family history of breast disease, according to a 1984 report in the *British Journal of Cancer*.

And regarding lung cancer, average serum vitamin E levels collected from 99 human subjects who developed lung cancer were lower than those of 196 matched controls, according to a 1986 study in the *New England Journal of Medicine*.

Folic Acid

Folic acid prevents smoking-related lung injury, according to research performed by Dr. Douglas Heimburger and colleagues at the University of Alabama. Dr. Passwater reports that the Heimburger team, "studied seventy-three male heavy smokers and found that fourteen of thirty-six volunteers given folic acid and vitamin B-12 supplements had reduced lung injury after four months. In the placebo control group, six of thirty-seven spontaneously improved."

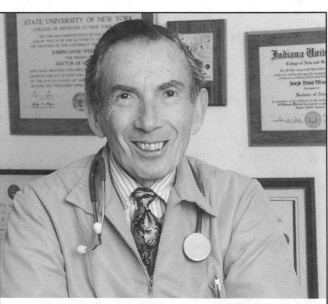

Glutathione

Some dietary nutrients are able to bind with cancer-causing substances and render them harmless. One such nutrient is glutathione. For example, the epoxide form of benzo(a)pyrene can cause cancer in humans. But benzo(a)pyrene, to-

Joseph Weissman, M.D., believes strongly in the value of dietary supplements to help prevent cancer, especially the use of selenium to prevent breast cancer. He also recommends supplementation with vitamins C and E, beta carotene and quercetin. Adequate fiber intake is also important for both quickening transit time of foods through the colon and for absorbing and purging carcinogenic chemicals from the body, he adds.

gether with its epoxide, can be bound by the nutrient glutathione and defused, Dr. Passwater reports "One study has been published in *Science* (May, 1981) showing that glutathione supplements cured liver cancer in laboratory animals."

Cysteine

An amino acid, cysteine can detoxify toxic chemicals that enter the body via smoking. "These compounds are called aldehydes," reports Dr. Passwater, "and they cause injury to body cells. Aldehydes are believed to cross-link healthy cells together in such a way as to impair their function. Although aldehydes may not be a direct cause of lung cancer, they do damage that impairs the body's defenses and prematurely ages the skins."

Fish Oil

Fish oil has shown some evidence of preventing and arresting the growth of breast, colon, prostate and pancreatic cancers, reports Dr. Passwater. One study demonstrated that eicosapentaenoic acid (EPA) could prevent the growth of transplanted mammary tumors in experimental animals. "After three weeks tumor growth was significantly less in the three MaxEPA groups than in the unsupplemented controls," reports Dr. Passwater.

Dimethylglycine

Known as DMG and among the smallest of the amino acids, this nutrient has helped improve human immune response increases by fourfold.

Quercetin

A potent anticancer nutrient and membrane stabilizer and potent inhibitor of bowel cancer, quercetin is found in onions, broccoli and squash and is available in supplements.

Magnesium

Animal studies have reported an increase in cancer incidence in those fed diets low in magnesium and a preventive effect in animals fed excess magnesium (Blondell 1980).

Zinc

This mineral is an important nutrient for the prevention of prostate cancer. In one study, 19 patients with prostatic tissue cancer had significantly lower zinc levels (Habib 1976).

Lactobacillus Acidophilus

Supplementation with *Lactobacillus acidophilus* has been demonstrated to help prevent cancer of the colon. In an experimental crossover study, 21 healthy young subjects were fed viable lactobacillus acidophilus cultures with milk in concentrations similar to those in commercial acidophilus milk and yogurt cultures. The fecal concentration of bacterial enzymes known to promote the formation of cancer-causing chemicals in the colon was markedly reduced (Goldin 1984).

Allium Sativum

Lower rates of cancer are associated with the highest intakes of this important sulfur-rich botanical. *Allium sativum* is rich in sulfur compounds and may be important in several detoxification pathways, reports *Clinical Pearls.*

Stearic Acid/Oleic Acid

Dr. Jonathon Wright reports that lower levels of red blood cell stearic/oleic acid appear to be a marker for malignancy. Dr. Wright reports that lower levels have been found in a variety of different types of cancers as compared to healthy controls.

Epigallocatechin Gallate

Also known as EGCG, Japanese people who ingest a lot of EGCG from their native diet have lower death rates from cancer of all types, especially cancer of the stomach. A nutrient found more commonly in Chinese and Japanese diets than those of Western nations, EGCG has demonstrated strong potential for inhibition of colon tumors. Japanese researcher Yoshihiro Fujita believes that EGCG may be a strong factor in lowering colon cancer risk. Putting EGCG into your daily diet could make an important contribution to the prevention of cancer—especially colon cancer.

"If the Japanese smoke more than Americans, than why do they have significantly lower rates of lung cancer?"

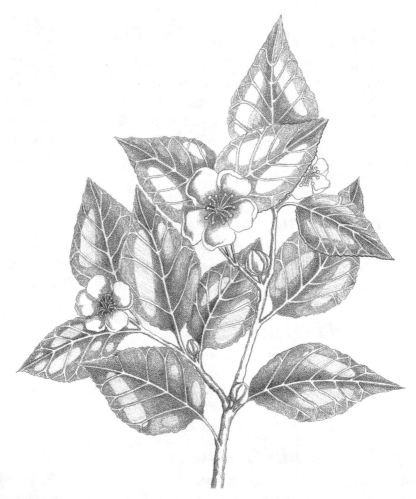

The powerful antioxidant EGCG is derived from the leaves of the plant Camellia sinensis. It is protective against a variety of cancers.

That's the question that researchers have pondered ever since the connection between smoking and lung cancer rates was correlated more than 40 years ago.

The answer finally came on August 28, 1991, when researchers reported during proceedings of the American Chemical Society that cigarette smokers who ingested epigallocatechin gallate (EGCG) had a 45 percent reduction in lung cancer rates. Not surprisingly, the Japanese obtain an abundant amount of EGCG through their diet, reported *Life Extension Update* in 1992. EGCG belongs to a family of chemicals known as catechins. EGCG prevents lung cancer!

EGCG prevents skin cancer! It's no secret that human exposure to harmful ultraviolet rays from the sun is causing increasing incidence of skin cancer. The depletion of the Earth's protective ozone layer appears to be a reality which is causing this increased exposure, not to mention the fact that so many Americans are sun worshippers who love being under the warmth of the golden eye in the sky. Why risk skin cancer when you can use EGCG to help in its prevention?

Life Extension reports: "Researchers at Rutgers University have described similar anti-cancer effects on skin cancer rates in lab animals. Animals given [EGCG] ten days before exposure to UV lights developed 50 percent fewer skin cancers."

"These effects of [EGCG] are quite interesting," says Rutgers study director Dr. Allan H. Conney. "There aren't that many things that have as broad a spectrum as [EGCG]."

The New Scientist reported in 1991 that Japanese and U.S. researchers have found that EGCG wards off several cancers, and one of the researchers went so far as to recommend its consumption daily.

Preventing Breast Cancer

Some vitamins, minerals, antioxidants and nutrients such as algin, fiber and other phytochemicals, that are readily available to women, have been demonstrated in experimental studies to offer some potential help in the prevention of breast cancer. In fact, researchers writing in the *Journal of the National Cancer Institute* assert that dietary intervention could prevent 24 percent of breast cancer in post menopausal women and 16 percent in premenopausal women.

Among the findings presented are the following:

•Researchers reporting in the *American Journal of Clinical Nutrition* report that low levels of beta carotene in the blood of women are associated with increased risk of breast cancer.

•A high fiber diet also appears to play an important role in the prevention of breast cancer, possibly by removing cancer-causing chemicals and excess estrogen.

•Omega-3 fatty acids, found in fatty cold-water fish, appear to have an inhibitory effect on mammary tumors, according to a report in *Medical Oncology and Tumor Pharmacotherapy*. A second study in *Nutrition and Cancer* shows that women with the highest consumption of fish tend to have the lowest incidence of breast cancer.

•Kelp has been conclusively proven to prevent breast cancer in women—especially Japanese women for whom kelp is viewed as a food not as a dietary supplement, reports Dr. Daniel Mowrey in his work *The Scientific Validation of Herbal Medicine*. The exact mode of action is not known but researchers have observed that kelp protects against radiation. Algin, the important ingredient in kelp, can prevent living tissue from absorbing radioactive materials including strontium-90, barium, mercury, zinc, tin, cadmium and manganese. The algin in kelp also increases fecal bulk and alters the nature of fecal contaminants and perhaps renders harmless bacteria that could be carcinogenic. It also appears to reduce cholesterol levels by inhibiting bile acid absorption.

•Selenium prevented or delayed the appearance of breast tumors in mice infected with a cancer-causing virus. Thirty-five breast cancer patients had significantly lower mean serum selenium levels than healthy controls.

•Soy protein reduced the risk of breast cancer in young women in Singapore. This is possibly because soy is low in iron and its addition to the diet displaces red meat which contains the most readily available form of dietary iron. There is evidence that increased body iron stores raise the risk of breast cancer, note researchers in *The Lancet*.

There is even more dramatic evidence of the importance of a soy-rich diet for breast cancer prevention, according to researchers writing in *The Lancet*. In women living in a small Japanese village and consuming the traditional low-fat Japanese diet, their urinary excretions were rich in phytoestrogens which are estrogenic substances derived from plants (as opposed to animals), the researchers reported.

The levels of plant estrogens in the urine of the Japense women were 12 to 107 times higher than in American and Finnish women. Interestingly, phytoestrogens have both estrogenic and anti-estrogenic activity in the human body—depending on the person's physiologicals needs. Such substances are known as *adaptogens*. This means that they *adapt* themselves to the physiological needs of the individual.

Similarly to more powerful and dangerous animal estrogens that are derived from meats and produced by the body itself, plant estrogens also bind to areas in each cell known as estrogen receptors. But that is where the similarities end. With plant estrogens, if the body is producing too much estrogen, their presence tends to depress excessive estrogen production. Conversely, if the body isn't producing enough estrogen, the amount of phytoestrogens consumed in traditional Japanese diets is large enough to have biological effects, especially in postmenopausal women with low estrogen levels.

•High intake of foods rich in phytoestrogens may partly explain why hot flushes and other menopausal symptoms are so infrequent in Japanese women. Their anti-estrogenic activity may explain in part why the risk of breast cancer is lower in Japanese women than in American women. Examples of foods rich in plant estrogens include soy products such as tofu, miso, aburage, atuage, koridofu, soybeans and other beans.

•An epidemiologic survey of 21 countries has suggested that high sucrose (sugar) intake is a major risk factor for the development of breast cancer in women over 45 years of age. In fact, we also know from a study published in *Nutrition and Cancer* that rats on high sugar diets developed significantly more mammary tumors than those on a high starch diet. Other studies have shown that human breast cancer mortality is positively correlated with dietary sugar intake but there is no such correlation with eating complex carbohydrates.

•Vegetarian diets may decrease the risk of breast cancer by lowering estrogen levels due to the low fat and high fiber content (Werbach 1988). In one study, ten vegetarian premenopausal women were found to excrete two to three times as much estrogen as 10 non-vegetarian controls and had lower serum estrogen levels, suggesting the fiber present in whole-grain, whole-vegetable diets absorbs estrogen and transports it out of the body .

The use of dietary supplements—especially antioxidants such as beta carotene and vitamins C and E and other minerals and nutrients—plays an important role in cancer prevention. For instance, various micronutrients may interact *synergistically* in the prevention of cancer. Ramesha and colleagues, reporting in the *Japanese Journal of Cancer,* found that the combined actions of selenium, magnesium, ascorbic acid and retinyl acetate prevented mammary cancer in experimental animal subjects exposed to the highly carcinogenic chemical 7,12-dimethylbenz[*a*]anthracene. Readers will also want to learn about other lesser known but extremely potent antioxidant nutrients such as superoxide dismutase, glutathione and Pycnogenol, discussed elsewhere in *Life Extenders and Memory Boosters.*

For more information about cancer prevention, readers should also contact the American Cancer Society at 1599 Clifton Road North East, Atlanta, Georgia 30329. Their telephone is (404) 320-3333.

---

11. *Shark Cartilage and Cancer Therapy*

If alternative still sounds far-out, consider the number of unorthodox procedures that were once outside the realm of "normal" practice. Louis Pasteur's germ theory of disease; antiseptic surgery, devised by Sir Joseph Lister; Edward Jenner's vaccine against smallpox. All were denounced as quackery. Even lumpectomy and radiation for patients with breast cancer were considered unacceptable treatments by American surgeons back in 1948 (Heimlich 1990). Sharks are probably the healthiest living creatures on earth. Scientists believe their powerful immune system can fight off virtually any disease that might afflict other living things. Now you can take advantage of their unique biolotical characteristics with a dietary supplement that holds dramatic potential to help in the prevention of cancer.

There is probably no disease more deserving of alternative therapy exploration than cancer. It is the second leading cause of death in this country. It claims more than 500,000 lives each year. Nearly 76 million Americans now living will eventually contract some form of the disease. And by the year 2000, the American Cancer Society (ACS) predicts that 1 out of every 2 people in the

U.S. will be cancer stricken (Lane 1992). Overall, traditional methods of treatment currently being prescribed do not seem to be providing the healthy picture of success we are all so desperately seeking. Avenues where there are ample hands-on scientific data available need to be examined.

That was exactly the mind-set of *60 Minutes* when their investigative reporters went on location in London, Mexico, Cuba, and Nicaragua. America's most widely watched news show was busy chronicling the dramatic success of shark cartilage used on cancer patients who were considered terminally ill. The famed TV show was also busy interviewing esteemed physicians such as Dr. Charles Simone, one of President Reagan's former oncologists, as well as Dr. I.W. Lane, whose book, *Sharks Don't Get Cancer*, brought shark cartilage to the attention of the American medical authorities.

We in the U.S. consider sharks either a fearful nuisance or an interesting object of curiosity. The Orient, however, considers it a popular delicacy. Shark fin soup, for example, is expensive Chinese fare. The shark fin is virtually pure cartilage. Its value, the Chinese believe, is in its purported ability to promote health, well being, and disease prevention. This may not be as fantastic as it sounds. After all, sharks rarely get ill. Even their most massive wounds heal quickly, free from infection.

Carl Luer, Ph.D., a biochemist at Mote Marine Laboratory in Sarasota, Florida, has conducted extensive research involving sharks and disease. Dr. Luer's research is based on a fact that has been well known for over a decade: That is, sharks rarely develop cancer, either naturally or when clinically induced. Even when sharks were exposed to high levels of aflatoxin B-1, which is carcinogenic, the sharks did not display an elevated incidence of tumors. In experiments conducted over a period of years, sharks were put into tanks containing strong concentrations of cancer-causing agents. Even then, not a single tumor occurred in any shark (Lane 1992).

Most of the shark cartilage research being conducted today began with a theory developed by Dr. Judah Folkman, world-renowned scientist, Harvard professor and physician at Children's Hospital and Harvard Medical Center. Back in the 1960s, Dr. Folkman was working on a hypothesis about the nature of tumors. Simply put, a tumor is new tissue made of cells that grow in an uncontrolled manner, suffocating and killing vital organs, and eventually, the host. Preventing cancer or cancer fatalities could depend on stopping the rampant growth of these runaway cells.

Dr. Folkman knew that tumors require a rich supply of blood to survive and feed their growth. Tumors implanted *in vitro* (outside the body), grew only a few millimeters in diameter. The same tumor implanted in mice, however, grew rapidly, eventually killing the mice. The difference between the two results is clear. In the mice, the tumor had a vibrant blood network from which to receive its nourishment. In the medium outside the body, it did not. When there is no fresh blood supply, the tumors cannot grow.

In 1971, Dr. Folkman published his hypothesis in *The New England Journal of Medicine*.

His primary conclusions were:

•Tumors cannot grow without a network of blood vessels to nourish them and remove waste products.

•The inhibition of the development of blood vessels could be a potential cancer therapy.

The process that Dr. Folkman hypothesized is known as *antiangiogenesis*. Angiogenesis, the formation of new blood vessels, usually occurs during ovulation and pregnancy, in the healing of wounds and fractures and in certain heart and/or circulatory conditions. The only other time angiogenesis (also called neovascularization) seems to occur is during the development of a tumor or other malady associated with the need for a new blood source.

Researchers began to look at cartilage as an angiogenesis inhibitor. They reasoned that since cartilage is avascular (without blood vessels) it could very well offer a path of keeping blood vessels from developing. Further support for this cartilage theory is offered by Patricia D'Amore, Ph.D., Laboratory of Surgical Research, Children's Hospital, Boston.

According to Dr. D'Amore, "The rationale for the use of avascular tissue extracts is that these tissues are devoid of vessels because they contain inhibitors of angiogenesis."

In the mid 1970s, a team of scientists working at the Massachusetts Institute of Technology submitted a study on cartilage to the journal *Science*. Robert Lange, Sc.D. and Anne Lee, Ph.D. reported that cartilage found in the shoulders of calves could inhibit the vascularization of solid tumors. Experiments were conducted with tumor bearing rabbits and mice receiving an extract of cartilage from the shoulders of calves (Lee 1983).

No toxicity was exhibited, and the growth of new blood vessels toward implanted tumors ceased while tumor growth stopped. However, further research was impeded due to a lack of a supply of cartilage. Mammals, having only a small amount of cartilage, were not an efficient source. Searching for a more abundant source, these researchers made a decision to turn to sharks. Researchers had already known about the tumor inhibiting potential of shark cartilage. Furthermore, since shark skeleton is composed entirely of cartilage, there is an ample supply. In addition to shark cartilage being far more abundant than mammalian cartilage, there are other advantages to justify its selection.

Shark cartilage is cleaner and purer than that of mammals because there is so little fat present; fat is an accumulator of environmental pollutants. Additionally, the cancer inhibiting extract from shark cartilage is vastly more prevalent than it is in mammals. For example, it takes 500 grams of calf cartilage to recover 1 milligram of cancer-inhibiting extract necessary to block vascular growth by 70 percent. Yet, the same amount of inhibitor can be processed from only .5 grams of shark cartilage. And this was still less inhibition than was achieved with one-thousandth as much material derived from a shark. Pound for pound, shark cartilage is 1,000 times more potent as a cancer inhibitor than cartilage obtained from cows and other mammals (Lane 1992). Compared to calves, reports the journal *Science*, sharks may contain as much as 100,000 times more angiogenesis inhibitory activity on a per animal basis (Lee 1983).

Use of Cartilage on Humans

Historically, the medical potential of cartilage utilization was proven by John Prudden, M.D., a Harvard-trained surgeon. He published a study regarding the treatment of cancer through the use of bovine cartilage extracts. Dr. Prudden's treatment was the result of his work using cartilage to accelerate wound healing. His work is of major import because it established the validity of using any kind of cartilage in medical applications.

Today's surgical texts routinely include discussions of how animal cartilage preparations can be used to accelerate wound healing, a treatment Dr. Prudden experimented with in 1960.

In a 1972 study, Dr. Prudden worked with cancer patients for whom standard radiation and chemotherapy were considered ineffective. Under rigorous test procedures, patients received a treatment regime of shark cartilage therapy, both orally and by injection. Toxicity tests, within stringent FDA standards, all proved negative.

There was a "complete response." This meant that all clinical evidence of an active tumor had disappeared for a minimum of twelve weeks and that skeletal radiographs clearly showed improvement. Dr. Prudden concluded that cartilage has a "major effect upon a wide spectrum of cancers." In 11 of 35 cases, a complete response with probable or possible cure was noted. These cases included cancer of the cervix, pancreatic carcinoma, and squamous cell cancer of the nose.

Dr. Prudden went on to conclude that in situations where traditional therapy is ineffective, such as certain cases of pancreatic cancer, the use of cartrix (powdered calf cartilage) therapy as a primary agent should be considered. One very strong argument in favor of this therapeutic regime is that, unlike chemotherapy, it does not burn any "immunological or hematological bridges."

According to an article published in 1988 by Dr. Patricia D'Amore, "The only event that stands between maintenance of metastatic cells in a dormant state and their establishment into a secondary tumor is the development of a vasculature. Thus, therapies aimed at interfering with vascularization represent viable strategies for anti-metastasis." It seems fair to conclude that shark cartilage, which *does* interfere with vascularization, would indeed be a viable therapeutic strategy in inhibiting tumor growth and its related spread.

Shark Cartilage and Cancer Patients

While many laboratory studies proved strong efficacy of shark cartilage therapy in an area where other cancer therapies were losing the battle, the time had come to put the therapeutic benefits of shark cartilage to use in a hospital environment with cancer patients.

One of the first trials of shark cartilage usage occurred in Costa Rica, which has both a large ocean shark population and the facilities for processing shark cartilage. There, in the late 1980s, Dr. Carlos Luis Alpizar, head of the geriatrics program in the social security hospital, was called upon to treat a patient with an inoperable abdominal tumor the size of a grapefruit. The patient was in a terminal stage and Dr. Alpizar was skeptical of the person's chance of survival.

With no other viable alternative open to him, he proceeded with experimental quantities of dry shark cartilage.

The patient took oral doses, three times a day, for one month. The routine was void of any other treatment and the doctor had no hope of patient survival. Using sonographic measuring procedures, the tumor ceased to grow within one month. After six months of continuous shark cartilage treatment, the grapefruit-size tumor was reduced to the size of a walnut. The patient regained his appetite, was able to function and after six months returned to normal life (Lane 1992).

In 1991, at the Ernesto Contreras Hospital in Tijuana, Mexico, eight patients with advanced, terminal cancer were selected for treatment with shark cartilage. After evaluation by Dr. Ernesto Contreras, Jr., each was taught to self-administer highly concentrated shark cartilage in pre-measured packets. Patients received weekly visits by a nurse and were given additional packets of cartilage material. In seven of the eight cases, every tumor disappeared. The proteins in the shark cartilage acted as an angiogenesis inhibitor, stopping the formation of replacement blood vessels causing rapid necrosis or death of the tumor.

In 1992, results were released from a preliminary clinical study by Dr. Roscoe L. Van Zandt, a gynecologist from Texas who practices part-time at the Hoxsey Clinic in Tijuana. He reported that eight women with advanced breast tumors had received daily doses of shark cartilage. After six to eight weeks, all eight patients had experienced significant reduction in their tumors.

Antiangiogenesis was a common factor in all these cases. In the June, 1981 issue of *Science*, an article written by Thomas H. Maugh III clearly states that angiogenesis inhibition is now a well-documented and fairly common phenomenon. Since this article was published, the exclusive angiogenesis inhibitor available commercially has been shark cartilage.

Shark Cartilage And Arthritis

Cancer may afflict over one million Americans annually. Arthritis, however, attacks 70 million people in the United States (Lane 1992). Sufferers battle constant pain in the lower back, arms, legs, fingers, knees, and shoulders. Both rheumatoid arthritis and osteoarthritis share symptoms of painful inflammation of the afflicted areas. Persistent angiogenesis appears to be at the root of the

Shark Cartilage
Personal Success Story

The ringing phone sounded like rattling bones. I knew it would be my sister, Florence, with the results of our father's prostate specific antigen (PSA) blood test for prostate cancer. My hand went electric as I picked up the receiver. I was anxious to get the most recent report of Dad's condition because of certain alarming changes in his health.

Julian Whitaker, M.D., editor of the medical newsletter *Health & Healing*, points out that the normal male PSA blood level is below four micrograms per liter. From four to ten micrograms is suspect of cancer, and above ten is consistent in most men with cancer that has grown outside the prostate capsule.

Dad had been operated on in December, 1991 for an enlarged prostate condition characterized by painful and difficult urination, along with fatigue. He had such a good recovery that the urologist did not recommend chemotherapy or radiation. Biopsy of the mass removed from the prostate showed only a low level presence of cancer cells.

Since the doctor had a base line on our father's cancer antigen level before surgery, he felt confident that he could track Dad's progress towards recovery with follow-up tests.

But the news that night from my sister was disastrous. The PSA blood result was 30, an indication that cancer cells were on the warpath! The doctor said we had to change our strategy and schedule radical prostate surgery.

Meanwhile, my sister had seen a report on *60 Minutes* about a marine biologist who noticed sharks never get cancer as do other fish. So the doctor decided to test the effect of shark cartilage given to animals with cancer to see if it would cure them. The rationale, of course, is that the shark cartilage inhibits the tumor from developing a network of blood vessels to bring it nourishment and it eventually dies.

The results in the laboratory test animals given shark cartilage were so dramatic that the doctor wanted to see if humans could be cured as well. Unable to get approval to test shark cartilage on human cancer patients in the U.S., he went to Cuba and conducted studies there with astounding results.

Shark Cartilage
Personal Success Story (continued)

Since that time, a survey of the popular literature will show shark cartilage being used with dramatic, if varying, results in people stricken with cancer.

In a turn of events that would later prove very fortunate, my father had also been scheduled for cataract surgery. The doctor decided to delay his prostate surgery a short time in order to let him go ahead with his eye procedure. This delay bought my father a precious month before his prostate surgery—just enough time, as we were all to learn, to allow shark cartilage and pineal gland extract to perform their healing.

Since there were no harmful side effects, I jumped on the band wagon and mailed off shark cartilage to my Dad the next day, along with pineal gland which has demonstrated cancer-fighting ability. Within three days, Dad was taking 800 milligrams of shark cartilage twice a day and 50 milligrams of pineal substance at night. (Pineal substance is most effective if absorbed by the body in the absence of light.)

We had Dad on shark cartilage one month before another PSA test was conducted.

We really had no way of knowing what would happen. We could only hope that shark cartilage was as effective as it seemed to be from the reports.

What followed was nothing short of a miracle. When the PSA screening test was done again on Dad's blood, his urologist was astounded at the results. His antigen level had dropped from 30 to 11 in only four weeks. His doctor agreed the shark cartilage/pineal gland supplement had made a positive difference. Dad continues using shark cartilage and pineal gland on a daily basis.

Dad is not out of the woods yet, and we are monitoring his situation closely, along with his doctor. But we do know that the combination of shark cartilage and pineal gland provided almost miraculous aid in his healing process.

Lynda L. Toth, Ph.D.

disease. The heart of shark cartilage is made up of central strands of protein and are among the largest produced by any cells. In addition to these powerful proteins, shark cartilage also contains complex carbohydrates known as mucopolysaccharides. Due to the large amount of mucopolysaccharides present in shark cartilage, a significant reduction of joint inflammation and pain seems to occur by blocking the angiogenesis process. Together, both the mucopolysaccharides and proteins are known to provide a stronger anti-inflammatory effect than each would separately. Dr. John Prudden, writing in the 1974 summer issue of *Seminars in Arthritis and Rheumatism* stated, "A material of such great potential benefit to so many millions of people should be made generally available as soon as possible."

Dr. Lane believed so much in the ability of shark cartilage to inhibit angiogenesis, he applied for a U.S. patent.

Since shark cartilage is considered a food, obtaining a patent was a tough uphill battle.

Dr. Lane spent years "knocking on doors, networking and nagging." But the evidence of shark cartilage's ability to inhibit angiogenesis was proven by formal scientific tests and studies conducted at the Institut Jules Bordet in Brussels. Concrete results, not hot air, provided the hard evidence needed to receive a patent. On Christmas eve, 1991, a patent was issued.

Today, shark cartilage is available as a food supplement. Studies have shown it to be successful in reducing pain in nearly 70 percent of osteoarthritis cases and 60 percent in rheumatoid arthritis cases.

Shark Cartilage Therapy Shows Great Promise

"More than 500,000 people this year will die in the U.S. from cancer," says Dr. Joe Weissman. "One in three Americans will be stricken in their lifetime. What intrigues me most about shark cartilage is the promise it has shown in the prevention of cancer. As Dr. Lane notes in the case of women who have had breast cancer, the chance of recurrence within two years is about 30 percent. Yet, among women who have used shark cartilage, 'it appears that seven to eight grams of shark cartilage daily may prevent reoccurence, especially if a sound lifestyle, including good nutrition is adopted and person is of normal body weight.'"

"Shark cartilage extract use daily may well be a prudent health strategy," continues Dr. Weissman who adds: "Yes, it will take years to confirm shark cartilage's potential. But I ask: can we, who seek health and longevity, afford to wait?"

Shark cartilage is already routinely used in skin grafts for burn victims because it is not rejected by the human body. In the past 20 years, shark cartilage has elicited a deep, dramatic response from terminally ill cancer patients. Yet, while the FDA continues to scrutinize the clinical data in support of shark cartilage therapy, preventing its use in traditional medical environments in this country, half a million people continue to die from cancer in the United States each year. Very often it is not the disease, but neglect of the remedy which may generally destroy life.

12. *Liver Protection*

It is amazing how well the liver survives the constant onslaught of toxic chemicals it is responsible for detoxifying. Some of the toxic chemicals known to pass through the liver include the polycyclic hydrocarbons that are components of various herbicides and pesticides, including DDT, dioxin, 2,4,5-T, 2,4-D and the halogenated compounds PCB and PCP. Although the exact degree of exposure of people to these compounds is not known, it is probably quite high, as yearly U.S. production of synthetic organic pesticides alone exceeds 600,000 tons (Regenstein 1982). The health effects of chronic exposure to these compounds are not well understood beyond the known ability in the case of certain chemicals to cause cancer in experimental animals and their association with cancers in various occupational groups such as farmers and forestry workers; their ability to cause birth defects and reproductive damage; and their damage to the kidney. As the liver is responsible for detoxifying these chemicals and many others, every effort should be made to promote optimal liver function.

The average human liver weighs about four pounds. It is the largest gland of the body and one of the few organs that will regenerate itself when part of it is damaged (up to 25 percent of the liver can be removed, and within a short period of time it will grow back to its original shape and size). The liver is the most important organ of metabolism.

The liver has four main functions including:

•*Vascular.* Its vascular functions include being a major blood reservoir and filtering over a liter of blood per minute.

•*Detoxification.* Additionally, the liver acts as a detoxifier; it effectively removes bacteria, endotoxins, antigen-antibody complexes and various other particles from the circulation. Protein metabolism and bacterial fermentation of food in the intestines produces the byproduct ammonia, which is detoxified by the liver. In addition to detoxifying ammonia, the liver also combines toxic substances—such as metabolic wastes, insecti-

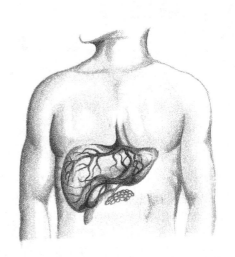

So essential is the liver to human health, that it can actually regenerate itself when damaged. Healing herbs can protect the liver and help it perform its detoxification function.

cide residues, drugs, alcohol and chemicals—with other substances that are less toxic. These substances are then excreted from our kidneys. Thus in order to have proper liver function, you must also have proper kidney function. Physicians have found that when either the liver or kidney appears to be malfunctioning, treating both organs produces the best health results.

•*Secretory.* The liver's secretory functions involve the synthesis and secretion of bile. Each day the liver manufactures about one liter of bile. Bile fluid is stored in the gallbladder for release when needed for digestion. Bile is necessary for the digestion of fats; it breaks fat down into small globules. Bile also assists in the absorption of the fat-soluble vitamins A, D, E, F and K and helps to assimilate calcium. In addition, bile converts beta-carotene to vitamin A. It promotes intestinal peristalsis helping to prevent constipation. Although the majority of the bile secreted into the intestines is reabsorbed, many toxic substances are effectively eliminated from the body by the bile.

    •*Metabolic.* The metabolic functions of the liver are immense; the liver is intricately involved in carbohydrate, fat and protein metabolism; the storage of vitamins and minerals; the formation of numerous physiological factors; and the detoxification or excretion into the bile of various chemical compounds including hormones such as throxine, cortisol, estrogen and aldosterone, histamine, drugs and pesticides.

Liver Health Problems

    The primary liver problems to affect people are congested liver, cirrhosis and hepatitis.

    Congested Liver. In the case of a congested liver, this probably reflects minimal impairment of liver function. Yet because of the liver's important role in numerous metabolic processes, even minor impairment of liver function has profound effects. One of the leading contributors to impaired liver function is *cholestasis*—diminished bile flow.

    Cholestasis can be caused by a great number of factors, including obstruction of the bile ducts. The most common cause of obstruction of the bile ducts is the presence of gallstones. Currently it is conservatively estimated that 20 million people in the U.S. have gallstones—nearly 20 percent of the female and eight percent of the male population over the age of 40 are found to have gallstones on biopsy, and approximately 500,000 gallbladders are removed because of stones each year. Both Petersdorf (1983) and Robbins (1984) assert that the prevalence of gallstones in the U.S. has been related to the high fat/low fiber diet consumed by the majority of Americans.

    Impairment of bile flow within the liver can be caused by a variety of agents and conditions. Cholestasis may be caused by such things presence of gallstones, alcohol, endotoxins, hereditary disorders such as Gilbert's syndrome, pregnancy, natural and synthetic steroidal hormones such as anabolic steroids, estrogens and oral contraceptives, certain drugs such as aminosalicylic acid, chloroethiazide, erythromycin estolate, mepazine, phenylbutazone, sulphadizine and thiouracil, hyperthyroidism or thyroxine supplementation and viral hepatitis (Dreisbach 1983).

These conditions are typically associated with alterations in laboratory tests of liver function. However, relying on these tests alone to evaluate hepatic function may not be adequate, as many of these conditions in the initial or subclinical stages may not show up within normal laboratory values. This is especially true in liver dysfunction related to oral contraceptive use and exposure to various drugs and chemicals (Petersdorf 1983, Robbins 1984).

At present, it appears that clinical judgment based on medical history remains the major diagnostic tool for the sluggish liver. Exposure to toxic chemicals, drugs, alcohol or hepatitis is usually apparent in individuals with a sluggish liver. Among the symptoms of this condition (Pizzorno 1988):

•Fatigue
•General malaise
•Digestive disturbances
•Allergies
•Chemical sensitivities
•Premenstrual syndrome
•Constipation

Cirrhosis. The second target area of liver therapy is cirrhosis, a degenerative, inflammatory disease in which damage and hardening of the liver cells occur. The liver is unable to function properly due to its scarred tissue, which can eventually prevent the passage of blood through the liver. The most common cause of cirrhosis of the liver is excessive alcohol consumption; a less frequent cause is viral hepatitis. Malnutrition and chronic inflammation can also lead to liver malfunction. In its early stages cirrhosis of the liver is characterized by constipation or diarrhea, fever, upset stomach and jaundice. Those people in the later stages of the disease may also exhibit anemia and bruising due to bleeding under the skin and edema.

Hepatitis.   Finally, there is hepatitis, which involves inflammation or enlargement of the liver. This disease has several primary causes including viruses and toxins. Among viruses, there is evidence that hepatitis can be caused by Epstein-Barr (Branch 1982). Hepatitis is most often transmitted by:
  •Person-to-person contact
  •Eating and drinking contaminated foods and beverages
  •Fecal contamination

Another form of hepatitis is more common among homosexuals and intravenous drug users. It is transmitted through the use of:

  •Contaminated syringes and needles
  •Bloodsucking insects
  •Blood transfusions
  •Sometimes through saliva
  •Sexual secretions

Symptoms of hepatitis include:

  •Fever
  •Weakness
  •Nausea
  •Vomiting
  •Muscle aches
  •Drowsiness
  •Headache
  •Abdominal discomfort
  •Jaundice

For reasons, not well understood, 10 to 40 percent of cases of hepatitis develop into chronic forms. It is surprising to most lay persons and even professionals that antibodies to the hepatitis A virus are detected in 50 to 60 percent of adults by age 50, indicating that most of us have immune systems which are strong enough to subdue this disease before it advances into more serious stages (Rubenstein 1988). Recently, a food server who neglected to wash his hands was responsible for at least 30 cases of hepatitis in the state of Colorado. Public officials' concern has been magnified by fears that afflicted children might infect playmates who would then infect their parents, thus turning the outbreak into an epidemic. You can see the insidious nature of this disease and why we believe it is so important that the immune system operate at optimal function in order to provide maximum liver protection.

Nutritional Liver Protection

The concept of liver therapy basically reflects an appreciation of the liver's critical role in all aspects of metabolism and an attempt to improve the liver's function by protecting it from damage. In terms of diet, one high in saturated fat increases the risk of developing fatty infiltration and stasis of bile in the liver and gall bladder.

Clinical experience indicates the value of a natural diet, low in saturated fats, simple carbohydrates (sugar, white flour, fruit juice, honey), oxidized fatty acids (fried oils) and animal fat. In contrast a diet rich in dietary fiber, particularly the water-soluble fibers, has a beneficial effect by promoting increased bile secretion, and has been shown to increase the elimination of bile acids, drugs and toxic bile substances from the system.

Several factors offer significant liver protection—lipotropins, antioxidants, membrane stabilizing compounds, choleretics and compounds that prevent the depletion within the liver of protein-sulfur compounds such as glutathione.

Additionally, hepatitis is a disease which greatly benefits from the use of natural therapies. Several nutrients and herbs—such as *Canna indica* and *Angelica sinensis* have been shown to inhibit viral reproduction, improve immune system function, and greatly stimulate regeneration of the damaged liver cells.

Liver Protectants and Lipotropic Factors

One aspect of optimizing liver function focuses on protecting the liver through the use of both liver protecting substances and lipotropic factors.

Liver protecting substances include many nutritional and herbal compounds which prevent damage to the liver associated with detoxifying harmful chemicals while lipotropic factors are by definition substances that hasten the removal

A Real Life Case for Liver Protectants to Save Lives

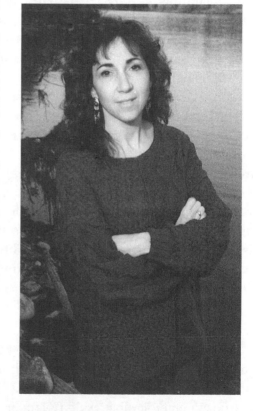

In 1991, Dr. Cynthia Watson faced one of the greatest challenges of her professional career when she was called upon to heal some 20 victims of a pesticide poisoning episode that occurred in the small California tourist town of Dunsmuir, Calif. A train derailment caused the spill of thousands of gallons of a highly toxic rice pesticide, metam sodium. Ultimately, an approximate 60 mile portion of the upper Sacramento River was completely destroyed with virtually all life disappearing—from insects to large wildlife such as bear and deer.

The human toll also was tremendous. One of the most significant maladies was liver damage as the victims' bodies tried to detoxify the highly toxic nerve gas.

Dr. Watson, a clinical faculty instructor at the University of Southern California, provided many of her patients with botanical liver protectants in order to save them from the highly toxic health effects of this pesticide.

One victim, Wayne Cunningham, is a barge operator who was asked to operate pumping and dispersing equipment at the headwaters of Lake Shasta as the spill worked its way south. He was exposed to the vapors and became deathly sick. He credits Dr. Watson's use of the same healing and protective botanicals such as *Silybum Marianum* described in this chapter with *saving his life.*

or decrease the deposit of fat in the liver through their interaction with fat metabolism. Compounds commonly employed as lipotropic agents include choline, methionine, betaine, folic acid and vitamin B-12, along with herbal cholagogues and choleretics. Cholagogues are agents that stimulate gallbladder contraction to promote bile flow, while choleretics are agents that stimulate bile secretion by the liver (as opposed to the expulsion of bile by the gallbladder.)

Formulas containing lipotropic agents have been used for a wide variety of liver conditions by physicians particularly in hepatic conditions such as hepatitis, cirrhosis and alcohol-induced fatty infiltration of the liver. They have also been used in treating premenstrual tension syndrome, as they are believed to aid the liver in its ability to conjugate and excrete estrogens.

Additionally, caring for your liver means stimulating the flow of bile, for bile contains many toxic substances. *Cholerectic* agents stimulate the secretion of bile by the liver thereby increasing the flow of bile. *Cholagogic* agents stimulate the flow of bile from the gall bladder and bile ducts into the duodenum. By stimulating the flow of bile, it is removed from the body and the body's circulatory system. That means fewer toxic substances will be returned to the liver. This is a very important nutritional principle; if the bile is not being transported adequately to the gallbladder, the liver is at increased risk of damage. Choleretics are very useful in the treatment of hepatitis and other diseases via the decongesting effect. Choleretics typically lower cholesterol levels, since they increase the excretion of cholesterol and decrease the synthesis of cholesterol in the liver.

Vitamin C

Large doses of vitamin C, at the rate of 40 to 100 grams orally or intravenously, were found to improve viral hepatitis greatly in two to four days with clearing of jaundice within six days (Cathcart 1981). Several other studies have documented similar results (Klenner 1971, Baetgen 1961, Baur 1954) and one controlled study failed to confirm this work (Knodell 1981). However Dr. Pauling claims that systematic errors invalidated this particularly study (Werbach 1987). Another controlled study found that two grams or more of vitamin C per day were dramatically able to prevent hepatitis B in hospitalized patients; while seven percent of the control patients (receiving less than 1.5 grams of vitamin

C per day) developed hepatitis, none of the treated patients did (Hasegaw 1975). A broad spectrum of antioxidants are essential in protecting the liver from free radical damage. Optimum tissue concentrations of these compounds should be maintained in the treatment of hepatic disease as well as the promotion of liver health.

Furthermore, because of the multiple benefits of vitamin C, its use at levels exceeding the RDA, is warranted for a number of other maladies, not the least of which is its ability to prevent the formation within the body of carcinogenic chemicals, and fight heart disease.

Choline

A fatty liver, similar in appearance to alcohol-induced fatty liver, has been produced in rats, guinea pigs, dogs, pigs, monkeys and several species of poultry when these animals have been placed on a diet deficient in choline and protein. These findings have promoted controversy concerning the role of choline in alcohol-induced fatty liver and cirrhosis in humans. Although these lesions may be similar to alcohol-induced lesions, choline itself has not been shown to be of any value in the treatment of alcohol-induced liver disease in humans (Baraona 1979, *Nutrition Review* 1984). Choline can be synthesized in humans by either methionine or serene. Choline may have some direct lipotropic effects in humans but research indicates that these effects may be more related to indirect effects via methionine metabolism. Dietary sources of choline include lecithin, egg yolk, liver and legumes (beans).

Methionine and SAM

Both Martin (1983) and Montgomery (1980) assert that methionine, an essential sulfur-containing amino acid, is a component of the major lipotropic compound in humans—S-adenosylmethionine (SAM). Methionine is a major source of numerous sulfur-containing compounds, including the amino acids cysteine and taurine. Methionine administered as SAM has been shown to be quite beneficial in two common conditions indicative of cholestasis, namely estrogen excess due to either oral contraceptive use or pregnancy and Gilbert's syndrome (Padova 1984, Frezza 1984, Bombardieri 1985).

SAM is able to inactivate estrogens through methylation, supporting the use of methionine in conditions of presumed estrogen excess such as PMS. Its effects in preventing estrogen-induced cholestasis have been demonstrated in pregnant women and those on oral contraceptives (Padova 1984, Frezza 1984). In addition to its role in promoting estrogen excretion, methionine has been shown to increase the membrane fluidity that is typically decreased by estrogens, thereby restoring several factors that promote bile flow.

Methionine levels are a major determinant in the liver's concentration of sulfur-containing compounds such as glutathione. Glutathione and other sulfur-containing small proteins, which are known as peptides, assume a critical role in defense against a variety of injurious agents by combining directly with these toxic substances, eventually to form water soluble compounds. As many toxic compounds are lipid soluble, conversion to water soluble compounds results in more efficient excretion via the kidneys. When increased levels of toxic compounds are present, more methionine is converted to cysteine and glutathione synthesis. Methionine itself has a protective effect on glutathione and prevents depletion during toxic overload. This, in turn, protects the liver from the damaging effects of toxic compounds (Montgomery 1980, Wisniewska-Knypl 1981).

Carnitine

Carnitine is a vitamin-like compound that people can manufacture within their own body. Since carnitine normally facilitates the conversion of fatty acids to energy, a high liver carnitine level is needed to handle the increased fatty acid load produced by alcohol consumption, a high fat diet and/or chemical exposure. While the use of lipotropic agents appears warranted in treating alcohol-induced fatty liver disease, many commonly used lipotropic agents such as choline, niacin, and cysteine, appear to have little value (Stanko 1978, Hartroft 1964). In contrast, carnitine significantly inhibits alcohol-induced fatty liver disease. It has been suggested that chronic ethanol (alcohol) consumption or chemical exposure results in a deficiency due to impaired synthesis (Sachan 1983,1984; Hosein 1975). By supplementing carnitine, this functional deficiency state is reversed, leading to normalization of fatty acid transport and alleviation of fatty acid infiltration within the liver. In other words, if you drink you need carnitine; it may be the best friend your liver has!

Liver Extracts

The oral administration of concentrated liver extracts has been used in the treatment of many chronic liver diseases since at least 1896 (Cavalieri 1974, Gilbert 1896). Numerous scientific investigations into the therapeutic efficacy of liver extracts have demonstrated that they possess a lipotropic effect, promote liver cell regeneration and prevent scarring (fibrosis) (Nagai 1970, Ohbayashi 1972, Hirayama 1978).

Clinical studies have also demonstrated that oral administration of concentrated liver extracts can be quite effective in the treatment of chronic liver disease, including chronic active hepatitis (Sanbe 1973).

Angelica Sinensis

Angelica sinensis root is also known as *Radix Angelica sinensis, Dong kwai, Tang-kuei,* and *Angelica dang dui.* *Angelica* nourishes and invigorates blood circulation, prevents decrease of liver glycogen and protects the liver, lowers blood cholesterol and has demonstrated anti-hypertensive effects. *Angelica* contains immunostimulating polysaccharides (Tsung 1986, Yamada 1987). Preliminary research reports suggest *Angelica* can increase red blood cell counts. This means the herb may prove beneficial in treating anemia. *Angelica* reportedly gives relief from colds, flu and bronchitis. It is sometimes used as a digestive aid (Castleman 1991). Inter-

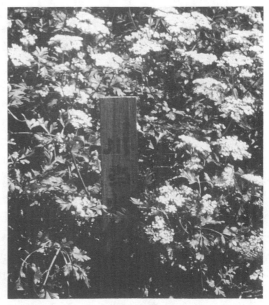

Angelica Sinensis

feron-inducing activity has also been demonstrated in *Angelica* extract (Yamada 1987). The most well-known function of interferons is their anti-viral activity. Additionally, 40 cases of a form of acute icteric hepatitis were effectively treated with an *Angelica* herbal formula, and *Angelica sinensis* reduced the thymol turbidity in 88 cases of persistent hepatitis, chronic hepatitis and cirrhosis of the liver (Chang 1986).

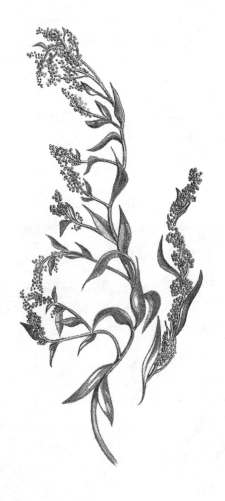

Artemisia capillaris

Artemisia Capillaris

Artemisia capillaris shoot has a bitter and pungent taste. This herb is noted for its ability to stimulate the flow of bile from the gall bladder and bile ducts into the duodenum as well as the secretion of bile by the liver. It is also known for its anti-jaundice effects. It is therefore used as a remedy for jaundice and hepatitis (Chang 1986).

Additionally, rats with carbon tetrachloride-induced liver damage, were given injections of *Artemisia capillaris;* histological examination on the eighth day revealed that swelling of hepatocytes, vacuolization, fatty degeneration, and necrosis were mild compared with the control group. The liver glycogen and RNA content were normalized or almost recovered, and the SGPT activity was markedly reduced. This evidence suggests the herb has a pronounced liver-protective effect.

Clinical studies of 32 cases of patients suffering icteric hepatitis given *Artemisia capillari* for seven days showed a rapid subsiding of jaundice and fever as well as marked decrease in the size of the liver. Additionally, there are several other studies demonstrating the positive anti-hepatitis activity of *Artemisia capillaris* in combination with other herbs (Chang 1986).

Bupleurum Chinense Root

In traditional Chinese herbal medicine *Bupleurum chinense* root is considered to be diaphoretic (*i.e.,* sweat inducing),which is important because perspiration is an essential excretory pathway and can help reduce the pressure of detoxification placed upon the liver; perhaps it is for this reason that *Bupleurum chinense* root is known for its liver-function restorative properties.

Bupleurum chinense root increased the total bile output and bile salt content in dogs. Another experiment indicated that *Bupleurum chinense* root stimulates bile secretions and flow with the fruit exhibiting the most potent effect, and the flower a weak activity. *Bupleurum chinense* root significantly checked experimental liver damage induced in animals by typhoid bacteria vaccines, carbon tetrachloride, and penicillin mold. *Bupleurum chinense* root with licorice markedly mitigated hepatic damage induced by carbon tetrachloride in rats. In clinical studies satisfactory therapeutic effects were obtained in 100 cases of infectious hepatitis treated with injection of *Bupleurum chinense* root (Chang 1986).

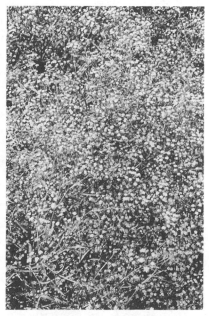

Bupleurum chinense

Canna Indica

Canna indica is taken from the root of the herb. Injections of *Canna indica*-based compounds administered to carbon tetrachloride-intoxicated mice for 10 days resulted in decreased damage. The herb alone given prophylactically for five days was also effective. These results indicate that *Canna indica* protects the liver from carbon tetrachloride-induced injuries. Additional studies have demonstrated the actions of *Canna indica* to protect the liver, increase bile flow and promote bilirubin excretion. *Canna indica* is used in the treatment of acute icteric hepatitis (Chang 1986).

Clinical studies have also shown beneficial effects. Out of 63 cases of acute icteric hepatitis treated with the oral decoction of the root of *Canna indica*, 58 were cured and three improved. Cures were generally achieved in about 20 days, 47 days at most. In another study where a *Canna indica* mixture was administered, out of 100

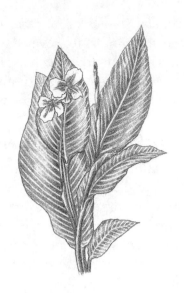

Canna indica

cases, 92 were cured and 8 basically cured. Symptoms and signs were rapidly improved and liver function was either improved or restored to normal (Chang 1986).

Curcuma Longa

A survey of the folklore literature of the world reveals that *Curcuma longa* has been employed in the medical systems of many nations. *Curcuma longa* has been found to provide liver-protection and it has anti-inflammatory properties. *Curcuma longa* stimulates the flow of bile. *Curcuma longa* has an anti-cholesterol action because it tends to bind cholesterolemic substances, thus rendering them incapable of absorption. *Curcuma longa* has antibiotic effects. In Chinese medicine, it is used to remove blood stasis, promote and normalize energy flow in the body, and relieve pain (Mowrey 1990).

Curcuma longa contains the yellow pigment *Curcumin* which has demonstrated liver protective effects similar to those of silymarin and cynarin (Kiso 1983). *Curcumin's* documented ability to stimulate bile flow supports its historical use in the treatment of liver and gallbladder disorders (Leung 1980).

Like cynarin, curcumin has also been shown to lower cholesterol levels (Wisniewska-Knypl 1981).

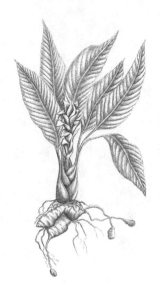

Curcuma longa

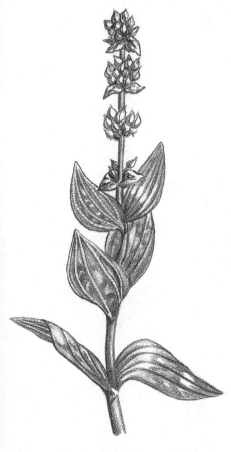

Gentiana Root/Rhizome

Gentiana Root Rhizome

Gentiana Root/Rhizome is used in the treatment of jaundice and hepatitis. A definite protective action on carbon tetra-chloride-intoxicated liver in mice was exhibited by injection (Chang 1986).

Clinical studies with a *Gentiana Root/Rhizome* combination decoction demonstrated that in 32 cases of liver dysfunction, a clinical cure was achieved in 27 cases and marked effects were observed in four cases; only one case was unchanged (Chang 1986).

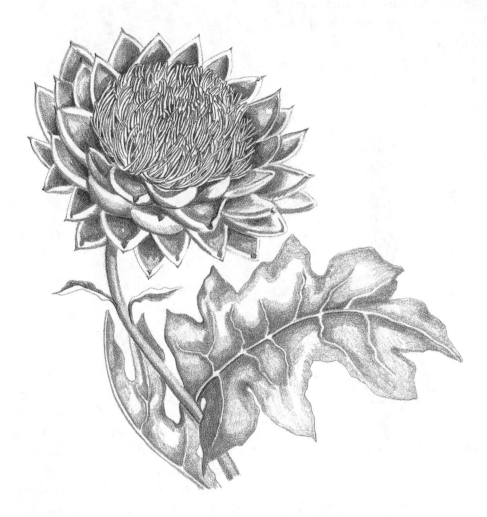

Cynara scolymus

Cynara Scolymus

Cynara scolymus has a long folk history in treating many liver diseases. Recent evidence supports this long-time use. *Cynara scolymus* is popular for its pleasantly bitter taste. One of its active ingredients is cynarin. *Cynara scolymus* has demonstrated significant liver-protecting and regenerating effects (Wagner 1981, Maros 1966, 1968). It also stimulates bile flow. Consistent with its choleretic effects, *Cynara scolymus* has been shown to lower blood cholesterol and triglyceride levels in both human animal studies (Maros 1966, Montini 1975, Pristautz 1975).

Glycyrrhiza Glabra

Glycyrrhiza glabra works synergistically by modulating and strengthening the activity of other herbs. Additionally, *Glycyrrhiza glabra* has been shown to have activities similar to that of cortisone. It induces the adrenal cortex to produce larger amounts of cortisone and aldosterone. *Glycyrrhiza glabra* has a positive effect on the adrenal-pituitary system as well as the thymus gland. *Glycy-rrhiza glabra* has anti-vi

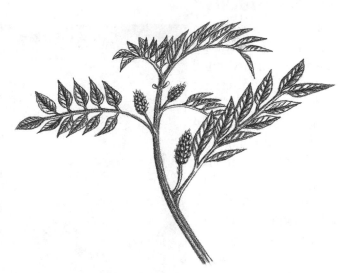

Glycyrrhiza glabra

ral and anti-atherosclerotic properties and has been observed to have a stimulating effect on immune response and production of immunological memory cells. *Glycyrrhiza glabra* has anti-viral (including anti-AIDS) activities; interferon-inducing activities; and T-cell activation effects (Abe 1982). *Glycyrrhiza glabra* prevents the suppression of immunity by stress and cortisone (Kumagai 1967). *Glycyrrhiza glabra* extracts have displayed antibiotic activity against staphylococcus, streptococcus and *Candida albicans* (Mitscher 1980).

The oral extract of *Glycyrrhiza glabra* significantly protected rats from liver injury due to carbon tetrachloride (Chang 1986).

Double blind studies have shown *Glycyrrhiza glabra* to be effective in treating viral hepatitis, particularly chronic active hepatitis (Suzuki 1984). This activity is probably due to its well-documented antiviral activity (Abe 1982, Pompeii 1980).

Lycium Chinense

Lycium chinense is used in traditional Chinese medicine for the deficiency of the liver and kidney. It is high in natural antioxidant factors and was found to decrease blood cholesterol in rats. It also inhibited the formation of experimental atherosclerosis in rabbits. The aqueous extract of this herb inhibited fat deposition in the hepatocytes due to liver damage induced by carbon tetrachloride and fostered the regeneration of the hepatocytes. Betaine aspartate also afforded protection against toxic hepatitis due to carbon tetrachloride. The liver-protective effect of betaine is probably due to its being a methyl donor (Chang 1986).

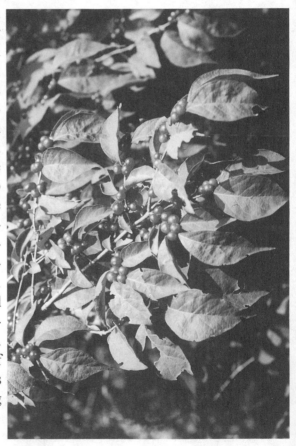

Lycium chinense

Schizandra Chinensis

Schizandra chinensis is an adaptogen which regulates various body functions and increases its ability to deal effectively with stress. *Schizandra chinensis* is an energy tonic which enhances mental activity and physical activity (Lucas 1991). The ethanol of *Schizandra chinensis* and its kernel markedly decreased the elevated SGPT of rabbits, rats and mice intoxicated by carbon tetrachloride.

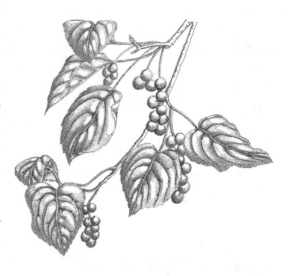

Schizandra Chinensis

More than 5,000 cases of various types of hepatitis have been treated with *Schizandra chinensis* preparations; the short-term effect for lowering the SGPT was quite good; the aggregate effective rate was 84 to 97.9 percent; SGPT was normalized in about 75 percent of the treated cases. The onset of action was about 20 days. Out of 86 cases with elevated SGPT due to drugs, 83 cases had normal SGPT after one to four weeks of treatment. What was most problematic was the re-rise of SGPT after discontinuation of the herb, usually in 1.5 to 3 months; the relapse rate was 46 to 69 percent and highest in chronic persistent hepatitis (Chang 1986).

Scutellaria Baicalensis

Scutellaria baicalensis (skullcap) is an excellent herb for almost any nervous system malfunction. It lowers blood cholesterol and blood sugar. It is a safe natural relaxant and nerve tonic. It strengthens circulatory tone and balances the nervous system. When *Scutellaria baicalensis* was given in intravenous injection it antagonized the toxic effects of strychnine in frogs, cats, and dogs, alleviated convulsion and lowered the mortality rate. When administered subcutaneously to mice, *Scutellaria baicalensis* reduced the toxic effects of strychnine (Chang 1986).

Clinically, *Scutellaria baicalensis* has been used to treat various forms of hepatitis, restored liver function and improved the clinical symptoms.

Sedum Sarmentosum

Sedum sarmentosum significantly protected rats from subacute liver damage due to carbon tetrachloride.

Silybum Marianum

Silybum marianum, also known more commonly as milk thistle, has become the plant therapeutic agent of choice for liver conditions. It can be given in acute stages of viral hepatitis and for all chronic liver disorders including fatty liver. *Silybum marianum* is perfectly safe and therefore does not carry the risks of many other major pharmaceutical liver drugs (Weiss 1988). Milk thistle is a large plant belonging to the daisy family (*Compositae*). It has been known for hundreds of years that the seeds of the *Silybum marianum* contain a principle with specific effects on the liver. Rademacher, a renowned German physician of the early 19th Century who was very interested in herbal medicine, gave his liver patients a tincture made from these seeds. This tincture today bears his name, *Tinctura Cardui Mariae Rademacher*, and is still listed in some pharmacopoeias today. A major advance came in recent years when the active principle was isolated and its chemical constitute established. The active isolate proved to be a flavonol not previously known and has been given the name silymarin (Weiss 1988). The concentration of silymarin is highest in the fruit but

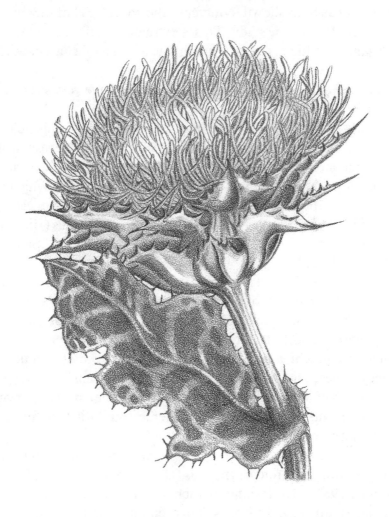

Silybum marianum

it is also found in the seeds and leaves.

Silymarin prevents free radical damage by acting as an antioxidant. Silymarin is many times more potent in antioxidant activity than vitamin E. Silymarin not only prevents the depletion of glutathione (GSH) induced by alcohol and other liver toxins, it has been shown to increase the basal GSH of the liver by 35 percent over controls in one study. This is extremely useful when exposure to toxic substances is high, due to glutathione's vital role in detoxification reactions.

Silybum marianum has flavonoid molecules that have very strong affinity for the liver (Vogel 1975, Hikino 1984).

Silymarin's effect in preventing liver destruction and enhancing liver function relates largely to its ability to inhibit the factors that are responsible for hepatic damage such as free radicals and leukotrienes, coupled with an ability to stimulate liver protein synthesis (Hikino 1984, Vogel 1975, Wagner 1986, Wagner 1981). The protective effect of silymarin against liver damage has been demonstrated in a number of experimental and clinical studies (Hikino 1984, Vogel 1975, Wagner 1981, 1986, Sarre 1971, Canini 1985, Salmi 1982, Scheiber 1978, Boari 1975).

Experimental liver damage in animals can be produced by such diverse toxic chemicals as carbon tetrachloride, amanita toxin, galactosamine and praseodymium nitrate. Silymarin has been shown to protect against liver damage by all of these agents (Hikino 1984, Vogel 1975, Wagner 1981, 1986.)

Another way in which the liver can be damaged is by the action of the leukotrienes. These compounds are produced by the transfer of oxygen to a polyunsaturated fatty acid. This reaction is catalyzed by the enzyme lipoxygenase. *Silybum* components inhibit this enzyme, thereby inhibiting the formation of these damaging compounds.

Perhaps the most interesting effect of *Silybum* components on the liver is their ability to stimulate protein synthesis (Hikino 1984, Vogel 1975, Wagner 1986, Wagner 1981.) The result is an increase in the production of new liver cells to replace the damaged old ones. This demonstrates that silymarin exerts both a protective and restorative effect on the liver.

In clinical studies, silymarin has been shown to have positive effects in treating liver disease of various kinds including cirrhosis, chronic hepatitis, fatty infiltration of the liver (chemical and alcohol induced fatty liver) and inflammation of the bile duct (Wagner 1981, 1986, Sarre 1971, Canini 1985, Salmi 1982, Scheiber 1978, Boari 1985). The therapeutic effect of silymarin in all of these disorders has been confirmed by histological (biopsy), clinical and laboratory data.

Silymarin is especially effective in the treatment and prevention of toxic chemical or alcohol induced liver damage (Wagner 1986, Wagner 1981, Sarre, 1971, Canini 1985, Salmi 1982, Scheiber 1978, Boari 1985).

Swertia Pseucochinensis

Swertia pseucochinensis is used in infectious hepatitis, acute and chronic bacillary dysentery and anorexia. Intragastric administration of the decoction of the herb to rabbits and subcutaneous injection of the total glycosides to rats, rendered protection against liver damage induced by carbon tetrachloride (Chang 1986).

Clinical results indicate that *Swertia pseucochinensis* is therapeutically effective in various stage of hepatitis (Chang 1986).

Taraxacum Officinale (Dandelion Root)

Taraxacum officinale is a familiar yellow flower found in lawns and in meadows. Actually, herbalists all over the world have revered this valuable herb for many centuries. Its common name, dandelion, is a corruption of the French for "tooth of the lion" (*dent de lion*) which describes the several large pointed teeth of the herb's leaves. Its scientific name *Taraxacum officinale,* from the Greek *taraxos* (disorder) and *akos* (remedy), alludes to dandelion's ability to correct a multitude of disorders.

Although generally regarded as a liver remedy, dandelion has a long folk use throughout the world for a variety of ailments. In Europe, dandelion was also used in the treatment of fevers, boils, eyes problems, diarrhea, fluid retention, liver congestion, heartburn and various skin problems. Its use in India, Russia and other parts of the world has revolved primarily around its action on the liver (Leung 1980, Duke 1985).   Until quite recently, the reason for cures from dandelion was not known, and they came to be regarded as thoroughly outdated. Yet when scientists became aware of the value of vitamins, this herb was found to be very rich in vitamins, minerals protein, choline, and pectins. Its carotenoid content is extremely high as reflected by a vitamin A content higher than that of carrots (dandelion has 14,000 IU of vitamin A per 100 grams

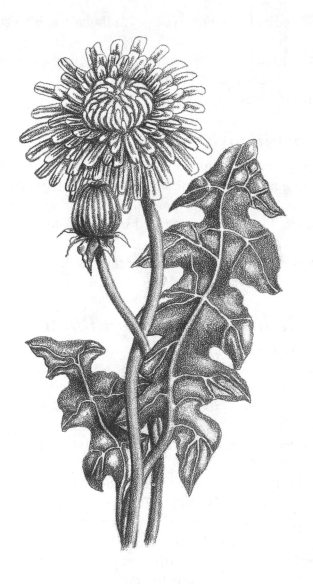

Taraxacum officinale

compared with 11,000 IU for carrots) (Leung 1985).

Initially, scientists believed that these beneficial effects were due to the high vitamin C content of dandelion; however, dandelion was found to additionally contain quite a large number of other different constituents that determine its therapeutic value. Not only was dandelion found to contain various bitters and vitamins, but also substances acting like enzymes, stimulating the function of the large glands, above all the liver and kidneys. In addition, these constituents stimulate cell metabolism as a whole, something that becomes particularly evident in those large glands, but which is effective also in other organic regions. Today, a connective tissue effect may also be assumed. This is responsible for the effect in chronic rheumatic conditions. Dandelion encourages kidney function (*i.e.*, has a diuretic action) as well as secretory function in the liver (showing cholagogue activity). This confirms the empirical findings of the past that it is a good remedy for biliary complaints. Its main influence is upon the liver and it is an excellent blood purifier. Because of its high content of minerals, it is used to treat anemia (Santillo 1991). Chinese physicians have prescribed dandelion since ancient times to treat colds, bronchitis, pneumonia, hepatitis, boils, ulcers, obesity. Animal studies demonstrate that dandelion has diuretic action and is recommended to help relieve the symptoms of premenstrual syndrome. In one study animals fed dandelion lost up to 30 percent of their weight. Because of its diuretic action, dandelion may be helpful in the treatment of high blood pressure and congestive heart failure. One study shows that dandelion inhibits the growth of *Candida albicans*. In Germany physicians routinely use dandelion to help stimulate bile flow and prevent gallstones. Some studies suggest dandelion root has anti-inflammatory properties. A Japanese study suggests some anti-tumor activity (Castleman, 1991).

Studies in humans and laboratory animals have shown that dandelion enhances the flow of bile, improving such conditions as liver congestion, bile duct inflammation, hepatitis, gallstones and jaundice (Mowrey 1986, Faber 1958). Dandelion's action on increasing bile flow is twofold—it has a direct effect on the liver, causing an increase in bile production and flow to the gallbladder (cholerectic effect); and a direct effect on the gallbladder causing contraction and release of stored bile (cholagogue effect). Dandelion's beneficial effect on such a wide variety of conditions is probably closedly related to its ability to improve the functional capacity of the liver.

Uncaria Gambier (Catechin)

An international workshop in 1981 on the use of *Uncaria gambier* in diseases of the liver concluded that this flavonoid has much promise for the treatment of many types of liver disease, particularly both acute and chronic viral hepatitis (Conn 1981).

Uncaria gambier has been shown, in numerous double-blind studies, to decrease serum bilirubin levels in patients with all types of acute viral hepatitis (Conn 1981, Suzuki 1986, Blum 1977, Berengo 1975, Theodoropoulos 1981, Demeulenaere 1981, Piazza 1983, Schomerus 1984). Furthermore, there is also more rapid relief of clinical symptoms (*i.e.*, loss of appetite, nausea, weakness, itching, and abdominal discomfort), more accelerated clearance of hepatitis virus antibodies from the blood, and greater reduction of liver enzyme levels than in control groups. One study of patients with chronic liver disease found that *Uncaria gambier* improved liver blood tests about twice as fast as compared to untreated controls (Suzuki 1986).

The liver-protecting effect of catechin is related to its free radical antioxidant properties, its anti-toxin effects in stimulation of immune system function, and its ability to stabilize membranes (Conn 1981, Abonyi 1984, Par 1984). Alcohol, and other toxic substance-induced liver damage (as evidenced by fatty infiltration), is usually unresponsive to commonly used lipotropic agents (choline, cysteine, inositol, niacin); but catechin, as well as silymarin, due to its wide range of actions, appears to prevent this hepatic damage.

You've got one liver. You can't live without it. Take care of it.

Recommended Amounts for Liver Protection

You should be sure to protect your liver daily—especially if you ingest alcohol regularly, are exposed to industrial chemicals at work or in the home environment *i.e.,* paint and cleaning solvents), use supplemental estrogen, or live in a polluted area. The following nutrients and herbal extracts, in suggested amounts to be used daily, should be the mainstay of promoting optimal liver function and health:

Vitamins, Amino Acids & Nutrients

Beta Carotene	10,000 IU
Phosphatidyl Choline	200 mg
Defatted/Dessicated Liver	500 mg
Thymus substance	200 mg
Lipoic Acid	15 mg
L-Methionine	400 mg
Free Form Amino Acids	100 mg
L-Carnitine Bitartrate	400 mg

Botanicals

Artemisia capillaris	15 mg
Angelica sinensis 4:1	25 mg
Cynara scolymus extract	500 mg
Gentiana root/rhizome	15 mg
Glycyrrhiza glabra	15 mg
Silybum marianum extract	500 mg
Uncaria gambier extract	400 mg
Schizandra chinensis extract 4:1	400 mg
Taraxacum officinale	300 mg
Swertia pseudochinensis	100 mg
Lycium chinense	100 mg
Bupleurum chinense root	100 mg
Curcuma longa extract	75 mg
Scutellaria root	50 mg
Canna indica	50 mg

Remember These Important Guidelines

For optimum liver function, a diet rich in dietary fiber and plant foods, low in refined sugar and fat, and as free from pesticides and pollutants as possible is preferred.

•Alcohol consumption is not advised. But if you choose to drink, you must be sure to use liver-protective dietary supplements.

•Liver protective substances appear to be indicated for many liver conditions, including minimal liver impairment (*i.e.*, sluggish or congested liver). The use of liver remedies may offer significant benefit (even in situations where only vague complaints, such as malaise and fatigue, are present).

•Lipotropic factors appear to be much indicated for those women who are taking oral contraceptive agents or those with increased estrogen levels (including pregnancy).

•Patients with a history of exposure to toxic compounds, especially organic solvents and polycyclic hydrocarbons such as pesticides and herbicides, may also benefit from liver-protective substances.

•When using cholerectic substances, a looser stool may be produced as a result of increased bile flow and secretion. If higher doses of choleretics are used it may be appropriate to use sequestering fiber compounds (*i.e.*, guar gum, pectin, psyllium, oat bran) to prevent irritation of the wall of the intestine and loose stools.

•Symptoms often associated with hepatitis—such as loss of appetite, nausea, vomiting, fatigue, flu-like symptoms, fever, enlarged tender liver, jaundice (yellowing of skin due to increased level of bilirubin in the blood), dark urine, elevated serum bile acids, signs of altered protein, carbohydrates or fat metabolism, or elevated liver enzymes in the blood—may all be markers that indicate the need for the use of liver support substances.

13. Relieving Arthritis

In 1858, London physician Sir Archibald Gerrod isolated and named the crippling ailment of arthritis. He suspected, but could not prove, that it was somehow related to nutrition. Today this relationship seems certain.

Rheumatoid arthritis is nicknamed The Great Crippler. The Arthritis Foundation has estimated the total annual cost of treating arthritic conditions in the U.S. at nearly five billion dollars with $690 million spent on prescription drugs and $575 million spent on non-prescription drugs. Approximately 32 million Americans—roughly one-seventh of our population—are affected by arthritis in its various forms with 6.5 million diagnosed as having rheumatoid arthritis and 16 million with osteoarthritis.

In its simplest definition, arthritis is an inflammatory affliction of a joint. Two versions of the disease—rheumatoid arthritis and osteoarthritis—are the most prevalent of some 100 different afflictions that have been discovered through research in rheumatology, the scientific name of the study of the entire disease we commonly call rheumatism or arthritis.

There are two primary forms of this disease:

•Osteoarthritis, says *The Bantam Medical Dictionary*, is a disease of joint cartilage, associated with secondary changes in the underlying bone which may ultimately cause pain and impair the function of the affected joint.
•Rheumatoid arthritis—sometimes called rheumatism—affects the joints of the fingers, wrists, feet and ankles and often the hips and shoulders, reports *The Bantam Medical Dictionary*. It is the second most common form of rheumatic disease.

Arthritis appears to be related to the body's immune system, asserts Lavon J. Dunne in the *Nutrition Almanac*, summarizing the nature of humankind's great affliction. Either the body is unable to produce enough antibodies to prevent viruses from entering the joints, or antibodies that are produced are unable to differentiate between viruses and healthy cells, thereby destroying both. Arthritis may also result from an allergy related to certain foods.
The joints are protected by synovium, which are membranes composed of mesothelium; connective tissue forms the sac enclosing a freely movable joint and secretes the lubricating synovial fluid. But when the synovium becomes inflamed—whether from a virus or malnutrition—the synovium begins eroding the bone. This situation is known as rheumatoid arthritis and as the inflamed tissue continues eroding the bones, the synovium thickens; chronic, sometimes deforming pain results. People suffering from rheumatism feel pain caused by the inflammation of the joints. Rheumatologists have recently discovered that the blood of arthritis sufferers shows a marked increase of antiglobulin antibodies called rheumatoid factors.

Symptoms listed by the American Rheumatism Foundation include:

•Morning stiffness
•Joint pain or tenderness
•Swelling of at least two joints
•Subcutaneous nodules (called arthritic nodules, usually found at pressure

points like the elbows and knees)

Statistics from the American Rheumatism Foundation show that the parts of the body most affected by rheumatoid arthritis, in descending order from the most prevalent locations, are:

1. Hip sockets
2. Elbows
3. Shoulders
4. Fingers and wrists
5. Knees
6. Sacrum
7. Heels
8. Toes

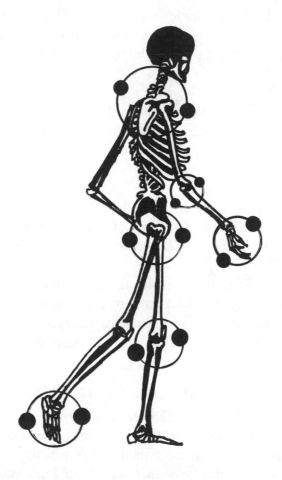

Immune System Connection

Rheumatoid arthritis's most popular victims are women aged 36 to 50, according to the National Rheumatism Foundation. The next major class of victims is men between the ages of 45 and 60.

The most prevalent form of crippling occurs when the hip sockets become so badly affected that complete incapacity occurs. Often a joint, which is infected, will freeze into a deformed position.

Rheumatoid arthritis usually first makes itself known by constitutional symptoms including fatigue, weakness and poor appetite. Other early signs include low-grade fever, anemia, and an increased erythrocyte rate (the rate at which red blood cells settle down in a test tube).

Advanced rheumatism shows up as structural changes in the joints that are apparent on X-rays, a positive rheumatoid factor agglutination test, decreased precipitation of mucin from synoval fluid, and characteristic histologic changes on pathological examination of the fluid.

Immune complexes are characteristically present in serum and joint fluid of most persons with rheumatoid arthritis. In many cases, rheumatoid arthritis spreads throughout the body and attacks one joint after another.

Treating Arthritis

Most physicians agree that the following steps make sense. The basic principles of treatment involve:

•Sufficient rest
•Exercises to maintain joint function
•Medication for the relief of pain and the reduction of inflammation
•Orthopedic intervention to prevent or correct deformities

Other treatments—including diathermy, ultrasound, warm paraffin applications, exercise under water, and applications of heat—are occasionally used. As rheumatoid arthritis is not always progressive, deforming, or debilitating, early treatment may help the patient to recover.

The Nutrition Connection

Every day, Dr. George A. Moore, a noted arthritis expert and head of six arthritis clinics in Southern California, sees that the majority of arthritic persons are usually undernourished. Many arthritic patients, he says, "have poor eating habits and need to be encouraged to obtain an adequate daily supply of nutrients . . . Appropriate vitamin and mineral supplementation is in order."

Usually the deficiencies are in minerals, he says—particularly zinc, as well as the B vitamins and Vitamin C.

One of the prime incentives for using optimal nutrition as your first health enhancing strategy is that nutrients are safer than prescription drugs.

In the case of arthritis, Dr. Pauling (1986) reports on the warnings associated with one such prescription drug which he calls Drug X. It is typical of the prescribed medications used to palliate this crippling disease.

Contraindications: Drug X should not be used in patients who have previously exhibited hypersensitivity to it or in individuals with the syndrome comprised of bronchospasm, nasal polyps and angioedema precipitated by aspirin or other nonsteroidal anti-inflammatory drugs.

Warnings: Peptic ulceration, perforation, and gastrointestinal bleeding — sometimes severe, and in some instances, fatal—have been reported with patients receiving Drug X. If Drug X must be given to patients with a history of upper gastrointestinal tract disease the patient should be under close supervision.

Precautions: As with other anti-inflammatory agents, long-term administration to animals results in renal papillary necrosis and related pathology in rats, mice, and dogs.

Acute renal failure and hyperkalemia as well as reversible elevations of BUN and serum creatinine have been reported with Drug X. In addition to reversible changes in renal function, interstitial nephritis, glomerulitis, papillary necrosis, and the nephrotic syndrome have been reported with Drug X.

Adverse Reactions, with incidence 20 percent to less than 1 percent: stomatitis, anorexia, gastric distress, nausea, constipation, abdominal pain, indigestion, pruritus, rash, dizziness, drowsiness, vertigo, headache, malaise, tinnitus, jaundice, hepatitis, vomiting, hematemesis, melena, gastrointestinal bleeding, bone marrow depression, aplastic anemia, colic, fever, swollen eyes, blurred vision, bronchospasm, urticaria, angioedema.

This particular drug has been administered to "millions of patients in eighty different countries," says Pauling.

He asks, "How many of these patients suffered from the side effects? How many read the foregoing contraindications before using Drug X?"

Drug X is probably very effective and its use in many cases medically justified. But we have to ask in how many cases it is being used as an expedient first resort before physicians have determined the optimal nutritional needs of their patients.

Optimal Nutrition Strategy

Why not first try the optimal nutrition strategy? More than 250,000 people have used supplements in arthritis treatment; they correct 80 to 90 percent of all arthritis cases, according to Robert Bingham, M.D., in the *Journal of the Academy of Rheumatoid Diseases*. Certainly nutritional therapy doesn't carry the extremely dangerous baggage of potential side effects that Drug X comes with.

Part of the reluctance of physicians and other health professionals to prescribe the use of nutritional supplements as a first or last resort or as a supplementary adjunct to other therapies in the treatment of arthritis is in part due to misinformation.

"As with other diseases," writes Dr. Pauling, "the question of the value of supplementary vitamins for the control of arthritis has been confused by misleading statements. Not long ago I read a brief report by a professor in a leading medical school about his trial of the value of unconventional treatments for arthritis. He stated that vitamin supplements were found to have no value. I wrote to him, asking how many patients he had studied, and how much vitamin supplement he had given them. His answer was that he had given an ordinary multivitamin tablet every day to a half-dozen patients, who seemed not to improve."

The patients whom Pauling describes in his work as receiving tremendous boosts in health from nutritional supplements "received one hundred and five hundred times the amounts in these tablets; it is the optimum intakes that have value in helping to control arthritis."

The following nutrients should be your first line of therapy for the treatment of arthritis.

DL-Phenylalanine

In 1973, neuroendocrinologists at the Johns Hopkins University School of Medicine discovered the existence of a brain structure which had a high affinity for opiate narcotics such as morphine. Subsequent research revealed the presence of brain hormonal substances which interacted with these "opiate receptors" and which themselves closely resembled morphine. Scientists named these brain hormones endorphins (*brain morphine*) and speculated that these endorphin hormones might constitute a built-in or endogenous pain relief system which might be activated by the body in times of extreme pain or injury. Subsequent research indicated that endorphins were indeed involved in such processes, and further that the administration of these substances into the central nervous system can elicit profound analgesia.

Administration of very small amounts (three milligrams) of endorphins in cancer patients and in women undergoing delivery has been reported to completely abolish pain sensations with a lack of adverse side effects. These analgesic effects tended to last for long periods of time (12 to 73 hours) while conventional narcotic analgesics have average durations of four to six hours. The authors of these studies concluded that endorphins "produced profound and long lasting analgesia." However, the clinical use of endorphins as pain relievers is not likely to occur because endorphins are small proteins and destroyed when swallowed by stomach acid and various digestive enzymes. Endorphins also cannot be used as injectable agents because they do not enter the brain from the peripheral circulation and must therefore be injected directly into the brain or the cerebrospinal fluid. Administration of exogenously derived endorphins tends to result in tolerance to the analgesic actions.

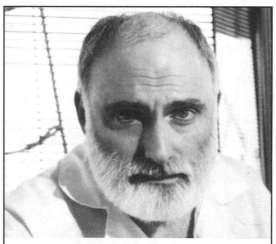

In light of these obstacles, another approach has been taken in order to utilize the endorphins as pain relievers. This strategy involves the inhibition of enzymes responsible for destruction of endorphins. D-phenylalanine, the active component of DLPA, has been found to inhibit at least two

Dr. Ron DiSalvo, Ph.D., is director of research and product development for Paul Mitchell Cosmetics. A believer in dietary supplements, Dr. DiSalvo notes that his mother, who has arthritis, regularly uses supplements containing DL-phenylalanine, yucca, *Equisetum arvense* and niacin.

enzymes believed to destroy endorphins. In strong support of this model is a study by Dr. Reuben Balagot, an anesthesiologist at the University of Chicago, which showed that a single dose of D-phenylalanine increased the activity of a small endorphin in a region of the brain believed to be intimately involved in analgesic mechanisms. This highly significant increase was extremely long lasting, persisting for up to six days and may be related to the extended duration of analgesic actions of DLPA in human patients. Thus the use of DLPA in the treatment of chronic pain syndromes constitutes a major advancement in the treatment of chronic pain in that it makes use of an intrinsic body system that has been shown in many specific investigations to possess extremely powerful analgesic properties.

Certain enzyme systems in the body continually destroy endorphins. DL-Phenylalanine effectively inhibits these enzymes and allows the pain-killing endorphins to do their job. *Research shows that chronic pain patients have lower levels of endorphin activity in their blood and cerebrospinal fluid.* With DL-Phenylalanine normal endorphin levels can be restored, thus assisting the body in reducing pain naturally, without the use of drugs.

Much of this pain is caused because arthritis sufferers have a lower level of endorphins, another of the body's natural pain killers.

Dr. Mindell (1983) reports that, "Dramatic results have been reported in patients suffering from a variety of chronic pain conditions, including rheumatoid arthritis and osteoarthritis, lower back pain, premenstrual cramps, migraine headaches, joint pains, whiplash, postoperative pain and neuralgia."

Why use a combination of the D and L forms (which form mirror images of themselves)?

Dr. Mindell (1983) points out that, "Pain researchers and health professionals . . . agree that the use of the D and L phenylalanine mixture has greater nutritive value to the body than the D form alone."

Does phenylalanine work? *Yes.*

Dr. Mindell (1983) reports, "The results of the first clinical study of D-Lphenylalanine in the treatment of chronic pain were published in 1978 by Dr. Seymour Ehrenpreis and other members of the Department of Pharmacology and Anesthesiology at the University of Chicago Medical School. This initial study was published in *Advances in Pain Research and Therapy* and was presented at the Second World Congress on Pain where experts from all over the world met to discuss current research findings in pain treatment. Patients

Phenylalanine Shown to Work Better than Conventional Pain Relievers

Condition	Duration	Prior Treatment	Time on DPA	Results
Whiplash	2 years	Empirin	3 days	Complete relief, 1 month
Osteoarthritis of fingers, thumbs of both hands	5 years	Empirin, aspirin	Maintained	Excellent relief, joint stiffness reduced
Rheumatoid arthritis (left knee); osteo-arthritis of hands	Several years	Empirin, codeine	1 week	Considerable relief
Low back pain; neck pain	Several years	90 acupunctures	3 days	Lower back pain gone; walked one mile
Low back pain	Several years	Spinal fusion; percutaneous nerve stimulation	3 days	Much less pain
Low back pain	Several years	Laminectomies; Depodrol; percutaneous nerve stimulation	3 days	Good to excellent relief
Fibrositis of muscle	Not known	Empirin	3 days	Pain gone; recurred after 2 days
Migraine headache	Several years	Not known	2 days	Good relief, may prevent recurrence
Cervical osteo-arthritis; postoperative pain	Not known	Not known	2 days	Very little pain
Severe lower back pain	Several years	Empirin, Valium	3 days	Excellent relief

selected for the study were those suffering from various conditions mentioned above who did not respond to other conventional pain treatments (*i.e.*, Empirin, Valium). Good to excellent pain relief was noted in every case. In addition, no adverse effects or tolerance to the analgesic action were observed Other scientific studies confirm the positive results of this initial study and showed DL-Phenylalanine to be particularly effective in treating the pain and inflammation associated with arthritis."

Because the patients that Dr. Ehrenpreis treated were unable to find relief with prescribed pain relievers, the use of phenylalanine is doubly significant as both a first and *last* resort.

The table on page 184 details the results of the Ehrenpreis study. Be sure to notice how ineffective prescribed medications were and how effective D-phenylalanine proved.

A follow-up study conducted at the University of Chicago and reported on in the journal of *Endogenous and Exogenous Opiate Agonists and Antagonists* found that statistically significant pain relief occurred within the fourth to fifth weeks after beginning D-phenylalanine therapy. By the fourth week of the study, 72.7 percent of the patients experienced significant pain relief. This increased to 78.9 percent by the fifth week. No adverse side effects were reported. A subset of these patients suffering from osteoarthritis were found to have a "much greater response" to D-phenylalanine compared to all other patients.

A double-blind controlled study was conducted at the department of anesthetics and pain relief service at the Royal Infirmary in England. All patients studied were resistant to previous treatment with drug and/or physical therapy and they were suffering from long-standing severe pain conditions such as post-herpetic neuralgia and lumbar fusion (post-operative) pain. Additionally, in assessing pain relief to D-phenylalanine (250 mg given three times daily) only those reductions which were rated as 50 percent or greater were regarded as significant. Approximately 32 percent of these patients "showed significant improvement" (50 percent relief) while taking D-phenylalanine. Further, "this improvement was not seen or maintained while the patients were receiving placebo." No significant adverse health side effects were noted.

Furthermore, DL-phenylalanine can be combined with any other existing therapy—drugs, aspirin, acupuncture, chiropractic—without adverse interactions and often with benefits greater than could be obtained by either therapy alone.

Perhaps most amazingly the pain relief can last far beyond the period in which it is taken. Some patients have reported that, following a week taking the product, pain relief continues for up to a month without medication of any kind. Clinicians have also confirmed that of all pain syndromes, those associated with osteoarthritis and rheumatoid arthritis are most receptive to treatment with DLPA.

Such effects originally reported in the research at the University of Chicago also seem to act in synergy with anti-arthritic medications such as Motrin, Naprosyn, Tolectin, Clinoril, Nalfon and Indocin. Thus, arthritic patients do not need to alter drug regimens prescribed by their physicians in order to benefit from DLPA. In this regard no negative interactions between DLPA and any prescription or nonprescription medication have been reported.

Studies indicate that proper dosage schedules are important to achieve results. Tablets generally available contain 375 mg of DL-phenylalanine and any recommendations made below are with reference to this standard form. Since many subjective factors (physical, mental and emotional) are involved in the individual's own experience of pain, the most effective dosages will vary with individuals or even from time to time with the same individuals.

Six tablets per day (two 375 mg tablets taken approximately 15 minutes before each meal) is a good way to begin your program. This schedule should be continued until a substantial amount of pain relief results. Preferably, take DLPA before meals for greater absorption. Some patients report feeling anxious or "pepped-up" after taking DLPA before meals. This may be the result of increased norepinephrine synthesis in the brain, and it can be eliminated by simply taking DLPA immediately after meals, thereby decreasing the ratio of increase of L-phenylalanine to other amino acids in the blood. Pain relief effects resulting from DLPA use generally require two to 20 days to develop. DLPA is not a fast-acting analgesic and is not intended to replace substances intended for such use. However, once pain relief effects are established, they can last for extremely long periods after discontinuing use. Most chronic pain patients studied to date have found that they do not need to continually use DLPA, and that they only need to take DLPA approximately two weeks out of the month. It is of great importance to emphasize that DLPA is of greatest benefit when it is added to ongoing therapeutic programs such as physical therapy, corrective procedures and even drug regimens aimed at reducing pain/inflammation symptoms. Like many pharmacologic treatments for arthritis and chronic pain such as aspirin, DLPA does not remove the cause of the primary disorder but does reduce symptoms to a level at which arthritis and chronic pain sufferers can regain functional capacities and experience lasting release from pain. DLPA is not recommended for use by patients with high blood pressure unless it is taken immediately following meals. Additionally, DLPA is not intended for use by phenylketonurics (PKUs) or during pregnancy.

If no substantial relief is noticed in the first three weeks, the initial dosage should be doubled for an additional two to three weeks. If there is still no response at this point, it should be noted that DLPA is not effective in about five to fifteen percent of all cases, and DLPA is contraindicated for people with phenylketonurea or during pregnancy. Persons with high blood pressure should take DLPA after meals. More likely pain will diminish within the first week of use. Dosages can then be reduced gradually until a minimum dosage requirement is determined. Whatever the daily ration, it should be spread throughout the day.

Dimethylglycine

Dr. Passwater (1991) reports that dimethylglycine can help *prevent* arthritis when its cause is related to immune dysfunction. "Injection of collagen into laboratory rats causes arthritis," Dr. Passwater says. "The animals produce antibodies to the collagen, which results in an inflammatory process and arthritis. DMG prevents the arthritis from forming."

Niacin

First discovered in 1937, vitamin B-3 is also known as niacin or niacinamide. In 1943, Dr. William Kaufman, a New England physician, published the first of several reports on the therapeutic benefits of the use niacin in the treatment of arthritis. In 1955 Dr. Kaufman told the American Geriatric Society that most of his patients enjoyed improvements when given one to five grams of niacinamide daily in doses of six to sixteen tablets. "I have had the opportunity to check the effectiveness of niacinamide, together with vitamin C, in controlling arthritis in a few patients, with results that support the conclusions stated by Kaufman," Dr. Pauling says.

Vitamin C

Cathcart (1981) asserts that severe depletion of vitamin C in the diet can lead to "disorders of the immune system such as secondary infection, rheumatoid arthritis and other collagen diseases."

Dr. Pauling (1986) says that, "In several diseases, including rheumatoid arthritis and cancer, substances are released by the diseased tissues into the blood that interfere with the mobility of phagocytes. Many investigators have reported that an increased intake of vitamin C improves the chemoactive response of phagocytes."

Dr. Pauling describes the successful fight that Norman Cousins, the former editor of the Saturday Review, waged against a particularly crippling form of arthritis known as ankylosing spondylitis. In severe cases the spine becomes completely rigid through fusions of its joints, reports *The Bantam Medical Dictionary*. "Cousins decided to try the effect of vitamin C and persuaded his physician to give him intravenous infusions of 35 grams of sodium ascorbate per day. This treatment, together with the psychosomatic aid of his determination to remain cheerful and to enjoy himself, achieved partially by leaving the hospital and receiving the treatment in a hotel room, led to his recovery."

Copper and Superoxide Dismutase

Dr. Passwater (1991) reports that researchers have found low tissue stores of copper cause pain and joint stiffness similar to that of arthritis. SOD, Dr. Passwater says, is one of the body's natural free-radical scavengers that reduces pain and inflammation. Despite its being quickly broken down upon oral administration, SOD levels in the body nevertheless experience a quick rise upon ingestion. Dr. Mindell also reports that a deficiency in copper can result in rheumatoid arthritis.

Yucca

Bellew and Bingham, of the National Arthritis Medical Clinic in Desert Hot Springs, CA, reported in 1975 in the *Journal of Applied Nutrition* that they used double-blind, controlled procedures to test the efficacy of yucca extracts in palliation of arthritic pain in 101 patients, giving half yucca tablets and the others placebos. Of the 50 receiving an average of 4 yucca tablets daily, 61 percent reported feeling less pain, stiffness and swelling in their arthritis than did those on the placebo.

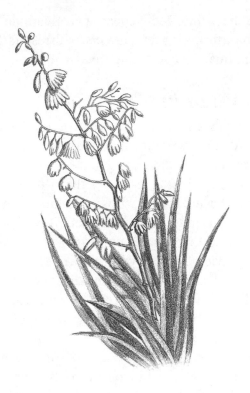

Yucca

L-Arginine

It has long been known that our bodies have a factor called human growth hormone. Since one effective cure for arthritis is to encourage the body to build healthy new bone and tendon cells, HGH is a strong part of any arthritis treatment. Clinical studies have demonstrated that increased HGH can reduce arthritis symptoms (Kotulak 1991). Recently scientists discovered that oral doses of arginine help increase circulation of HGH. A study in *Current Medical Research and Opinion* reports that 15 healthy male volunteers, aged 15 to 20, free of all endocrine or metabolic abnormalities and who were not receiving any kind of medical treatment, received a single oral dose of 2400 mg of amino acids including arginine. In each case—often as fast as 30 minutes—the amino acids were rushing HGH throughout their bodies. There is no doubt that the amino acids stimulated circulation of HGH, concludes the report.

Equisetum Arvense

There are 25 known species of *Equisetum arvense*, also known as horsetail. The plant is considered an excellent source of natural silica, needed in the creation of bone. Mowrey (1986) reports that horsetail supplies calcium, the primary mineral required for the healing of bones and that it is "rich in several other minerals that the body uses to rebuild injured tissue."

Green-Lipped Mussel

Traditionally, plants and other organisms, both from land and sea, have proven valuable sources of pharmacological agents for the treatment of chronic diseases, most recently and notably, of course,

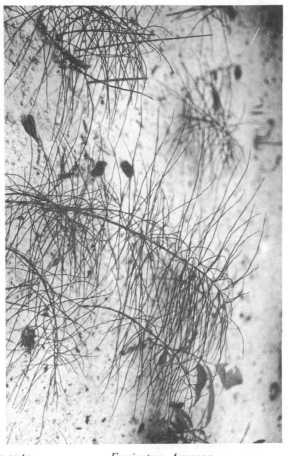

Equisetum Arvense

taxol from the Pacific yew tree and kelp--for the cure and prevention of various cancers. In fact, it was during the screening of marine molluscs for possible anti-tumor activities that scientists first discovered that the sea harbors special agents offering promise of relief from arthritis-related pain (Miller 1992). For example, take the rich waters of New Zealand where *Perna canaliculus*, more commonly known as the green-lipped mussel, resides. "There is some evidence that the green-lipped mussel may be of benefit in the treatment of inflammatory joint disease," notes Takuo Kosuge, of the Shizwoka College of Pharmacy in Japan (Kosuge 1986). It possesses moderate anti-inflammatory activity and contains an ingredient that inhibits the body's synthesis of prostaglandins, some of which may be harmful and can aggravate the painful arthritic condition, says K.D. Rainsford of the Tasmania Medical School, in Hobart Australia (1980).

At the Glasgow Homeopathic Hospital in England, extract of the green-lipped mussel is achieving very positive results in helping arthritis sufferers. "In our experience of treating over 500 patients, green-lipped mussel extract has proved to be the single most effective preparation which we have yet encountered for the treatment of both rheumatoid arthritis and osteoarthritis," note medical professionals Robin G. Gibson and Sheila L.M. Gibson (1981).

"We have been using [green-lipped mussels] for about seven years . . . Not only have we had consistently good results, particularly in rheumatoid arthritis, but we have also obtained X-ray evidence of reversal of rheumatoid joint pathology, an effect which has not, to our knowledge, previously been reported. We now also have a number of rheumatoid patients who have been able to discontinue all therapy . . . While we certainly do not claim that these patients have been 'cured', it is obvious that much of the symptomatology and disability associated with rheumatoid arthritis is more reversible than is generally realized. The fact that many disabled and crippled patients can return to an active, working life, speaks for itself" (Gibson 1981). If you suffer arthritis, green-lipped mussels offer the potential for dramatic relief. But there's more.

Ganoderma

Many people are familiar with the traditional nutritional adjuncts for arthritis relief such as DL-phenylalanine (DLPA), *Allium sativum, Equisetum arvense*, yucca, *Chiang huo, Clerodendron* and Chinese quince. Now, people who have arthritis will be learning about *Ganoderma Japonicum*, a Japanese anti-inflammatory botanical that researchers from Gifu College of Pharmacy in Japan demonstrated offers strong relief from inflammation (Ukai 1983).

A Final Word on Arthritis

Arthritis is a complex disease with a simple treatment. Sadly, too many Americans are ignoring the most simple cure. Arthritis cannot be treated outside the body. We must fight it where it lives--deep inside the cell.

What cures arthritis? Doctors can prescribe certain drugs but many have potentially harmful side-effects. If drugs don't work, arthritic joints—like hips and knees—can be replaced by surgeons.

Or, as is being proven every day, you can control arthritis by watching what you eat and taking daily supplements to help keep your joints healthy.

Optimal Nutrients for Fighting Arthritis

DL-Phenylalanine
L-Arginine
Dimethylglycine
Yucca
Allium sativum
Superoxide Dismutase
Niacin
Clerodendron
Equisetum arvense
Chinese Quince
Safflower Oil
Evening Primrose Oil
Vitamin C
Chiang hou
Pycnogenol
Green-Lipped Mussel
Ganoderma
Fish Oil

Where to Find the Formula
Editor's Note: Readers should also know that a formula containing most of the ingredients reported on in this chapter is now also available from an American Company, Gero Vita International. That product is called Arthril and can be ordered by calling (800) 825-8482.

For more information on arthritis, readers should contact the National Arthritis Foundation, 1314 Spring Street NW, Atlanta, Georgia 30309. Their telephone is (404) 872-7100.

14. Super Vision

How much would you give to learn about nutrients that can not only improve your night vision but preserve your eye sight throughout your life—perhaps even prevent the onset of cataracts? How precious is your vision? Do you love looking at the natural world—giant trees of the California Coast, a New Hampshire Maple, a redtailed hawk, or soaring eagle above a placid Alaskan inlet? How about reading the newspaper on Sunday morning? Even gazing on your spouse, children and other loved ones? If so, you know how precious your vision is and you assuredly want the proverbial vision of an eagle throughout your life.

If there were supplements containing such health-enhancing nutrients that could protect your vision, how much do you think they would cost? Where would you find them? Certainly not at the local prescription counter! Until recently, about the best you could do was use eye drops to take away the red. But while eye drops may have their benefits, they won't strengthen your eyes or prevent the blurry vision and throbbing that accompanies eye strain. And most important of all as you age—eye drops certainly don't protect you from cataracts.

We know something that can do both—and more . . .

   In fact, the cost for the vision of an eagle and a life free from cataracts is only pennies a day! Throughout the United States office workers and senior citizens are discovering that little known nutritional supplements finally available in this country have ingredients with demonstrated potential not only to fight the effects of stress on the eyes but also help prevent cataracts.

   These remarkable compounds are found in the leaves of a shrubby perennial plant found in portions of Europe and Asia.

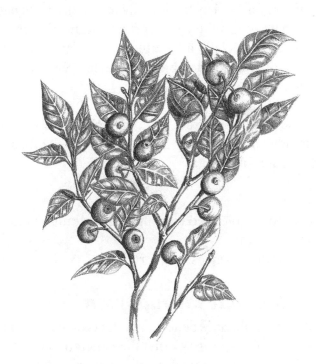

Vaccinium myrtillus

Vaccinium myrtillus

One area of especially promising research has been concerned with the eye-related curative properties of the bilberry plant, *Vaccinium myrtillus*, a shrubby perennial that grows in areas of northern Europe and Asia.

Bilberry has been used for centuries to reduce blood sugar levels in diabetics (Bever 1979). More recently, scientists have been fascinated by its ability to improve the healthy functioning of the eye, as well as visual acuity.

It was the amazing claims of World War II British Royal Air Force pilots that triggered an entirely new research direction for this herb.

At that time in aviation history, pilots controlled their craft visually. They did not have computers and radars to direct them. Their vision had to be keen. RAF pilots swore that eating bilberry jam prior to night missions significantly improved their vision, especially adaptation to the dark and visual acuity.

Such reports stimulated considerable research interest in bilberry throughout Europe and in South America.

Over the course of several years, following World War II, studies were published that demonstrated bilberry fruit extract was an effective treatment for a variety of visual problems:

•Night blindness.
•Visual fatigue from prolonged reading and working in dim light.
•Severe nearsightedness.
•Various vascular disturbances of the retina.

Bilberry Stimulates Rhodopsin

One explanation for bilberry's beneficial effects on the eye stems from our present theory of vision. Experts say that the generation of neural impulses from the retina of the eye to the brain depends on the presence of visual purple in the eye's rods. Visual purple is known as rhodopsin. Each time light strikes a rod, rhodopsin is depleted. In very bright light, the eye's stores of rhodopsin are used up faster than can be regenerated. As the day wanes and darkness nears, stores of rhodopsin build, the rods regenerate and prepare themselves for the difficult task of night vision. The more saturated with rhodopsin rods become the better they are at adapting to the dark.

Following up on the claims of the RAF pilots, laboratory researchers discovered that a certain family of phytochemicals, known as anthocyanosides, found in bilberry dramatically speeded up regeneration of rhodopsin in experimental animals and produced remarkably fast dark adaptation (Alfieri 1964).

Repeated trials with a variety of experimental animal species produced similar results (Jayle 1965).

Claims from pilots and truck drivers and studies of experimental animals are one thing but the real test comes with clinical trials involving human subjects.

One of the first published clinical trials was a simple attempt to demonstrate dark adaptation and improvements in visual acuity under controlled conditions in normal human adults. The study was carried out in 1964 by French scientists. Their subjects' adaptation to dark, following prolonged exposure to bright light, was significantly accelerated (Jayle 1965). Furthermore, a slight improvement in visual acuity in dim light was also observed.

Additional clinical trials followed that demonstrated the power of bilberry in the treatment of:

•Night blindness (Bailliart 1969).
•Severe myopia (Ala El Din Barradah 1967).
•Chronic visual fatigue (Gil Del Rio 1968).

By 1980, more than 50 scientific articles had been published on the extraordinary benefits of bilberry for optimal vision and healthy functioning of the eye.

Tired Eyes Need Bilberry

The practical side of this research can be demonstrated in instances like night driving when the bright flash of an oncoming headlight can be temporarily blinding. Bilberry can accelerate adjustment to darkness following exposure to bright light flashes.

Bilberry does much more. Spending your day typing in front of an office computer screen or even doing a lot of driving can be very tiring to your eyes. Indeed, if you're one of 65 million American office workers doing what you have to everyday to survive and you're working hard—you know that by the end of some days your eyes are burning, scratchy, blurry and fatigued. You don't see well at night and you may even suffer redness and a dull throbbing ocular ache. Persons suffering eye strain of almost any kind will benefit from long-term daily use of bilberry: students, truck drivers, pilots, those who must stare at computer monitors for extended periods of time, and people who constantly work in very dim light or very bright light.

Since its introduction this vision-saving nutrient has begun to gain a steady and loyal following among office workers who're suffering eye-related stress as well as senior citizens who are especially interested in doing all they can to help prevent cataracts and just about anybody else whose eyes are under strain.

In addition, research has shown that bilberry is particularly helpful as an effective treatment for cataracts and other chronic eye diseases; in France, it is used in countering developing myopia, as well as fighting eye diseases associated with hypertension and diabetic-induced glaucoma (Bever, 1979).

In fact, in Europe, standardized bilberry extracts are listed as the primary ingredient in a wide range of over-the-counter preparations designed specifically for the treatment or relief of a variety of eye problems. Bilberry is a firmly established part of European pharmacology. It is completely nontoxic when administered orally.

Cataract Protection

A cataract is basically any opacity of the eye, causing blurring or preventing vision. Cataracts are often caused by the accumulation of protein molecules into particles large enough to scatter light.

Literally millions are at high risk for cataracts. Nearly 20 percent of Americans aged 65 and older are victims of cataracts. What a shame! Because it doesn't have to be this way.

Any nutritional supplement that is designed to help improve the health and optimal functioning of the eye must include a number of additional vitamins and minerals that can help prevent cataracts, in addition to extracts such as bilberry.

The following nutrients have demonstrated strong potential in the prevention of cataracts and other eye-related disorders.

Vitamin C

Vitamin C appears to be the key to cataract prevention. There is much evidence linking a low intake of vitamin C to cataract formation. "The importance of vitamin C for good eye health is suggested by the fact that concentration of this vitamin in the aqueous humor is very high, twenty-five times that in the blood plasma," says Pauling (1986). "Many investigators beginning as long ago as 1935 with Monjukowa and Fradkin have reported that there is very little vitamin C in the aqueous humor of cataractous eyes and that patients with cataracts often have a low level of vitamin C in their blood plasma . . . Monjukowa and Fradkin reported that the low concentration of vitamin C in the lens preceded the formation of the cataract and concluded that low vitamin C is the cause, not the consequence, of cataract formation. They suggested that in old age there is a decreased permeability of the eye to vitamin C and suggested it might be overcome by a high intake of the vitamin."

Vitamin E

A cataract-prevention supplement should also contain vitamin E. Why? Vitamin E also helps prevent cataracts, according to researchers at the University of Western Ontario. In fact, supplements of vitamin E at 400 IU and vitamin C at 300 milligrams daily have proven largely successful in freeing people of cataracts, Dr. Passwater reports. The results indicate that both vitamins should be combined for an even more profound effect. *Time* magazine (Toufexis 1992) reports, "Patients taking high doses of both vitamins (C and E) appear to reduce the risk of cataracts by at least 50 percent." This news is especially important in light of the more than one million cataract operations performed annually in the United States (Passwater 1991).

Adequate intake of vitamins C and E helps prevent cellular damage to the eye caused by oxygen free radicals, as well as cataract formation (Roberts 1991). Researchers writing in the *American Journal of Clinical Nutrition* report, "Fair to good evidence for causal association between supplementary vitamin C and E consumption and freedom from senile cataracts." Their study, they say, "suggests that the consumption of supplementary vitamins C and E may reduce the risk of senile cataracts by about 50 to 70 percent" (Robertson 1991).

Beta Carotene

Beta carotene (the safety tested precursor of vitamin A) can help prevent night blindness as well as corneal lesions (Milkie 1972).

Zinc

Evidence has been presented that inadequate dietary zinc plays a role in poor dark adaptation (Milkie 1972). In addition Indian researcher Dr. K Seetharam Bhat has found that the zinc and copper levels in the eyes may influence the onset of cataracts.

Euphrasia officialism

Eyebright

Eyebright, *Euphrasia officialism*, is a wild European herb that appears to help alleviate acute or chronic inflammations of the eye as well as light sensitivity (Jameson 1988). Indeed, as its very name indicates, it is one of the primary herbal sources of eye care (Mowrey 1986). For some 2,000 years or longer, eyebright has been used for the treatment of eye problems. As Mowrey (1986) states, "Most cases involve sore and/or inflamed eyes in which there is considerable stinging and irritation associated with watery-to-thick discharges, or conjunctivitis (pink eye). The herb may help to relieve other symptoms that often accompany inflamed eyes, such as runny nose, earache and sneezing. Science has been remiss in not investigating this herb." Eyebright may be procured and used by itself as a topical eyewash or compress to potentiate its effects. Be sure to use the whole herb for any topical applications.

Goldenseal Root

A potent antibiotic and antiseptic (Gibbs 1947, Nandkarni, 1954), goldenseal root, *Hydrastis canadenis*, can greatly reduce infections and inflam-

Top Nine Nutrients for Healthy Eyes

Vitamins	Recommended Amount
Beta Carotene	5,000-15,000IU
Vitamin C	500-2,000 mg
Vitamin E	200-600 IU
Minerals	
Copper	2 mg
Selenium	50 mg
Zinc	40 mcg
Botanicals	
Eyebright	200-400 mg
Bilberry	200-400 mg
Goldenseal	
Bovine Eye Substance	20-40 mg

mation of the eyes. Its use goes back more than 100 years for curing conjunctivitis (Felter 1983). The American Indians used goldenseal for sore eyes, according to Mowrey (1986).

Bovine Eye Tissue

Bovine eye factor is a rich source of flavonoids that are most helpful to the eye. The reason for this is based on the theory that like organs have an affinity for each other. Therefore, by introducing bovine eye factor, rich in flavonoids, one would expect that its nutrients would be most readily available for use by the human eye. Additionally, medical researchers have demonstrated that flavonoids also can help delay onset of cataracts (Pautler 1986). Thus, bovine eye factor appears to be a potent supplement.

So if you want to protect your vision for the long run, be sure to combine the nutrients discussed in this chapter.

A supplement that is designed to care for the eye should contain the nutrients listed in the following table on the next page.

If you want to ensure that you are doing everything possible to prevent the formation of cataracts or if you have loved ones who labor at jobs that produce substantial eye strain or are otherwise at risk for cataracts, you should look to the protective buffer offered by a nutritional supplement specifically designed for the care and protection of the eyes.

15. Memory Boosters and Smart Pills

The human brain continues to fascinate and mesmerize scientists. It is a warehouse of information that some researchers compare to a highly sophisticated computer. With its super conductor qualities the brain continuously collects, sorts, and recalls data. It has the ability to process information creatively as well as, logically. Although it only weighs only about three pounds, the human brain is one of the most complex structures known to humanity. Like all other organs, the brain is affected by nutrition. But, can the brain's elaborate biochemical functions and structure be enhanced by vitamins, amino acids, and herbs? Medical research is uncovering powerful data that is leading researchers to believe that brain performance can be enhanced and that the prevention of senility is possible. Ask any smart pill taker if their brain is functioning at optimum levels. Most likely they will respond with stories of increased mental energy, greater concentration, and memory recall abilities. Science is just beginning to tap into human kind's unlimited intelligence and potential. Biological and chronological aging no longer need *to happen in the same breath. Biological aging may be slowed down and even reversed, starting with the brain.*

The brain is responsible for motivating every thought, action, and movement. Signals are sent to nerve endings or neurons and in turn, stimulate the release of "chemical messengers" known as neurotransmitters. Neurotransmitters spark impulses which lead the body to create, think and move. In order for neurons to keep up their proper stimulation of neurotransmitters, they need a heavy supply of chemical precursors. The two most important and commonly known neurotransmitters are acetylcholine and norepinephrine. Both rely on the precursor choline, a lipotropic B vitamin and phenylalanine, an amino acid that is converted into norephinephrine and dopaine, two excitatory brain transmitters that are known to enhance overall alertness. By supplementing the body with these ingredients, along with other known brain nutrients, many believe the brain's activity will increase its ability to receive and process information.

When a business associate handed a well-known author, whom we will call D., a bottle of a dietary supplement containing dimethylaminoethanol (DMAE) and told him to try it and see if he liked its effects, D. entered his smart pill experience not knowing quite what to expect. He did not know that DMAE is actually what is today known as a "smart drug". But D. took the DMAE and began using it primarily because he'd had the feeling for some time that he could be living life more intensely, could become more focused, and feel his inner creative flame burning more brightly. Says D.: "I guess I was willing to take a chance to see if there is truly something new under the sun."

After ingesting two to six tablets daily for about three weeks, something very wonderful and unexpected began to occur.

First, D. began experiencing dreams with tremendous lucidity. Even though D. would be asleep, he was extraordinarily conscious of his dreams. Yet, he was sleeping more deeply than ever.

Second, his attitude became superbly positive. He began waking ready to seize the morning. In the past he never was a good early riser, worried over the seeming walls of tasks everyday befalling him. Now, D. woke knowing he could handle the day. He was making lots of good humored remarks.

Third, at work, D. was producing a much greater amount of material. He wasn't speedy or hyped up or electrified as though he were using an amphet-amine or drinking lots of coffee. "How can I explain this?" says D. "It was no drug high that I was experiencing. I wasn't stoned. There were no munchies, slurred speech, or irritability. I was happy in a way that I never was before. I was enjoying challenges in my work. Let's say the candle was burning more brightly and intensely."

At this point, we must stress, that it was only after these experiences that Bob began to research the ingredients. We say this because if it were the other way around, you might suddenly become skeptical and say it was simply the power of suggestion that brought on these experiences. We assure you it was not. D. did not know that he was using a "smart pill." Ultimately, however, D. discovered he was experiencing the subtle effects of a substance that truly used to be available by prescription. That substance is called DMAE (dimethyl-amino-ethanol).

DMAE was once known as the prescription drug Deaner, which was manufactured by Riker Laboratories for helping hyperactive children. In the early 1980s, when the Food and Drug Administration requested Riker to perform a whole new series of studies on Deaner to prove its efficacy. The company declined and discontinued marketing DMAE in 1983, primarily because Ritalin emerged as the drug of choice for such disorders. The market was not large enough. And since DMAE is not a patented drug, but occurs naturally, there was no possibility for Riker to maintain propietary rights.

In fact, DMAE is a *nutrient* that we have a hard time supplying to our bodies from everyday diets. Although the natural presence of DMAE in living organisms has been demonstrated in scientific studies, its concentrations are minute due to its very quick conversion in the body to another important chemical: choline. DMAE is found most abundantly in those foods which the public tends to thinks of as "brain" foods such as anchovies and sardines. But you would have to eat a whole lot of sardines and anchovies to approximate the dosage Bob was ingesting on a daily basis.

The choline connection is important. Choline is used in the body for rebuilding cell membranes as well as producing the important brain neurotransmitter acetylcholine, responsible for mental alertness, learning and memory. Plenty of foods such as green leafy vegetables, legumes, wheat germ and egg yolks, contain choline. Yet, medical scientists believe strongly that DMAE is in many ways the superior nutrient. A 1973 report in *Experimental Gerontology* asserts that choline does not readily cross cell membranes. DMAE does. In fact, DMAE easily crosses the protective blood-brain barrier. That means it is more available to the body.

Unfortunately, as we age, our bodies produce less and less acetylcholine. By ingesting DMAE in generous amounts D. was rejuvenating his nervous system. In addition, the DMAE he was ingesting has demonstrated a beneficial yet mild stimulant effect. Researchers, studying DMAE under grants from Riker Laboratories and the U.S. Public Health Service Mental Health Institute, reported in a 1959 issue of the journal *Clinical Pharmacology and Therapeutics* that human subjects showed increases in muscle tone, better mental concentration, and changes in sleep habits including:

•*Less sleep needed*
•*Sound sleep*
•*Absence of a customary period of inefficiency in the morning*

The users of DMAE also generally reported favorable effects such as "improved mood," "relief of headaches," and "clearer thinking," the research team reported.

D. felt absolutely no side effects and pretty soon he was learning all he could about smart pills and nutrients from experienced users, doctors and researchers. Some were available in natural food markets, others by prescription.

This experience may make some readers recall the sixties and seventies when individuals smoked marijuana, snorted cocaine, or popped LSD. They may wonder whether what he was doing was nothing more than a nineties version of this earlier drug era. Certainly, the substances D. was using were not "drugs" in the sense that they are addictive, highly toxic, or narcotic. Yet, if we think of a drug as any substance which affects the structure or functioning of a living organism, these so-called smart drugs are indeed *drugs. But they aren't like marijuana, cocaine or other recreation drugs.* "The drugs that were used in the sixties like marijuana and cocaine depleted the brain's neurotransmitting chemicals," explains John Morgenthaler, coauthor of *Smart*

Drugs & Nutrients (B&J Publications 1991). "Smart drugs do precisely the opposite; they increase the activity and production of neurotransmitting chemicals." Morgenthaler says he prefers calling smart drugs *nootropics*, derived from the Greek word meaning: "acting on your mind."

There are now more than 200 "smart" bars in the U.S. Jim English, owner of Smart Products in San Francisco which distributes smart drink mixes to these bars, says his company is adding five or six bars a day to his list of purchasers. The drinks served to patrons at smart bars like the Nutrient Cafe in San Francisco contain ingredients such as choline and the amino acid phenylalanine (which is turned into norephinephrine and dopamine, two excitory brain transmitters that can help keep you awake and alert). Although these so-called smart bars themselves may be a fad whose longevity is likely to fade, the idea that dietary supplements and smart drugs can add extra intensity and creativity to our human experience and that more and more people will be willing to experience their effects will not fade. According to *Forbes* magazine, the first company to get FDA approval for a smart drug will earn a billion dollars in the first year alone, science reporter Michael Guillen told the nation on ABC News *Nightline* last year.

All of this burgeoning excitement, coupled with the enormous popularity of the book *Smart Drugs & Nutrients* has gotten the U.S. Food & Drug Administration to declare a war of sorts on smart drug use.

FDA spokesman Mike Shaffer says that:

•There simply is no evidence that drugs and nutrients can help mental functioning in healthy individuals nor that drugs originally tested to help correct dysfunctional brain conditions such as epilelpsy or dementia can somehow elevate normal brain function to a smarter and better-than-normal state.

•None of the claims for smart drugs have been subjected to testing in controlled clinical trial—the standard regularly accepted by health officials and researchers.

•There are risks in using prescription drugs without the supervision of a physician and even ordinary nutrients such as vitamins and amino acids can be highly toxic when taken at excessive doses, although Shaffer also concedes, "No injuries have been reported."

We strongly believe that Shaffer's first two statements are plainly exaggerations: Reports do appear in the medical literature (one which we cited about

DMAE), that smart drugs and nutrients can increase brain function of healthy people; furthermore these studies have employed scientific protocols that would satisfy all but the most prejudiced and skeptical mainstream researchers. On the other hand, some risks accompany smart drug use. Uninformed users of deprenyl may not know it can be fatal when ingested with cocaine, Ecstasy or even over-the-counter decongestants. Yet, it is available without prescription from overseas suppliers. A poster at the Nutrient Cafe warns patrons that the smart drug elixir *Renew You* (containing DMAE, phenylalanine, pyroglutamic acid and tyrosine) is not for use by pregnant women, people with the genetic disorder known as PKU, or individuals using blood pressure medication or certain drugs for Parkinson's disease and cancer.

The FDA by law cannot evaluate or allow labeling claims to be made for dietary substances or drugs which claim to enhance mental performance in healthy people since they are not suffering a disease. Yet, despite its official antipathy towards smart drugs and nutrients, FDA watch dogs are having a difficult time gaining the upper hand on stopping the flow of goods across the nation and past its borders. Physicians can legally prescribe medications such as Hydergine and Vasopression for their smart drug clients, and smart drugs not available in the U.S. can be legally imported from overseas suppliers for personal use as long as physicians include prescriptions and letters accompanying the shipment stating that the user is under their medical care.

The question isd: to what extent smart drugs and nutients can help improve brain function and intelligence in healthy people? Dr. Ross Pelton, R.Ph., Ph.D., reports in *Mind Food and Smart Pills* (Doubleday 1989) that in a double blind, short-term memory test of healthy volunteers, subjects receiving *Ginkgo* "showed a significant improvement in short-term memory." Meanwhile, high doses of choline significantly enhanced the ability of college students to recall lengthy word sequences, reports Dr. Richard Passwater in his book *The New Supernutrition* (Pocket Books 1991). An English study of the effects of Hydergine on 10 normal volunteers demonstrated that its use produced dramatic increases in alertness and high-level cognitive function, says Dr. Pelton.

Proponents of smart drugs and nutrients assert that they appear to be helpful in ameliorating three processes that can result in accelerated aging of the brain:
    •*Poor blood flow to the brain*. Without enough blood, the brain is deprived

of adequate amounts of oxygen and nutrients required for normal functioning. Botanical extracts such as *Ginkgo biloba* promote blood flow especially microcirculation in the tiny capillaries of the brain.

•*Diminished ability to produce neurotransmitting chemicals.* As you age, your central nervous system function decreases in many ways. Your brain produces less neurotransmitting chemicals which can lead to cell degradation and loss, slow information processing, and less efficiency. Molecular substances—known as oxygen free radicals which are produced by the body during energy production and when the immune system subdues toxins such as bacteria, viruses and environmental pollutants—damage cellular function. Such damage becomes cumulative. When the branches of nerve cells, (known as dendrites, which are tiny extensions that branch out from brain cells) deteriorate, nerve impulses become delayed and inefficient. Production of acetylcholine decreases; meanwhile, nerve receptors, that pass along acetylcholine, decrease in function. Most ominously, the production of enzymes that destroy acetycholine increases. Dr. Passwater asserts that aging individuals require additional dietary choline-forming nutrients such as DMAE and phosphatidylcholine, to maintain optimal brain function. Other smart "drugs" such as deprenyl seem to stimulate activity of other important brain neurotransmitters. Finally, the smart drug, Hydergine, seems to mimic the effect of a substance called nerve growth factor which stimulates the growth of dendrites, potentially enhancing communcation connections between nerve and brain cells, say Dean and Morgenthaler.

•*Production of lipofuscins.* Literally "cellular garbage," lipofuscins are composed of excess fats and wastes from portions of cells damaged by oxygen free radicals; (age spots on your skin are lipofuscins). By the time a person is nearing the end of his or her life, nearly 30 percent of cellular materials may be lipofuscins. Some smart drugs such as Centrophenoxine remove lipofuscins and help repair nerve synapses, which form the connections between nerve cells. Botanicals, such as *Ginkgo,* can also help prevent lipofuscin from accumulating in brain cells.

Is it smart to tamper with seemingly natural aging processes? Should we be using chemical—both nutrients and drug—to ostensibly make ourselves smarter or slow down the aging process? Most of us would love to have a sharper memory, enhanced creativity, and increased IQ—if only we knew how to achieve such goals. Smart drugs are not saviors of the mind. But they probably can create greater human potential and very possibly increase IQ and sustain powers of creativity. They definitely can extend mental powers of concentration and create greater intensity in life and work.

And there are spiritual aspects to smart drugs. "I'll tell you something most smart drug takers don't mention," says Los Angeles screenwriter Jeff Mandel, supervising producer of the syndicated science fiction television show *Super Force*. "When your brain is working more efficiently, all of *it* is working better including your level of intuition and spirituality. Many smart drug users report an incredible increase in precognitive events. It is sort of like *remembering the future*. Things happen like you may be thinking that the phone is about to ring and that an old friend is calling and then the phone does ring and *it is your old friend.*"

Other experts remain skeptical. "If you take a pill and say, 'Now I'm smarter,' am I just supposed to take your word for it?" asks Dr. James L. McGaugh, Ph.D., director of the Center for the Neurobiology of Learning and Memory at the University of California, Irvine.

Still other physicians such as Dr. Elias Tsambis, medical director of the New York Institute of Medical Research, in Tarrytown, acknowledges, "There are several compounds that I've worked with, one of them being an extract from a plant, the *Gingko* tree, that seem to have some beneficial effect on human intellectual functioning." On the other hand, Dr. Tsambis asserts that, "It's a funny thing to say, but I firmly believe that the less you do as far as injecting substances or taking megadoses of vitamins is best. I tell people to try to allow nature to do what it is suppose to do normally. You should live a balanced life, exercise cerebrally and physically, get enough sleep, and play as much as you work. The key is striking a balance—emotionally, physically and spiritually. If you're healthy, leave it alone."

Dr. Tsambis says he is by no means categorically opposed to the use of smart drugs and nutrients. But he is concerned that individuals using them are self-diagnosing and that they may really be suffering from an underlying condition that requires an expert's care. "A lot of people have approached me about their use of smart drugs," he says " I think they're in the situation where they are potentially treating themselves for a correctable condition with a nutrient that may have no value at all in their individual situation. If you just supplement without really understanding what is wrong, you could supplement with the wrong item and deprive yourself of the best treatment. If there is something wrong, get an evaluation." On the other hand, smarts drugs and nutrients are part of the future of preventive medicine, he adds. "At my neurological clinic we're doing brain function assessments that are really sensitive in terms of measuring brain function decline and determining when somebody should begin treatment. We measure brain activity from a variety of parameters—IQ tests, brain mapping, scans. Certain characteristics should alert you if you need such an evaluation—a family history with a genetic predisposition towards diseases such as Alzheimer's, hypertension or diabetes, or if you're beginning to experience some subtle changes. We have a whole host of people coming into our clinic who are telling us they have memory impairment. About 50 percent of them have a reversible condition caused by sleep deprivation, nutritional deficiencies or seasonal affective disorders. Your brain reflects how the rest of your body is doing. If you're not sleeping you're going to have cognitive difficulties. It's important to find out the reason why people are feeling a decline in mental function because finding out the reason determines the treatment. If I see declining alpha activity and increased beta and theta brain activity; first it is important to rule out causes like thryoid conditions, sleep patterns and even electrolyte imbalances. Then I might suggest that a person start using dietary supplements.

Furthermore, says Dr. Tsambis and other experts, people desiring increased brain function should engage in a diversity of mind challenging activities for making ourselves smarter. "Take up activities that stimulate activities in your brain," he says. Certainly an active lifestyle, that emphasizes both exercise and intellectual improvement—including activities that challenge the mind— is vitally important, he says. Some people take up crossword puzzles, others learn new languages or take music lessons. Still others return to school, entering new fields of study. Dr. Tsambis says that the work of Harvard University researchers demonstrates how important these recommendations are. In their research Harvard, physicians injected small doses of radioactive glucose into human test subjects, then used a device called a positron emission tomography scanner to monitor the glucose as it traveled through the brain. The subjects were subjected to different stimuli. When a question was asked, blood rushed to one part of the brain. When music was played, the blood rushed to another part of the brain. This, says Dr. Tsambis, is strong proof that engaging in a variety of intellectually stimulating activities, from listening to music, singing, drawing, writing, reading and other educational activities, is an important part of mental fitness. The adage that your brain is like a muscle and needs to be exercised to stay in shape, is more true than we may have imagined. "Those studies were accurate," he says. "They have been replicated several times. When someone is utilizing a different aspect of their brain, they are developing it. By learning mathematics or to play piano, you're laying down new memory traces, and that's important for maintaining good mental function."

Beginner's Guide to Smart Pills and Nutrients

Always consult a knowledgeable physician before using any of the smart drugs and nutrients listed below. For a list of knowledgeable physicians write to the Cognitive Enhancement Research Institute, P.O. Box 4029, Menlo Park, CA 94026.

•*Choline.* I use the form of choline known as phosphatidyl choline which appears to be most readily used by the brain, being able to cross the blood-brain barrier. It is my daily *brain fuel.* I ingest capsules at intervals during the day and they seem to enhance my powers of concentration and endurance. Dr. Passwater recommends that to improve their test performance, students should ingest 2,000 milligrams of phosphatidyl choline immediately before the exam. Morgenthaler recommends a dosage of about three grams of choline per day. He adds that all forms of choline should be taken with one gram per day of vitamin B-5 so that the choline can be converted into acetylcholine. Choline should not be used by people who are manic depressive; it can deepen the depressive state.

•*Dimethylaminoethanol.* A gentle stimulant, its effects may require three weeks to build-up. Its worst side effect seems to be a tightening of the jaw which will disappear with a lowering of the dosage. DMAE is available at natural food markets. Dosages range from 250 to 1,000 milligrams daily.

•*Ginkgo Biloba.* Even skeptical medical professionals are fascinated by the scientific findings regarding *Ginkgo biloba*, a tree native to China, occassionally found in the U.S., often in botanical gardens because of its strange appearance. It is unique because it is the last surviving species of an otherwise extinct family of prehistoric trees. One of its main effects is to increase blood flow throughout the body—especially to the brain—which is important because brain function is dependent on the nutrients it receives through the blood. *Ginkgo* also stimulates micro-circulation in the brain and helps prevent damage caused by free radicals. Dosages range from 100 to 1,000 milligrams daily. It is nontoxic.

•*Pyroglutamate.* Steve Fowkes, editor of *Smart Drug News,* published by the Cognitive Enhancement Research Institute, reports that in using the pyrglutamate, "There is a general heightening of mental functions—a sense of fullness; my skin felt a little bit stretched. I was facing a deadline at the time and I got a lot of writing done. It has a global effect on brain metabolism." Dosages range from 500 to 1,000 milligrams. It is nontoxic.

•*Lecithin.* As the aging process begins, the brain produces less and less neurotransmitting chemicals. This can lead to memory loss, cell degradation, and to a limited or a much slower rate of the brain being able to process information. Healthy brains normally contain 30% lecithin. Lecithin is source of choline, and because it is a precursor of acetylcholine it is considered to be an excellent "brain supplement". Choline is derived from at least 3 known sources: a small amount is synthesized by the brain some comes from the breakdown of phosphatidylcholine in membranes, and some is transported into the brain by plasma. Plasma choline fluctuates as a function of lecithin intake. (Lieberman 1986) With diminishing supplies of acetylcholine the brain cannot store and recall information properly. According to Dr. Pelton, author of *Mind Food and Smart Pills*, "lecithin functions as a source of structural material for every cell in the human body, particularly those of the brain and nerves". Studies have shown that "symptoms of tardive dyskinesia (involuntary twitching and movement of the face and tongue) and Alzheimer's, disease have been ameliorated in some patients" (Wood 1982).

Both lecithin and choline are important compounds of cell membranes. They help the liver to metabolize fat. A study (Etienne 1978) reported on the clinical effects of choline on seven patients suffering from Alzheimer's disease. Increasing the amount of choline in the blood of the seven patients suffering from Alzheimer's resulted in improvements in cognition and speech in three of the seven. The results were replicated in a similar clinical study carried out by Mesulam and Weintraub (1979) in which two of six Alzheimer's-afflicted patients improved after administration of lecithin. Although only two of six patients improved, this is significant, for it demonstrates a marginal, if not greater, nutritional basis for the prevention and onset of one of our nation's most devastating diseases.

Commenting on the Mesulam/Weintraub study author Stuart Bell noted in 1982, "This may not seem like much, but imagine yourself as one of the two clinical effects of choline on seven patients suffering from Alzheimer's disease. Increasing the amount of choline in the blood of the seven patients suffering from Alzheimer's resulted in improvements in cognition and speech in three of the seven. The results were replicated in a similar clinical study carried out by Mesulam and Weintraub (1979) in which two of six Alzheimer's-afflicted patients improved after administration of lecithin. Although only two of six patients improved, this is significant, for it demonstrates a marginal, if not greater, nutritional basis for the prevention and onset of one of our nation's most devastating diseases.

Commenting on the Mesulam/Weintraub study author Stuart Bell noted in 1982, "This may not seem like much, but imagine yourself as one of the two patients, especially considering that there is no other useful treatment. After treatment with lecithin, memory improved considerably—as did speech and the entire mode of daily living. One patient, who could not perform activities alone before treatment, became able to lead a relatively normal life. Another patient, who was very slow in thought, speech and movement before treatment, became more alert and able to interact with other people. Both of these people, as a result of treatment with lecithin, were able to lead more normal lives. This leads one to believe that people suffering from Alzheimers may be aggravating their situation more because of a choline deficiency. By increasing their daily intake of lecithin, it may be possible to boost IQ levels and help alleviate the suffering of Alzheimer's. In his book *The New Supernutrition,* Dr. Passwater writes that high doses of choline, when administered to college students, improved their ability to recall lengthy word sequences.

Amino Acids: Tyrosine, L-Glutamine, and L-Carnitine

Tyrosine is a semi-essential amino acid that is a natural anti-depressant.

Tyrosine has been used to help alleviate stress, anxiety, mood deterioration and low performance levels while serving extended amounts of time in military service. Research shows that tyrosine is a precursor of the neurotransmitter norepinephrine. Various forms of stress (depression, anxiety, etc.) have been shown to deplete the brain's supply of norepinephrine in animals; hence, "The administration of tyrosine may minimize or reverse stress-induced performance decrement by increasing brain depleted brain norepinephrine levels" (Owasoyo 1992). Tyrosine users report that tyrosine gives them a feeling of "calmness and well-being."

Tyrosine has also been shown to lower blood pressure. When hypertensive laboratory animals were injected with tyrosine their blood pressure was reduced to normal levels within 2 hours. "It appears that tyrosine's antihypertensive action is mediated by an acceleration in norepinephrine's release within the central nervous system" (Sved 1979).

Tyrosine has also been used to increase a low sex drive and for treatment in Parkinson's disease (Haas 1992*).*

L-Glutamine, another cognitive enhancing amino acid, when taken is turned into glutamic acid by the brain. Dr. Earl Mindell reports that "glutamic acid serves primarily as brain fuel". It has the ability to pick up excess ammonia-which can inhibit high-performance brain function—and convert it into the buffer glutamine." "Since glutamine produces marked elevation of glutamic acid, a shortage of the former in the diet can result in a glutamic acid shortage in the brain." Dr. H.L. Newbold, in his book *Mega Nutrients For Your Nerves* writes, "L-Glutamine relieves depression, impotence, and helps fight fatigue."

Acetyl-L-Carnitine is a molecule that is naturally found in milk and other foods. Acetyl-L-carnitine is similar to choline, in that, one of its primary functions is to aid in supplying the cells' mitochondria (the source of the body's energy production) with fuels such as fat. Acetyl-l-carnitine may have some anti-aging benefits for the brain by fighting the build up of lipofuscin which reduces mental ability. No observable side effects have been noted.

Panax Ginseng

Almost as old of a remedy and as widely used as *Ginkgo,* is Panax ginseng. Panax ginseng's use was first recorded by the ancient Chinese. These records say that Panax ginseng "restores the five internal organs, tranquilizes the spirit, calms agitation of the mind, allays excitement, and wards off harmful influences, while its continual makes for long life with light weight of the body" (Pelton 1989).

Because of Panax ginseng's adaptogen qualities, it has the ability to stabilize excessive amounts of glucose in the blood, by lowering blood sugar levels. Low blood sugar is often associated with mental fatigue and confusion accompanied by a low attention span. Panax ginseng has also been found to stimulate long and short-term memories. The Institute of Physiology of the Bulgarian Academy of Sciences found that, "Ginseng stimulates the adrenal cortex, improves the ability to remember, accelerates learning, and even regulates the brain's activity, placing it at a higher level." It is no wonder that Panax ginseng is called "the root of life." It is not a panacea but is widely used and known for its abilities to balance both physical and mental stress.

AntioxidantVitamins

Antioxidant vitamins are important to mental fitness, since they help intercept and protect the brain cells against free radical damage. Important free-radical fighters are vitamins A, C, and E. Vitamin C is a necessary antioxidant vitamin, because it is needed in order to manufacture neurotransmitters. In his book, *Mental and Elemental Nutrients*, the late Dr. Carl Pfeiffer writes, "vitamin C is an essential constituent in the specific metabolism of the amino acids phenylalanine and tyrosine." Dr. Pfieffer reports that "during stress, vitamin C is depleted from the tissues, particularly the adrenal cortex."

Meanwhile, vitamin E, "may retard the aging process," writes John Morgenthaler in his book, *Smart Drugs and Nutrients*. It can hinder the rate in which the cells age and since it is a fat soluble vitamin, vitamin E guards against free radical attack on essential fatty acids (Pelton 1989).

Vitamin A has antioxidant properties that neutralize free radicals and fight against stress. Schizophrenics, who show skin alterations due to large amounts of stress, may benefit from taking vitamin A (Pfieffer 1975).

Xanthinol Nicotinate

A form of niacin (vitamin B-3) that is easier for cells to metabolize than niacin, xanthinol nicotinate helps stimulate blood flow to the brain and creates an "increase in glucose metabolism." This, in turn, supplies the cells with more energy.

Smart Drugs By Prescription

•*Hydergine.* Hydergine is a good mental focusing agent. It is derived from the same ergot fungus found on rye and other grains as lysergic acid. "It allows me to involve myself with a project for a long period of time," says Fowkes. "It didn't matter whether I was writing a book or cleaning the garage. It also enhanced my visual fields. It made it easier for me to see shapes and forms; colors were brighter as well. I would use it for several days at a time and at other times intermittently." Pelton reports it is known to stimulate increased blood and oxygen supplies to the brain, slow lipfouscin deposits, protect the brain from damage during periods of insufficient oxygen supply, in addition to increasing intelligence, memory, learning, and recall. Recommended dosage in the U.S. is three milligrams, in Europe nine milligrams.

•*Vasopressin.* A hormone secreted by the pituitary gland, vasopressin has been used to treat people with impaired memory. "Vasopressin is necessary for imprinting new information in your memory," says Morgenthaler in the book *Smart Drugs & Nutrients.* "Vasopressin is very useful when learning large amounts of new information. It can increase your ability to memorize and recall." Vasopressin is a good first drug to try because its effects can be felt within seconds. It has not been proven safe during pregnancy and Dean and Morgenthaler warn sufferers of hypertension and epilepsy that caution is required. Other side effects include nasal congestion, runny nose, itch or irritation of the nasal passages, abdominal cramps, headache and increased bowel movements. It is available in the U.S. with a doctor's prescription.

•*Piracetam.* "I wrote 20 scripts in 14 weeks for *Super Force* using a combination of piracetam, hydergine and vasopression," screenwriter Jeff Mandel says. Many users report that piracetam works well with other smart drugs and nutrients such as DMAE, choline and hydergine. One of the unique findings on Piracetam is that it promotes nerve transmission flow between the right and left brain hemispheres. It also effects the cerebral cortex portion of the brain associated with human thought and reasoning—which may be one of the reasons why creative artists and spiritual seekers like its effects. Piracetam is available only from overseas suppliers. It is nontoxic.

For more information about the causes and prevention and treatment of Alzheimer's disease, readers shoulder contact the National Alzheimers Foundation, 919 North Michigan Avenue, suite 1000, Chicogo, Illinois 60611-1676. Their telephone is (312) 335-8700.

16. The Healthy Prostate

What do ABC News President Roone Arledge, Supreme Court Justice John Paul Stevens, U.S. Senator Robert Dole, Time Warner Chairman Steven Ross, actor Bill Bixby and rock star Frank Zappa all have in common? All of these prominent men have suffered bouts with prostate cancer. And Steven Ross, Bill Bixby, and Frank Zappa recently passed away, after losing their battle with the disease. They deserve a lot of credit, however, for going public with their illnesses.

The prostate is the most common site of disorders in the male genito-urinary system. Yet, for all too long, men have shown fear and cowardness in dealing with the pain of prostate disorders.

We want you to live a healthy, vital life all through your golden years. That's why we want to discuss the disease every man needs to know about and the dietary supplements that many experts believe every man should be using.

If there is a single leading reason why middle-aged men dread going to the doctor, it is the fear of prostate disease. Yet the fact is that as the male population ages, the number of cases of prostate cancer and other disorders is rising significantly. Whereas in 1970, some 60 men out of every 100,000 were struck with prostate cancer annually, by 1990 that number was 120 men out of every 100,000. Clearly, men need to do something on a personal level about preventing this chilling disease.

The New York Times reported recently that each year, 400,000 American men spend at least $3 billion on prostate surgery (Altman 1992). Unfortunately for many men, they have to repeat the procedure within five years to once again ameliorate the often painful conditions of an enlarged prostate (known as benign prostatic hypertrophy). *Complications from surgery include impotence and incontinence* (Freudenheim 1992). Obviously, if there were a better way, you'd want to know about it. We know a better way. But before we tell you about the dietary supplements you should be using daily as a prostate health insurance policy, you should be forewarned about the latest ballyhooed treatment being brought to you by the pharmaceutical industry.

Of course, now we have the newest prescription—the relatively untested medication known as Proscar, from Merck. Proscar was recently approved by the Food and Drug Administration. Proscar has raised hopes among the medical community that surgery will become less necessary. The drug, however, which became available in July, was only effective for about half the men it was tested on. Furthermore prostate shrinkage and symptom relief—if they are to occur at all—will occur only after taking the drug for six months to a year. The annual cost is $638.75, and the drug must be taken for life. The full range of Proscar's side effects will not be known for some time but unclude impotence in five percent of users. That doesn't sound all that promising for right now. Who wants to be a guinea pig? Well, you do if you start taking Proscar!

Men of all ages can help themselves for the long haul, protecting both their health and sexual potency by simply taking the correct supplements.

There are three significant disorders affecting the prostate:

•*Prostatitis.* Prostatitis is common in men of all ages. It is the acute or chronic inflammation of the prostate gland. The usual cause is a bacterial infection from another area of the body which has invaded the prostate. Prostatitis can partially or totally block the flow of urine out of the bladder, resulting in urine retention. As prostatitis becomes more advanced, urination becomes more difficult. This causes the bladder to become distended, weak, tender and susceptible to infection as a result of the increased amount of bacteria in the retained urine. Infection in the bladder is easily transmitted up the ureters to the kidneys.

Symptoms of prostatitis include:
•Pain between the scrotum and rectum
•Frequent and burning urination with blood in the urine
•Lower back pain
•Temperature
•Impotency

•*Benign Prostatic Hyperplasia.* Benign prostatic hyperplasia (BPH) is the result of gradual enlargement of the prostate. While not cancerous, this enlargement can cause disability and even serious illness if left untreated. *Taber's Cyclopedia Medical Dictionary* defines prostatic hypertrophy as, "enlargement of the prostate gland due to the aging process rather than inflammation or neoplasm (cancer)."

If enlargement progresses to cause obstruction of the urethra, surgical intervention may be indicated. Nearly 60 percent of men between the ages of 40 and 59 years of age have an enlarged prostate gland. Other researchers believe that figure may be higher. In fact, Barry (1990) notes that, "a high proportion of the 12 million men in the U.S. over age 65 must have clinical BPH, meaning literally millions of men may be putting up with at least some symptoms of BPH." The cost of hospital care and surgery for BPH in the United States alone is more than one billion dollars annually (Horton 1984).

When the prostate becomes too large, it presses against the urethral canal. This interferes with normal urination and backs up in the kidneys. As a result, the kidneys become damaged by both the pressure and the contaminated urine. Kidney infection is likely to occur when the kidneys are filled with this contaminated urine. Bladder infections such as cystitis are associated with prostatitis.

The normal male aging process favors the development of BPH due to a variety of factors, including age-related alterations in men's hormone levels. As men age there are many significant changes in hormone levels (Horton 1984). BPH represents a male hormone-dependent disorder of metabolism. Testosterone and, particularly, free testosterone levels decrease with age after the fifth decade, while other hormones such as prolactin, estradiol, sex hormone-binding ligand, lutenizing hormone, and follicle stimulating hormone levels are all increased.

These changes create an increased amount of dihydrotestosterone within the prostate. Dihydrotestosterone, a very potent androgen derived from testosterone, causes the overproduction or hyperplasia of prostate cells which ultimately results in prostate enlargement.

Additionally there is an increase in the uptake of testosterone by the prostate which appears to be caused by yet another hormone, prolactin. Drugs that reduce prolactin levels reduce many of the symptoms of BPH; however, these drugs have severe side effects and they are not widely used.

Symptoms of enlargement of the prostate include the need to pass urine frequently during the night, with frequency increasing as time goes on. There can be pain, burning, and difficulty in starting and stopping urination.

Many physicians believe that surgery is the only solution to the problem, yet the surgical procedure often results in complications. *However, benign prostatic hyperplasia will often respond to nutritional and herbal support. Furthermore, nutritional factors may offer significant protection against developing prostatic enlargement.*

•*Prostate Cancer.* The most common male genito-urinary disorder is cancer of the prostate. Prostatic cancer is also the third most common type of cancer found in males, following lung and colon cancer. A history of venereal disease or repeated prostatic infections has been linked to developing cancer of the prostate. Family history does not appear to play a part. It rarely occurs in men under sixty years of age. Because symptoms are vague, nearly 90 percent of prostatic cancer remains undetected until it has spread beyond the most easily treated stage.

Symptoms of early cancer of the prostate are blood in the urine, or reddish or pink urine; difficulty in starting urination; increasing frequency of arising at night to pass urine; and a burning sensation during urination. These are also BPH symptoms. That is why digital rectal exams are absolutely necessary. Cancer of the prostate changes the way the prostate feels when it is examined rectally. The usual rubbery firm consistency hardens to a wood-like firmness. All men over forty-five years of age should have a thorough prostate examination every three years. Cancer of the prostate may require surgery.

Because impotency and incontinence are just two of the troubling side effects of prostate surgery, it is imperative that men take a proactive approach to the health of this all important gland.

Zinc

All the research points to the fact that one of the most common zinc deficiency diseases is prostate enlargement. Chronic prostatitis, where inflammation of the gland is often combined with infection, has been found to respond to treatment with zinc. (The prostate gland normally contains about ten times more zinc than any other organ in the body.)

A zinc deficiency may "adversely affect cell division and restrict testicular growth," says Ananda Prasad, M.D., of Wayne State University School of Medicine. But, he adds, zinc "supplementation resulted in reversal of testicular failure in such cases."

So why would we tell you that you need a dietary supplement to obtain this nutrient? "Most of the zinc in food is lost in processing, or never exists in substantial amount due to nutrient-poor soil," says Dr. Mindell.

Indeed, Dr. Mindell's assertion is backed by no less than Dr. Denham Harman, M.D., Ph.D., professor emeritus at the University of Nebraska School of Medicine and founder of the free radical theory of aging. "A significant percentage of the male population

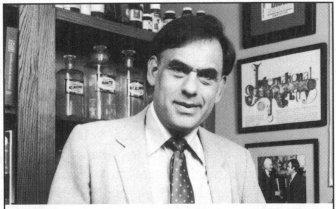

Earl Mindell, author of the best seller *Vitamin Bible*, says that men risk the complications of prostate surgery when they neglect their prostate's health. To protect this vital gland, Dr. Mindell advises that all men use a daily supplement containing many of the ingredients discussed in this chapter. He says that the amino acid combination of alanine, glycine and glutamic acid, combined with zinc, is especially helpful.

consumes diets deficient in zinc," Dr. Harman says.

"Men with prostate problems—and even men without them—would be well advised to keep their zinc levels up," says Dr. Mindell. "In many cases, symptoms have completely disappeared. I have even seen success in cases of impotence with a supplement program of B6 and zinc. And as an added bonus, elderly people, concerned about senility, might find a zinc supplement beneficial."

Paramount to an effective BPH prevention and treatment plan is adequate zinc intake and absorption. Zinc has been shown to reduce the size of the prostate—as determined by rectal examination, X-ray and endoscopy—and to reduce symptoms in the majority of patients (Fahim 1976). The clinical efficacy of zinc is probably due to its critical involvement in many aspects of hormonal metabolism.

Zinc has been shown to inhibit the activity of 5-alpha-reductase, the enzyme that irreversibly converts testosterone to dihydrotestosterone (Leake 1984a, Wallae 1975, Lahtonen 1985, Sinquin 1984). Zinc also inhibits the binding of both male hormones to cellular receptor molecules, thereby allowing for increased excretion of these hormones (Leake 1984b).

The net result of all of zinc's actions is very apparent in BPH—a reduction in the dihydrotestosterone content of the prostate, which in turn causes a reduction in both the size of the prostate, and the symptoms of BPH.

The efficacy of oral zinc supplementation is dependent on absorption of the ingested zinc. Probably most important from a therapeutic standpoint is the choice of zinc chelate (or salt) used. Zinc picolinate and perhaps zinc citrate are the best. Our recommendation that you use zinc picolinate is based on our knowledge of zinc absorption in humans. Following ingestion of zinc, the pancreas secretes picolinic acid into the intestine; the picolinic acid forms a complex with zinc that enhances the absorption of zinc from the intestine. In humans and animals, the quantity of zinc transported across the absorptive cells of the intestine is directly related to the availability of picolinic acid (Evans 1980). Inborn errors in metabolism that affect the conversion of tryptophan to picolinic acid or a vitamin B-6 deficiency will result in impaired zinc absorption (Evans 1981). A decrease in the output of secretions by the pancreas would result in impaired zinc absorption. This is probably a major factor responsible for the decreased zinc levels in the elderly. Pancreatic insufficiency is a common condition with increasing age. This means that, even though an individual may be consuming high levels of zinc, a deficiency may result due to decreased absorption. Supplementation with zinc picolinate appears to be particularly indicated in individuals with even mild pancreatic insufficiency (Boosalis 1983). Picolinic acid is synthesized in our bodies from the amino acid tryptophan. Vitamin B-6 is needed for this reaction to occur. But if vitamin B-6 is lacking, zinc absorption can be limited. Providing zinc as zinc picolinate bypasses the need for picolinic secretion by the pancreas (Evans 1980, 1981; Krieger 1984).

Several other factors in BPH suggest the use of zinc picolinate. Intestinal uptake of zinc is impaired by estrogens. Since estrogen levels are increased in men with BPH, zinc uptake may be low despite adequate dietary intake. Providing zinc as zinc picolinate may compensate for estrogen depression of zinc uptake.

Alcohol is another dietary anti-nutrient that reduces zinc uptake and increases zinc excretion, leading to relative zinc deficiency. In addition, alcohol reduces active vitamin B-6 levels which may further reduce zinc stores. Indeed all the research points to the fact that one of the most common zinc deficiency diseases is prostate enlargement. Chronic prostatitis, where inflammation of the gland is often combined with infection, has been found to respond to treatment with zinc.

Vitamin B-6

Zinc's helpful effects on prostate health are enhanced by vitamin B6 which can also help reduce harmful levels of prolactin (Judd 1984). As zinc and vitamin B-6 are intricately involved in hormone metabolism, deficiency of one or both of these nutrients may be a contributing factor in the cause of prostate disorders. In addition, vitamin B-6 supplementation may also enhance zinc absorption (Evans 1981).

Essential Fatty Acids

Linseed (flax) oil is the most beneficial oil to add to the diet to ensure the essential fatty acid requirement is being met. One to two teaspoons (four to eight grams) per day is usually a sufficient amount. The administration of an essential fatty acid (EFA) complex containing linoleic, linolenic and arachidonic acids has resulted in significant improvement for many BPH patients. All 19 subjects in an uncontrolled study showed diminution of residual urine, with 12 of the 19 having no residual urine by the end of several weeks of treatment. These effects appear to be due to the correction of an underlying essential fatty acid deficiency, since these patients' prostatic and seminal lipid levels and ratios are often abnormal (Scott 1945, Boyd 1939). Based on this evidence alone, supplementation with an essential fatty acid complex appears important.

Amino Acids

By accident, two doctors discovered three amino acids which are very important to the health of the prostate. According to Donsbach (1989): The physicians were treating a group of allergic patients with a mixture of three amino acids—glycine, alanine and glutamic acid. One of the patients volunteered the information that his urinary symptoms had disappeared while he took the amino acid mixture. This led to a trial of the same compounds on non-allergic patients with urinary symptoms. Patients with enlarged prostates and associated urinary symptoms experienced prompt and rather spectacular relief. They remained free of the symptoms while taking the compounds, but often after discontinuing the medication, the symptoms returned. The combination of glycine, alanine and glutamic acid has been shown in several studies to relieve many of the symptoms of BPH (Feinblatt 1958).

Serenoa Repens

One of the best botanical helpers for curing prostate disorders is *Serenoa repens* (also known as *Serenoa serrulata*), which has been demonstrated to act directly on the enlarged prostate to reduce inflammation, pain and throb (Mowrey 1986). Also important: *Serenoa repens* inhibits the production of dihydrotestosterone (Pizzorno 1989).

The most astute physicians, in fact, like the use of *Serenoa repens* not only for maintenance but for preventing potentially sexually damaging, unneeded surgery. "I've had real success with *Serenoa repens* in relieving an enlarged prostate in some patients who were candidates for surgery," says Dr. Andrew

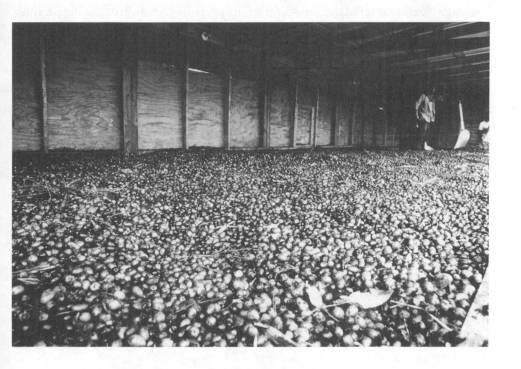

Serenoa repens

Weil, a physician who practices in Tucson, Arizona.

Another great side benefit of *Serenoa Repens* is that it has been used for years to increase sperm production and sexual vigor.

Originally, the American Indians consumed *Serenoa repens* as part of their diet. Later, naturopathic physicians also used *Serenoa repens* as a tonic to naturally support the body in the treatment of genito-urinary tract disturbances—in men to increase testicle function and in women with mammary gland disorders. Many herbalists have regarded *Serenoa repens* as a mild aphrodisiac. These historical uses prompted European researchers to investigate the clinical use of *Serenoa repens* extracts in BPH. They discovered the fat and sterol portion of the berry offers the greatest therapeutic benefit in treating BPH. A standardized extract of the fat-soluble (liposterolic) fraction of the berries has shown remarkably consistent pharmacological effects (Pizzorno 1989). This effect appears to be due to its inhibition of dihydrotestosterone, the compound which causes the prostate cells to multiply excessively. This antagonism of dihydrotestosterone by *Serenoa repens* extract has been demonstrated in experimental studies and further supports the therapeutic effect seen in clinical trials as well as the long folk use for this condition (Carilla 1984, Champault 1984).

Panax Ginseng

In experimental animal studies, *Panax Ginseng* increases testosterone levels while decreasing prostate weight (Fahim 1982). This suggests that ginseng should have favorable effects in BPH, since increased tes-

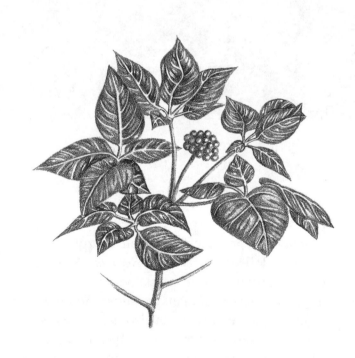

Panax Ginseng

tosterone would improve intestinal zinc absorption, and decreased prostatic size would help alleviate the symptoms of BPH.

"Long revered in the East for its recuperative and revitalizing powers, *Panax ginseng* is one of a handful of herbal remedies studied by modern science," reports Kirk Johnson, editor of the *Journal of Health Care for the Poor and Underserved* at Mcharry Medical College, Nashville, Tennessee in a recent issue of *East West Natural Health* magazine. "One study conducted at the Department of Biochemistry at The Chinese University of Hong Kong concluded that ginseng preparations have been found to increase performance capability in university-age athletes; to improve vitality, mood, and ability to concentrate in middle-age subjects; and to increase alertness and motor control in elderly subjects." Johnson adds that when ginseng extracts were given to mice, researchers "found that the animals were protected from the deterioration in sexual behavior that often accompanies stress."

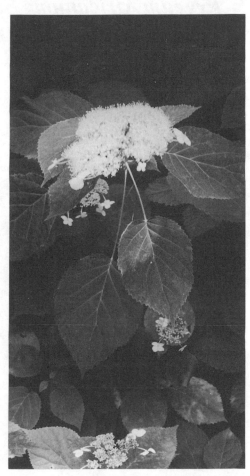

Equisetum Arvense

Equisetum arvense is commonly known as horsetail and it can help you maintain your stallion status! It is noted for its help in reducing inflammation or benign enlargement of the prostate (Hoffmann 1991). *Equisetum arvense* is often used in tandem with *Hydrangea arborescens*, commonly known as hydrangea, which is also highly effective in the treatment of inflamed or enlarged prostate glands (Hoffmann 1991).

Hydrangea arborescens

Bee Pollen

Bee pollen from flowers has been used to treat prostatitis and BPH in Europe since at least the early 1960s (Ask-Upmark 1967). It has been shown to be effective in several double-blind clinical studies. Its effect may be related to its high content of plant flavonoids. In any event, there is good evidence of its powers in this area of male health. It also supplies necessary nutrients for sexual reproduction.

Pygeum Africanum: *Superior Therapy for Prostate Healing and Disease Prevention*

A large African evergreen only recently available in the U.S., *Pygeum africanum* has been studied for more than 20 years. In double-blind, controlled trialsi, *Pygeum* has been demonstrated to be highly effective in reducing prostate enlargement and inflammation. The key symptoms of BPH are also effectively relieved. Unlike prescription drugs for the prostate, which cause birth defects and possibly cancer, *Pygeum* is completely devoid of side effects—except that it is known for stimulaing sexual libido.

In both France and Italty, extract of *Pygeum* is recognized for prostate therapy and available by prescription.

Its primary active ingredients include:

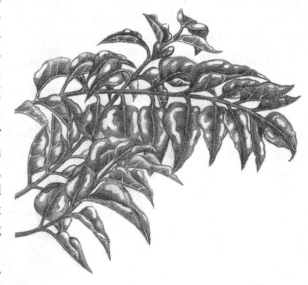

Pygeum Africanum

•Plant sterols which are anti-inflammatory
•Triterpenoids which are also anti-inflammatory
•Linear long chain alcohols which may act by reducing levels of cholesterol in the prostate.

For younger men who are more likely to suffer prostate infections rather than BPH, *Pygeum* is an excellent natural antibiotic.

Interestingly, throughout the world, *Pygeum* is available only by prescription at an exceedingly high cost. However, an American company has recently made a more potent form of extract of *Pygeum Africanum* available to American men at a fraction of the international cost.

Dietary Tips

Pay attention to these lifestyle factors:

•*Cholesterol.* If men would only radically cut down the fat in their diet, the numbers afflicted with prostate maladies would be greatly reduced, according to Dr. Carl P. Schaffner, Ph.D., professor of microbial chemistry at Rutgers University.

Male canines also suffer a disproportionately high number of prostate-related disorders. Dr. Schaffner discovered that by reducing cholesterol levels in aged dogs, he was also able to reduce the size of the animals' enlarged prostates.

Another study, reported to the American Urological Association, corroborates the possibly harmful effects related to high cholesterol levels on prostate disease. Dr. Cammille Mallouh, M.D., Chief of Urology at Metropolitan Hospital in New York, examined 100 prostates from men of all ages and found an 80 percent increase in cholesterol content of prostates with BPH.

Additionally, cholesterol metabolites are damaging to cells and they are carcinogenic. Cholesterol has been shown to accumulate in enlarged or cancerous human prostate.

Cancer of the prostate, which accounts for a frightening proportion of deaths due to cancer, may also be associated with the Western diet. Observing that rural, black South Africans—who eat a low-fat, whole-food diet—are a low-risk group for prostate cancer, Dr. Peter Hill, Ph.D., of the American Health Foundation in New York City, conducted a study to test whether diet was responsible for their relative immunity. Dr. Hill and his associates placed a group of black South African volunteers on a typical Western diet with lots of fats and meats. At the same time, a group of North American volunteers, black and whites, were put on a low-fat diet. Dr. Hill and his colleagues tested for diet-induced hormonal changes that are associated with the development of prostatic cancer.

After three weeks, Dr. Hill found that the South Africans eating the Western diet were excreting notably more hormones, while the reverse occurred with the North Americans eating the low-fat diet. The metabolic profile of the North American now resembled that of the low-risk group (*Cancer Research* 1979). Dr. Hill states, "This study is a preliminary indication that a low-fat diet is one of the factors which can lower the risk of prostatic cancer. By reducing total calorie intake, and substituting fruit and vegetable calories for animal calories, a high-risk prostatic cancer group has switched to a low-risk one."

•*Drugs and Pesticides.* The diet should be as free as possible from pesticides and other contaminants, since many of these compounds such as dioxin, polyhalogenated biphenyls, hexachlorobenzene and dibenzofurans can increase the formation of dihydrotestosterone in the prostate (Ask-Upmark 1967).

It is quite possible that the tremendous increase in the occurrence of BPH in the last few decades reflects the ever-increasing effect that toxic chemicals have on our health. BPH is just one of many health problems that may be due to these toxic substances. A diet rich in natural whole foods may offer some protection due to the presence of many protective substances. In particular, minerals (such as calcium, magnesium, zinc, selenium, germanium), vitamins, plant pigments (flavonoids, carotenes, chlorophyll), fiber (especially gel-forming and muci-laginous types) and sulfur-containing compounds all possess actions which help the body deal with toxic chemicals and heavy metals.

Top Seven Tips for Prostate Health

The following guidelines are of critical importance to protect your prostate from serious maladies:

1. Adequate zinc intake and absorption are required for normal prostatic function and hormonal metabolism.

2. Adequate vitamin B-6 intake is essential.

3. Elimination or reduction in the amount of beer and other alcohol consumed is advisable.

4. Maintain serum cholesterol below 220 mg/dl.

5. Consume an adequate intake of at least one to two teaspoons daily of essential fatty acids such as linseed/flax oil.

6. Limit dietary and environmental exposure to pesticides and other environmental contaminants.

7. Increase your fluid intake. Drink two to three quarts of pure water daily to stimulate urine flow. This helps prevent retention, cystitis and kidney infection. Purity is essential. Water should be filtered or from a nonpolluted source; even the chlorination process used to disinfect municipal water supplies produces cancer-chemicals known as trihalomethanes which cause bladder cancer.

It is important for all men to pay attention to the health of their prostate gland beginning at an early age and throughout their lives, so that they may enjoy all of the benefits of lifelong sexual potency and vigor, while avoiding all of the pain involved in traditional surgical treatments. Regular digital exams are critical—especially after age 45. Also, eating a low-fat diet will be very beneficial for your body. But for extra insurance, a dietary supplement designed for prostate health can become an important part of the health maintenance program for this sexually important part of the male body.

Nutrients For Prostate Health

The following nutrients should be emphasized in a prostate-health program:

Amino Acids
Alanine: 200 mg per day
Glutamic Acid: 200 mg per day
Glycine: 200 mg per day

Vitamins
Beta Carotene: 25,000 IU daily
Vitamin B6 (pyridoxine): 100 mg per day
Vitamin E: 400 IU daily

Oils
EPA/DHA; Flaxseed; and Borage

Minerals
Zinc Picolinate: 50 mg per day

Herbs/Plants
Bee Pollen Extract: Two tablespoons of bee pollen equivalent daily.
Equisetum arvense: 250 mg daily
Hydrangea arborescens: 250 mg daily
Panax ginseng: Equivalent to 25-50 mg ginsenosides daily
Pygeum Africanum Extract: 400 mg daily
Serenoa repens: 850 mg daily

17. Preventing Osteoporosis

An older woman falls due to a bone fracture. Her hip simply gave way, but her family and her doctor assume that she lost her balance. She knows that she doesn't "lose her balance" so easily, but because of her age, her own version of the accident is not given much credibility. This scenario is far more widespread than imagined. But it doesn't have to happen, and that's what's so important about what you're about to read—especially for mature men and women.

These are the facts that men and especially women need to know about the crippling bone disease, osteoporosis:

•Osteoporosis causes 1.2 million fractures per year, primarily among women.

•One out of three women will demineralize their bones enough to cause fracture during their lifetime.

•From one to two million fractures occur in postmenopausal women in our nation every year.

•In 1980, a study conducted in Knox County, Tennessee, revealed that the incidence of fractures requiring hospitalization doubled every five years after the age of 50.

•One-third of women who live to the age of 90 break a hip (Kamen 1989).

Osteoporosis, which literally means porous bones, is widespread in the United States. Osteoporosis, also known as the "brittle bone disease," has reached epidemic proportions. At the International Symposium on Osteoporosis held in Denmark in 1988, researchers announced that: "More women die from osteoporosis-related fractures than from cancer of the breast, cervix and uterus combined, and in the United States hip fracture health care costs up to $10 billion annually, causing 200,000 deaths (about one-tenth of all deaths)."

Fractures may be caused by a fall that normal bones can easily resist. But sometimes the bone actually breaks first—before the fall—and the break is the reason for the fall.

The fact that bone is more than a collection of calcium crystals is often overlooked by medical experts. Bone is active living tissue continually remodeling itself through osteoblastic (bone forming) and osteoclastic (bone resorbing) activity, and constantly participating in a wide range of biochemical reactions.

Although the entire skeleton may be involved, bone loss is usually greatest in the spine, hips and ribs. Since these bones bear a great deal of weight, they are then susceptible to pain, deformity or fracture.

Normally there is a decline in bone mass after the age of 40. This bone loss is accelerated in patients with osteoporosis. Bone mass reaches its peak around age 30 to 35, then declines steadily through life in both men and women. Menopausal acceleration of bone loss begins even before the last menstrual period, and this accelerated loss continues for approximately 10 years. The danger of osteoporosis, or bone demineralization, after menopause is well known. *What is not known is that a significant amount of bone mass may be lost swiftly in the first two years after menstruation ends; in fact, some research indicates that this initial bone loss may be as much as 10 percent per year with a two to four percent average annual loss of bone mass each successive year for the first eight to ten years after menopause. Serious problems occur when 30 to 40 percent of bone mass has been lost.*

However, this bone demineralization often remains undetected until a woman suffers a fracture 20 or 30 years later. Current management of bone loss in women consists primarily of estrogen therapy and calcium supplements. This approach is helpful, but its success is limited to about 25 percent of the cases.

What is Osteoporosis?

Osteoporosis involves both the mineral (inorganic) and non-mineral (organic matrix) components of bone. This is the first clue that there is more to osteoporosis than a lack of dietary calcium. In fact, lack of dietary calcium in the adult results in a separate condition known as osteomalacia or softening of the bone. The two conditions, osteomalacia and osteoporosis, are different. Osteomalacia is only a deficiency of calcium in the bone. In contrast, osteoporosis is a lack of both calcium and other minerals, as well as a decrease in the non-mineral, organic matrix, framework of bone (primarily composed of collagen and other proteins). The evidence points to the importance of taking all possible precautions to avoid osteoporosis, the earlier the better, preferably before the actual onset of menopause.

Causes of Osteoporosis

Pizzorno (1985) reports that many dietary factors cause osteoporosis: low calcium, high phosphorous intake, high protein diets; high acid-ash diets and trace mineral deficiencies. Tooth loss may be due to loss of bone around the roots of the teeth and Wical (1974) asserts that patients without teeth have been consumers of low-calcium, high phosphorous diets. Indeed, 44 percent of patients with osteoporosis require complete dentures before the age of 60, as compared with only 15 percent of non-osteoporotic patients, and one of the initial symptoms of a calcium/phosphorous imbalance is periodontal (gum) disease.

Other researchers assert that bone problems are not caused so much by a lack of calcium as by overconsumption of protein. Research has shown that the rate of urinary calcium excretion is significantly increased after the consumption of a high protein meal. Vegetarians have more bone density than age-matched meat eaters (Holl 1988).

Ellis (1972) asserts that vegetarian diets are associated with a lower risk of osteoporosis. Marsh (1983) says that although bone mass in vegetarians does not differ significantly from omnivores in the third, fourth and fifth decades, there are significant differences in the later decades. This appears to indicate that the decreased incidence of osteoporosis in vegetarians is not due to increased initial bone mass but rather decreased bone loss in the later years of life.

Pizzorno (1985) asserts that decreased bone loss observed in vegetarians is probably due to a lowered intake of protein and phosphorous. Raising daily protein intake from 47 to 142 grams doubles the excretion of calcium in the urine. A diet this high in protein is common in the West and may be a significant factor in the increased number of people suffering from osteoporosis.

Many people believe that consumption of dairy products will help prevent osteoporosis. But the data does not support this assertion. The fact is that Americans drink more milk than the people of any other nation; yet they also have the highest incidence of bone problems.

Because it is so rich in protein, milk can cause greater calcium loss than gain (Recker 1985). Lewis (1989) reports that in a recent study from the Department of Nutritional Sciences at the University of Wisconsin the ingestion of milk—or ordinary calcium supplements—had no overall effect on calcium retention. Subjects were fed typical American diets and were given recommended levels of calcium supplementation in divided doses with meals. They adjusted rapidly to the calcium supplements and the milk by decreasing the efficiency of calcium absorption in the intestines, and the necessary reabsorption of calcium in the kidneys.

Sugar intake increases the urinary excretion of calcium and reduces the amount of phosphorous so that these minerals may be too low for bone formation (Thom 1978).

Preventing Osteoporosis

Osteoporosis is preventable through optimal nutrition. But one must do more than supplement their diet with calcium. Osteoporosis is a complex condition involving hormonal, lifestyle, nutritional and environmental factors. A wide range of nutrients is needed to maintain a healthy skeleton. The vitamins B-6, C, D, K and folic acid are essential; and the minerals calcium, phosphorous, magnesium, manganese, boron, zinc, copper, strontium and silicon are all needed. There is substantial scientific evidence that supplementation with a balanced combination of the proper nutrients can be effective in maintaining good skeletal health.

Estrogen: Risks Vs. Benefits

In 1984 the National Institutes of Health Consensus Development Conference on Osteoporosis concluded that the risk for endometrial cancer increased with the use of estrogen therapy. But the group stipulated that, "Estrogen-associated endometrial cancer is usually manifested at an early stage and is rarely fatal when managed appropriately." In other words women were told that it was perfectly all right to turn themselves over to their physicians for estrogen treatment and that if they were stricken with cancer as a result that their physicians knew how to keep them from dying (National Institutes of Health Consensus Conference 1984).

Synthetic estrogen was first isolated in the 1920s but did not become widespread in popularity until the 1960s when it was touted in *Feminine Forever* by Robert Wilson as the antidote to aging in women. By 1975, more than half of the 30 million post-menopausal women in the U.S. were being prescribed estrogen. Then in the mid-1970s reports began to show that these women were five times more likely to develop uterine cancer and the fad rapidly waned. Recently with studies showing that adding progesterone for at least 10 days each month to the estrogen replacement therapy exerts a protective effect against uterine cancer, estrogen replacement therapy (ERT) has again become the treatment of choice for many women. ERT offers the allure of remaining youthful well beyond the reproductive years. ERT seems to be preventive against osteoporosis and helps control hot flashes, although the hot flashes return, at least mildly, when the ERT is

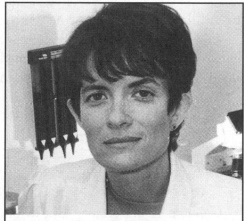

Megan Shields, M.D., is a strong believer in the use of nutritional supplements to help her patients prevent osteoporosis—especially the use of boron and calcium citrate in combination with other nutrients discussed in this chapter.

discontinued. ERT also appears to be protective against heart disease. But this advantage is offset when it is combined with progesterone. Estrogen also helps alleviate vaginal dryness, particularly when used as a cream. For many women, ERT seems to be the answer to their dreams. Estrogen and progesterone replacement are not without their drawbacks, however. The most common complications are uterine and breast cancer and liver and gallbladder disease. Estrogen, in any form, must be broken down by the liver, and thus a nutritional supplement that exerts a protective and stimulatory effect on the liver is desirable for women who use prescription hormone therapy.

Research has shown that although estrogen retards bone loss, it does not completely prevent it. Fractures do occur, although less frequently, in estrogen treated women. The benefits of estrogen must be weighed against its risks, particularly the increased risk of endometrial cancer. Although many physicians recommend estrogen replacement for post-menopausal women, at present it seems that the risks may outweigh the benefits in the majority of women who are at risk for osteoporosis. We recommend that a strong emphasis be placed on nutritional and lifestyle factors. It is important to realize, however, that, while estrogen and calcium are of value in some cases, a superior job can be done when all nutrients proven to be significant to bone metabolism are utilized.

Like any living tissue, bone has diverse nutritional needs and serious consequences occur when these needs are not met. Following are the minerals, vitamins, and botanicals recommended for optimal skeletal health and maintenance.

Although we will start with a discussion of calcium simply using a calcium supplement is not enough.

Calcium

Calcium is important. But to understand why using just any calcium supplement is not enough, one must know how calcium is absorbed by the body.

The absorption of calcium and other minerals is dependent on the level of stomach acid, particularly in the elderly. People with low stomach acid usually absorb calcium and other minerals poorly.

In studies with post-menopausal women, about 40 percent are severely deficient in stomach acid (Grossman 1963). Patients with insufficient stomach acid output can absorb only about 4 percent of an oral dose of calcium carbonate while a person with normal stomach acid can typically absorb about 22 percent (Recker 1985). Patients with low stomach acid need a form of calcium already in a soluble and ionized state like calcium citrate. About 45 percent of the calcium will be absorbed from calcium citrate in patients with reduced stomach acid (Recker 1985). Calcium citrate is more bioavailable in subjects with normal stomach acid as well (Nicar 1985). Thus calcium citrate is the form of calcium required for optimal nutritional performance from a supplement.

The RDA for calcium is 1,000 mg daily. Studies show that the average calcium intake for women is only 650 mg daily, and that one-third of women receive 500 mg or less daily. The National Institutes of Health has recommended a minimum intake of 1,000 mg for most people, and 1,500 mg for women who are pregnant, lactating or post-menstrual; and for men over age 65. Calcium 2-aminoethanol phosphate and calcium citrate appear to be the very best forms of calcium for better absorption and decreased risk of developing kidney stones (Recker 1985, Nicar 1985, Lancet 1986).

Calcium citrate fulfills every requirement for an optimum calcium supplement because it is easily ionized, it is almost completely degraded, it has virtually no toxicity, and it has been shown to result in increased absorption of calcium. In addition, citrate has some properties that suggest further benefits (*i.e.*, its ability to chelate out heavy metals, prevent recurrent kidney stones, augment treatment of urinary tract infection, and promote urination). There is no question that calcium deficiency can cause osteoporosis, yet skeletal calcium depletion is present in only about 25 percent of osteoporotic women. Calcium supplements were found to increase bone mass in these women, but had no effect in the other 75 percent who were not calcium deficient.

Magnesium

Various studies make it clear that magnesium deficiency is widespread in the U.S. Diet surveys have shown that 80 to 85 percent of American women consume less than the RDA for this mineral. Daily magnesium intake in two other studies was only 1/3 of the RDA. Magnesium participates in many biochemical reactions that take place in the bone, and is apparently as important as calcium supplementation. Whole body content and bone concentrations of magnesium were below normal in 16 of 19 osteoporotic women. Alkaline phosphatase, an enzyme involved in forming new calcium crystals, is activated by magnesium. All 16 women with low magnesium levels also had abnormal crystal formation in their bones, increasing their risk of fracture (Cohen 1981). It is important that magnesium be in at least a one-to-two ratio with calcium respectively. That is, that for every 500 mg of magnesium, one should ingest 1,000 mg of calcium.

Manganese

Manganese is required for bone mineralization and for the synthesis of connective tissue in cartilage and bone. The optimal intake of manganese is not known but at least half of the manganese in a typical diet is lost when whole grains are replaced by refined flour. Rats fed a manganese deficient diet had smaller, less dense bone with less resistance to fractures than those fed adequate amounts of manganese. Many humans may also be sensitive to a marginal or severe deficiency of manganese.

Boron

The evidence for boron's key role in bone formation is astoundingly strong. A paper expounding the value of this trace element was published as early as 1910. The article describes boron as being essential for the growth of higher plants, even though it appears in such exceptionally minute quantities. Indeed, boron was initially thought to be essential only for plants but now appears to play a key role in human nutrition, particularly in bone health.

In the early 1980s studies showed that boron might affect calcium, phosphorous or magnesium metabolism. Boron appears to work like an adaptogen in that if the diet is optimal it has little benefit but in deficient diets it proves to be very advantageous. In a 1986 study to examine the effects of boron along with a few other minerals on major mineral metabolism in post-menopausal women, subjects were fed a standard diet for 119 days supplying about 0.25 milligrams of boron per day. Supplementation of this diet with 3 mg boron per day reduced urinary calcium excretion by 44 percent and markedly increased serum concentration of the active estrogenic hormone estradiol. *Amazingly, the levels of estradiol in boron-supplemented women were the same as in women receiving estrogen therapy.* An increase in hormone concentration may be very important since estradiol is the most biologically active form of estrogen.

Boron's action in the body is not yet known but seems required in order for vitamin D to be converted to its most active form within the kidney. Boron deficiency accentuates vitamin D deficiency in chicks resulting in abnormal bone formation and elevation of alkaline phosphatase (Nielsen 1988). Nielsen's animal studies estimated the human boron requirement to be approximately one to two milligrams per day. Fruits, vegetables, and nuts are the main dietary sources of boron, but at this time it would appear that most diets do not deliver optimal amounts of boron, possibly due to soil depletion through the use of chemical fertilization methods and a resulting short fall in the food itself.

Toxicity studies in animals have shown a very comfortable margin of safety for supplemental doses of boron of one to three milligrams per day. Moreover, there were no adverse effects seen in dogs and rats fed intravenously with 350 parts per million of boron which corresponds to approximately 117 milligrams per day in humans. There are areas of the world where the diet contains as much as 41 milligrams of boron per day and no complications have been reported.

It is important to realize that while boron may raise blood levels of estradiol, this does not suggest it poses the same risk as supplemental estrogen therapy itself. The carcinogenic effect of estrogen is dose related. Most orally administered estrogen is converted to estrone rather than the more desirable estradiol; therefore large amounts of estrogen must be given to achieve clinically useful serum levels of estradiol. Therefore, boron appears capable of producing an estrogenic effect without exposing the body to dangerously high amounts of estrogen.

Zinc

Zinc is also important in the prevention of osteoporosis. Zinc participates in normal bone function by enhancing the biochemical actions of vitamin D. Zinc levels were low in serum and bone of elderly patients with osteoporosis as well as in individuals with accelerated forms of bone loss. Dr. Harman believes that Americans suffer widespread and significant zinc deficiency in their diets. In fact, widespread dietary zinc deficiency has been reported in several studies. In some surveys, 68 percent of the adults consumed less than two-thirds of the RDA for zinc. The picolinic acid salts of zinc, manganese and chromium seem to have a greater degree of bioavailability than other forms of these minerals Picolinic acid is a naturally occurring metabolite of tryptophan which is believed to enhance zinc absorption and transport in humans.

Copper

Rats fed a diet deficient in copper had reduced bone mineral content and reduced bone strength. Copper supplementation inhibited bone resorption. The mechanism of action of copper is not known; however this mineral is a co-factor for the enzyme lysyl oxidase which strengthens connective tissue by cross-linking collagen strands. Collagen is the connective tissue that binds everything together and gives bones flexibility. Since the typical American diet contains only about 50 percent of the RDA for copper, deficiency of this mineral may be very widespread.

Strontium

Don't be afraid of strontium!
Your body can benefit from strontium.

Strontium occurs in high concentration in bones and teeth where it is thought to replace a small fraction of the calcium crystals (the form of calcium found in bone tissue). Awareness of the nutritional significance of strontium in the past has been overshadowed by fear of radioactive strontium, a component of nuclear fallout. Because strontium tends to accumulate in bone tissue, radioactive strontium might be particularly hazardous to humans. On the other hand, non-radioactive strontium occurs naturally in food. This mineral is apparently quite safe even with long-term administration in doses hundreds of times greater than the usual dietary intake. Beneficial effects of strontium on calcified tissues is suggested by several studies. The incidence of cavities was significantly reduced in geographic regions with high levels of strontium in drinking water. Furthermore, in mice, the addition of strontium to their drinking water reduced bone resorbing activity by more than 11 percent.

The effect of strontium on osteoporosis has been studied in 32 patients given pharmacologic doses of strontium for periods ranging from three months to three years. Ten patients received estrogen and testosterone as well. Twenty-seven (84 percent) of the patients experienced marked reduction in bone pain. Radiologic examination showed improvement in bone density in 78 percent of the strontium-treated patients (McCaslin 1959).

Equisetum Arvense

Equisetum arvense, commonly known as horsetail, is a botanical source of valuable silica. Silicon's participation as an essential trace element for connective tissue in bone and cartilage has been noted in recent years. Silicon is found in high concentration at calcification sites in growing bone. This mineral appears to strengthen the connective tissue matrix by cross linking collagen strands. Chicks fed a silicon-deficient diet developed gross skull abnormalities and had unusually thin leg

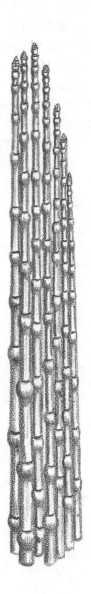

Horsetail

bones with evidence of impaired calcification. Silicon also may counteract the deleterious effects of aluminum, in both osteoporosis and Alzheimer's disease (Birchall 1986, Carlisle 1986).

It is not known whether the typical American diet provides adequate silicon. As with other nutrients, sub-clinical deficiency could result from over-consumption of refined foods. In patients with osteoporosis, where accelerated bone regeneration is desirable, silicon requirement may be increased and supplementation may be needed. This is a nutrient that is virtually nontoxic and therefore supplementation could function as an insurance policy until there are better means of assessing patients' needs.

Vitamin B-6

Vitamin B-6 deficient diets have produced osteoporosis in rats. Diet surveys indicate B-6 intake by American women is frequently less than the RDA. Biochemical evidence of B-6 deficiency was found in more than half of a group of presumably healthy volunteers. Birth control pills can induce B-6 deficiency, so whenever birth control pills are taken, at least 50 mg of B-6 daily should be added to protect the body from serious side effects associated with long-term B-6 deficiency.

Low levels of vitamins B-6, B-12 and folic acid are quite common in the elderly population and may contribute to osteoporosis (Barker 1979, Infante-Rivard 1986). The effect of B-6 upon bone health involves several different mechanisms. This vitamin is the co-factor in the enzymatic cross-linking of collagen strands which increases the strength of connective tissue. Vitamin B-6 also helps break down homocysteine, a metabolite of the amino acid methionine, which has been implicated in a variety of conditions including heart disease and osteoporosis. Increased homocysteine concentrations in the blood have been demonstrated in post-menstrual women and are thought to play a role in osteoporosis by interfering with collagen cross-linking leading to a defective bone matrix (Brattstrom 1985).

Folic Acid

Clinical folic acid deficiency is relatively common, occurring in up to 22 percent of individuals 65 years of age and older. Typically, American diets often contain only half the RDA for folic acid. Tobacco smoking, alcohol consumption, and oral contraceptives tend to promote folic acid deficiency.

Folic acid and the vitamins B-6 and B-12 are important in the conversion of the essential amino acid methionine to cysteine. If there is a deficiency in these vitamins, or if a defect exists in the enzymes responsible for this conversion, there will be an increase in the production of homocysteine, a potentially toxic compound (Brattstrom 1985).

Folic acid supplementation has been shown to reduce homocysteine levels, but vitamin B-6 and B-12 are necessary for this to occur. The danger of homocysteine was discovered by studying individuals with a genetic disorder in which abnormally large amounts of homocysteine accumulate. These individuals develop severe osteoporosis at an early age possibly due to the adverse effect of homocysteine on bone. Before menopause, women are especially efficient at converting homocysteine to less toxic compounds which may account, in part, for their resistance to bone loss. At the time of menopause, however, a breakdown in homocysteine metabolism occurs which can be partially corrected by folic acid supplementation. Serum homocysteine levels were measured in female volunteers after administration of methionine. The levels of homocysteine were substantially greater in post menstrual than in premenopausal women, with no overlap between the two groups. Treatment with folic acid partially prevented the methionine-induced rise in serum homocysteine even though none of the women were deficient in folic acid by standard laboratory criteria. It appears that menopause is associated with an increased requirement for folic acid which, when inadequate, may result in an elevation of serum homocysteine.

Vitamin C

Osteoporosis can result from vitamin C defiency. Bone cannot be built without calcium, and the matrix to build bone with calcium cannot be formed without vitamin C. About 90 percent of bone matrix is made of collagen, which depends heavily on this water-soluble nutrient (water-soluble nutrients are not stored in the body; they need to be replaced daily). Although scurvy is rare in the United States, subclinical ascorbic acid deficiency appears to be common. Vitamin C levels in the white blood cells of elderly women are often half those of young adults. Available vitamin C is drastically reduced by smoking. Biochemical evidence of vitamin C deficiency was found in 20 percent of elderly women even though they were consuming more than the RDA of 60 mg per day of vitamin C. Lack of vitamin C can cause aching in the joints.

Vitamin D

Levels of vitamin D in American women decrease by about 50 percent in the course of a lifetime. This nutrient correlates directly with calcium absorption. One would expect to see little change in the blood content of vitamin D in older people in the U.S. because our foods are so heavily fortified with vitamin D. However, a study of a group of Americans demonstrated a 47 percent reduction in vitamin D levels in healthy elderly subjects as compared with younger people. The reduction was significant enough to contribute to the decline in calcium absorption with age. Low concentrations of vitamin D may lead to malabsorption of calcium and bone loss to an even greater degree in older house-bound people (Francis 1987).

Vitamin D is required for intestinal calcium absorption. Factors that lower vitamin D levels in the elderly include reduced exposure to sunlight, decreased dietary intake and malabsorption.

Fortunately, people afflicted with osteoporosis can be treated with the 1, 25 dihydroxy form of vitamin D for improved calcium absorption and calcium balance. Unfortunately, it is expensive and testing is necessary to prevent the risk of hypercalcemia which can be associated with long-term use.

The first step in vitamin D management should always be to enhance the conversion of vitamin D precursors to the biologically active form known as 1, 25 dihydroxyvitamin D3. This conversion may be facilitated by treatment with magnesium and boron.

Vitamin K

Sixteen patients with osteoporosis had average Vitamin K concentrations that were only 35 percent that of age-matched controls. This strongly suggests that vitamin K deficiency is probably more common than previously believed due to low vegetable intake or antibiotics which may destroy naturally occurring vitamin K producing bacteria in the intestine.

The major non-collagen protein in bone is osteocalcin. This protein is dependent on vitamin K in order to occur in its active form (*Nutrition Reviews* 1984). Vitamin K is necessary so that the osteocalcin can chelate the calcium and hold it in place within the bone. A deficiency of vitamin K could therefore lead to impaired mineralization of the bone due to inadequate osteocalcin levels.

Rats fed a vitamin K deficient diet had significantly increased urinary calcium excretion. Interestingly, vitamin K supplementation accelerated healing of experimental fractures in rabbits even though they were already receiving supposedly adequate levels in their diet. In a preliminary study of osteoporotic patients, treatment with vitamin K reduced urinary excretion of calcium by 18 to 50 percent. The evidence suggests that when accelerated bone formation is desirable, as in osteoporosis or after a fracture, a greater amount of vitamin K is required.

Vitamin K is found in green leafy vegetables and may be one of the protective factors of a vegetarian diet. Fat soluble chlorophyll capsules are an excellent source of naturally occurring vitamin K. Vitamin K deficiency is prevalent in individuals with chronic gastrointestinal disorders or poor fat absorption (Krasinski 1985). This group is also at greater risk of developing osteoporosis.

Kelp

A trace element is defined as one occurring in amounts less than 0.01 percent of the human body. The role of trace elements in health and disease is currently an extremely important area of research. Present understanding is increasing at a rapid rate. Researchers are continuing to uncover evidence demonstrating the profound impact which the presence or absence of trace quantities of these substances have on metabolic processes. Despite their minuscule amounts, trace elements have very significant biological functions. Kelp is a good source of boron (see boron *above*).

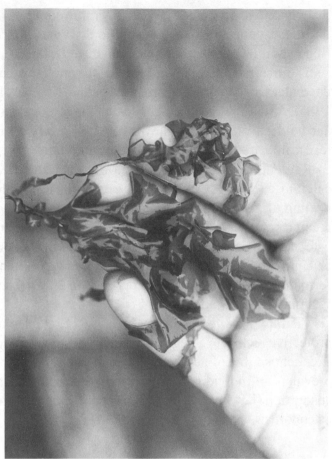

Kelp

Both kelp and alfalfa are excellent sources of all trace minerals, thus providing both known and as yet undiscovered benefits.

Proanthocyanidins and Anthocyanidins

These types of flavonoids are responsible for the deep red-blue color of many berries including hawthorn berries, blackberries, blueberries, cherries

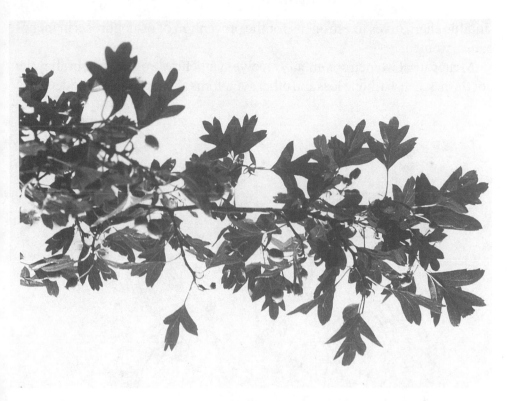

Hawthorn Berry

and raspberries. Proanthocyanidins and anthocyanidins are remarkable in their ability to stabilize collagen structures (Rao 1981). Since collagen is the major protein structure in bone, stabilization of its integrity and structure is strongly indicated. Supplementation with extracts or eating plenty of those berries rich in these flavonoids may offer significant benefit in preventing osteoporosis. Hawthorn and bilberry extract are excellent sources of proanthocyanosides and anthocyanosides.

Phytoestrogens

Plant estrogenic substances or phytoestrogens are components of many medicinal herbs with historical use in conditions that are now treated by synthetic estrogens. Many physicians have found that these botanicals are

suitable alternatives to estrogens for the prevention of osteoporosis in menopausal women.

Menopausal women commonly receive synthetic estrogens to help allay the
hot flashes, nausea, bone loss and other symptoms associated with the decrease

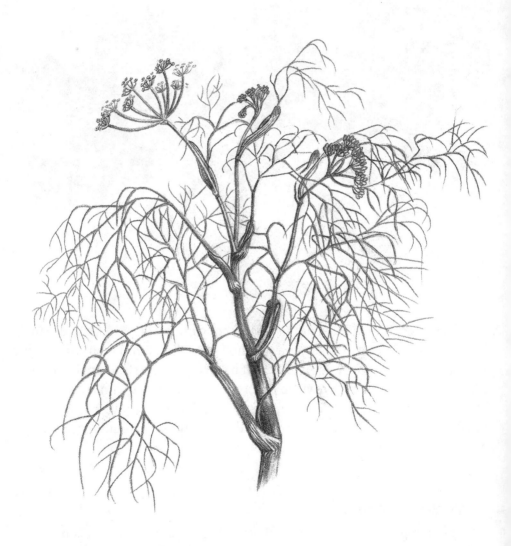

Foeniculum vulgare

in the body's own natural hormone level. While generally effective, both synthetic and natural animal estrogens may pose significant health risks, including increasing the risk of cancer, gallbladder disease, strokes and heart attacks. *Phytoestrogens have not been associated with these side effects.*

Phytoestrogens are capable of exerting estrogenic effects, although the activity compared to estrogen is only 1:400. Because of this, phytoestrogens tend to counteract extreme estrogen levels. If estrogen levels are low, since phytoestrogens have some estrogenic activity they will cause an increase in estrogen effect; if estrogen levels are high, the phytoestrogens, which bind to estrogen receptor binding sites, thereby competing with estrogen, will cause a decrease in estrogen effects.

Because of the balancing action of phytoestrogens on estrogen levels, it is common to find the same plant recommended for conditions of estrogen excess (*i.e.,* premenstrual syndrome) as well as conditions of estrogen deficiency (*i.e.,* menopause, menstrual abnormalities). Many of these herbs are referred to as uterine tonics.

Some of the prominent herbs that possess both proven estrogenic activities and long-standing historical use in treating various female complaints include

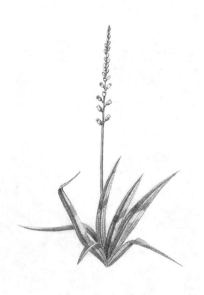

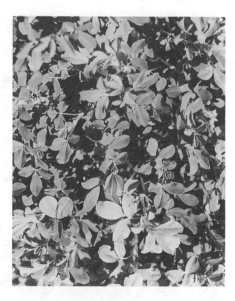

Aletris farinosa   *Medicago sativa*

(Duke 1985, Leung 1980, Albert-Uelo 1980, Costello 1950):

- *Aletris farinosa* (Unicorn root)
- *Angelica sinensis* (Dong quai)
- *Cimicifuga racemosa* (Black cohosh)
- *Foeniculum vulgare* (Fennel)
- *Glycyrrhiza glabra* (Licorice)
- *Medicago sativa* (Alfalfa)

A Final Word on Osteoporosis

Unfortunately, today's food supply has an 80 percent or more reduction in zinc, magnesium and other minerals essential to good bone health.   All adults—especially women after age 35—

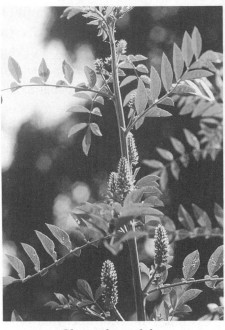

Glycyrrhiza glabra

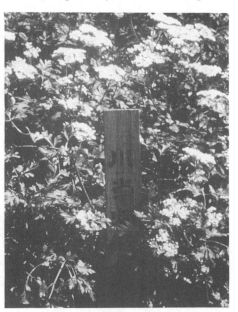

Angelica sinensis

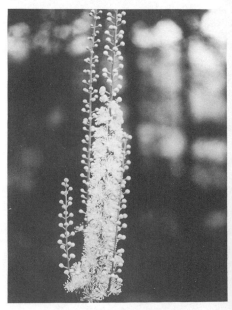

Cimicifuga racemosa

need good mineral supplementation. We have provided you with the nutritional tools to prevent osteoporosis.

The time to start is *now*. If you are a post-menopausal woman, you need to start on such a program immediately. But if you are menstruating, you still need to start supplementation. The greatest bone loss occurs immediately during the transition from menstruation to menopause. Osteoporosis is much more easily prevented than treated.

Your best health program will involve exercise and dietary supplements. This combination, whether begun prior to menopause or after its commencement, will offer you the best chance possible of maintaining a strong, active physique throughout your life.

18. *Easing Menopause*

*Many of our nation's most progressive and caring physi-
cians believe that the use of phytoestrogens is one of the
brightest, most positive breakthroughs for women who are
going through what can be a trying period of life known as
menopause.   But perhaps most important is that the
phytoestrogens found in botanicals are effective and appear
to be safer than synthetic estrogens.*

Hot flashes, night sweats, sleeplessness, irritability, mood swings, short-term memory loss, migraine headaches, vaginal dryness, urinary incontinence and weight gain—these are some of the difficult experiences that women go through during this change in their lives (Beck 1992).

Even today tranquilizers are often prescribed for women who are going through menopause. "One patient of mine came in having been prescribed multiple anti-depressants and tranquilizers by a physician who neglected to see if she was having trouble with her hormones," says Cynthia Watson, M.D., clinical faculty member of the University of Southern California. "That certainly wasn't the proper therapy!"

But the mainstream medical community has not always understood that women have special needs—that the symptoms of menopause are not "just in your head"—that they are real and that they deserve more and better medical attention than simply tranquilizing suffering women.

"It's disgraceful that in our sophisticated world of medicine, with our phenomenal track record, we still can't answer simple questions about menopause," says Dr. Bernardine Healy, director of the National Institutes of Health (Beck 1992).

Says Dr. Richard Passwater (1992), "Physicians used to ignore the subject or treat it very superficially. One lady who had been in nursing school during the 1940s reported that male physicians told her that menopause was all in the woman's head—that it didn't exist. Other women told me that they suffered as silently as possible because of the lack of understanding of their husband and the disinterest of their doctors."

Then after the publication of *Feminine Forever* by Robert Wilson, estrogen replacement therapy spread through the medical community like wild fire. By 1975 more than half of the 30 million post-menstrual women in the United States were being prescribed estrogen. However, in the mid-1970s, when reports began to show that these women were five times more likely to develop uterine cancer, the fad waned.

Today, about 15 percent of women going through menopause are given estrogen replacement therapy which can help relieve hot flashes, vaginal dryness and even smooth out mental discomforts such as swings in emotions and moods. Estrogen replacement therapy may even help combat the risk of heart attacks and bone loss which can also accompany menopause. Estrogen is sometimes administered as a cream to combat vaginal dryness, but "the drawback to this method is that the precise dosage is hard to regulate" (Beck 1992).

Risks vs. Benefits

For some women on hormonal replacement therapy there may be some increased risk of breast cancer, related to the length of time that they are on such therapy and the dosage.

Studies have found breast cancer incidence rates rise slightly with estrogen replacement therapy. And although the breast cancer data are controversial less so are the data surrounding the role of estrogen in causing increased risk of cancer of the uterine lining. Without the protective effects of progesterone, the risk of uterine cancer is clearly established. That's why women are also given progesterone orally for approximately 10 days a month along with estrogen. But progesterone reduces the protection from heart attacks provided by estrogen. It can also cause bloating. Sometimes women become uptight when taking progesterone. Beck (1992) reports, "Because [progesterone] breaks down the uterine lining, it also brings on 'withdrawal' bleeding for a few days each month."

If you are a mature woman and you are using one of the estrogen replacement hormones as part of post-menstrual therapy *you may be placing yourself at an increased risk for cancer.* If you want to receive the benefits of hormone replacement therapy while avoiding the risk, you should consider using phytoestrogens.

Risky Drug!

Have you read the label for Premarin? It is one of the most frequently prescribed estrogen replacement drugs for post-menstrual women who are suffering menopausal symptoms. Recently we examined the label for Premarin and became quite concerned.

Premarin's manufacturers warn, "The risk of cancer of the uterus increases the longer estrogens are used . . . *the persistence of risk was demonstrated for 10 years after stopping estrogen treatment . . . Some studies have suggested a possible increased incidence of breast cancer in those woman taking estrogens for prolonged periods of time and especially if higher doses are used.*"

They further warn that side effects include nausea, vomiting, pain, cramps, swelling, abdominal tenderness, yellowing of the skin and/or whites of the eyes, breast tenderness, enlargement of benign tumors of the uterus, bleeding or spotting, vaginal yeast infections, headaches, migraines, dizziness, faintness, mental depression, involuntary muscle spasms, hair loss, changes in sex drive, and worsening of pre-existing conditions of heart disease.

Out of Balance

Ultimately, all of these powerful estrogens throw the body way off balance. So doctors give their patients progestogens, and that can really cause problems! One of the problems with synthetic progestogens is that they inhibit a woman's concentration of natural progesterone in the blood and, in fact, worsen the imbalance of the female hormones. Some of the synthetic progestogens are actually 2,000 times more potent than progesterone, which is why certain progestogens can make women feel more out of sorts than others, and they also appear to increase the risk of certain cancers. When a woman is treated with synthetic progestogens, her body becomes confused, producing less natural progesterone. Eventually women may suffer salt build up, fluid retention and blood sugar imbalances.

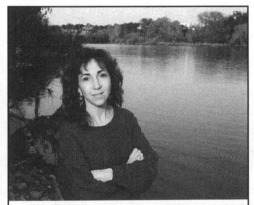

Cynthia Watson, M.D., a clinical faculty instructor at the University of Southern California, has used plant estrogens in her medical practice and has found that they are as effective as synthetic or animal estrogens in easing symptoms of menopause without the complications of conventional therapy.

Although it is true that one of the benefits of estrogen therapy is its help in preventing osteoporosis and heart disease, there may be safer alternatives. "To put it plainly," says Dr. Watson, "I have found in my medical practice that some women have a lot of side effects from synthetic estrogen therapy. They suffer weight gain, fluid retention and breast tenderness. Many continue to have hot flashes and vaginal dryness. Estrogen therapy simply doesn't serve them well."

Although synthetic and animal-derived estrogens may be suitable for some patients, Dr. Watson says that she has found through her clinical work that the plant estrogens are much milder in their effect. "As physicians we recognize the extra burden that estrogen replacement therapy puts on the liver," Dr. Watson says. "However, I believe that the estrogens derived from plants will be metabolized more easily by the liver. I simply haven't seen the severe side effects with the plant estrogens that I do with the synthetic versions.

"I've been using botanical estrogen therapy for about a year now and I'm finding that my patients like it much better. Some of my patients have had serious depression, night sweats and mood disorders; yet, once they go on the plant estrogens those symptoms are much improved."

Vitamin E

All too often we find that the medical community sometimes overlooks what worked in the past and that some of our old time physicians may have known a thing or two that their modern brethren have forgotten. Why is this? Dr. Passwater offers this explanation, "Drug salesmen known as 'detail' men call upon doctors to inform them of the wonders of their products, but there are no salesmen calling upon physicians to sell them on the virtues of vitamins. Vitamins are not patented and are inexpensive. Thus, there is not enough of a profit margin or monopoly to warrant salesmen to call on doctors."

In 1945 Dr. C.J. Christy reported in the *American Journal of Gynecology* that an "entire" group of menopausal women responded to vitamin E treatment and showed either complete relief or very marked improvement. No untoward after-effects were noted. In some cases, relief was more easily obtained with vitamin E than with the use of estrogen; however, the chief advantage of vitamin E over estrogens was its freedom from a stimulative effect on the genital system or the breasts. And because vitamin E has no carcinogenic (cancer-causing) effect, it may be used quite freely in menopausal patients suffering from neoplasm.

In 1948, Dr. H. Ferguson reported in the *Virginia Medical Monthly* that "sixty of sixty-six patients with severe menopausal symptoms were completely relieved with 15 to 30 IU of vitamin E daily."

Dr. Passwater conducted his own survey on vitamin E; here's what he reported in *Prevention* magazine from respondents:
• "Vitamin E stopped my hot flashes."
• "Vitamin E prevented hysterectomy in 1958."
• "Vitamin E eliminated the need for estrogen shots."
• "Corrected vaginal dryness. It's *great—GREAT!!!*"

•"Vitamin E took care of the hot flashes and night sweats completely. I ran out of vitamin E for two months and started having heavy night sweats again. I started back again with vitamin E and have had no symptoms since. I will never be without vitamin E again."

Safer Phytoestrogens

So now you know there is a safer alternative to estrogens. You should certainly consult a physician before stopping synthetic or animal-based estrogen replacement therapy, although some physicians may not be familiar with the medical literature on plant estrogens, meaning they will need *you* to educate them. Bring them this section of your book and they can start their education.

Nevertheless, the fact remains that plants have a long and documented history of use for their estrogenic influences that is once again gaining popularity.

•Werbach (1988) reports that naturally occurring bioflavonoids found in some botanical extracts have estrogenic influences that were much more effective than sub-therapeutic doses of estrogen for the control of vaso-motor flushing.

•Mowrey (1986) reports that *Cimicifuga racemosa* was introduced to American medicine by the Indians who called it squaw root with reference to one of its common uses in treating uterine disorders. "Among clinical findings are the following: it promotes and/or restores healthy menstrual activity; it soothes irritation and congestion of the uterus, cervix and vagina."

•The estrogenic activity of *Glycyrrhiza glabra* has been clearly documented (Sharaf 1975, Costello, 1950, Pointet-Guillot 1958, Murav'ev 1972). In infantile and sexually stunted experimental animals, administration of *Glycyrrhiza glabra* increased uterine weight (Mowrey 1986). It has helped induce ovulation in women who could otherwise not ovulate (Yaginuma 1982).

•Other estrogenic-active botanicals include *Aletris farinosa, Angelica sinensis,* and *Foeniculum vulgare.*

•For a balancing effect, *Dioscorea villosa* is important because it is rich in progesterone precursors. *Agnus castus* contains essential oils and flavonoids that help increase the production of progesterone.

Follow the Japanese Lead

There is dramatic evidence for the importance of a diet rich in plant estrogens for both the easing of menopausal symptoms and breast cancer prevention, according to researchers writing in 1992 in *The Lancet*. In women living in a small Japanese village and consuming the traditional low-fat Japanese diet, their urinary excretions were rich in phytoestrogens which are estrogenic substances derived from plants (as opposed to animals), the researchers reported.

The levels of plant estrogens in the urine of the Japanese women were higher by 12 to 107 times than American and Finnish women. Interestingly, phytoestrogens have both estrogenic and anti-estrogenic activity in the human body—depending on the individual. Such substances are known also as *adaptogens*. This means that they *adapt* themselves to the physiological needs of the individual.

If the body is producing too much estrogen, their presence tends to depress excessive estrogen production. Conversely if the body isn't producing enough estrogen, the amount of phytoestrogens consumed in traditional Japanese diets is probably large enough to have biological effects, especially in postmenstrual women with low estrogen levels.

Eases Hot Flushes

High intake of foods rich in phytoestrogens may partly explain why hot flushes and other menopausal symptoms are so infrequent in Japanese women. Their anti-estrogenic activity may explain in part why the risk of breast cancer is lower in Japanese women than in American women. Examples of foods rich in plant estrogens include soy products such as tofu, miso, aburage, atuage, koridofu, soybeans and other beans. But these are not the traditional foods of American women. That's why a dietary supplement containing plant estrogens can be so essential for post-menstrual women who are considering hormone replacement therapy.

Although other kinds of synthetic and natural estrogens may pose significant health risks, including increasing the risk of cancer and gallbladder disease, phytoestrogens have not been associated with these side effects.

Plant Progesterone via Wild Yam

A study by Dr. John Lee, a physician in California, over the last 11 years with 100 postmenopausal women, aged 38 to 83, showed that 97 of them had five percent to forty percent new bone density within 6 to 48 months after using a wild yam cream with natural progsterone. Some women attained as much as 105 percent of the average bone structure of a 35-year-old female. The incidence of pathological fractures was zero among this group.

Typically, a progesterone cream should be used on a 28 day cycle. For those who have already experienced bone loss, fractures, or have been diagnosed with osteoporosis, use of the cream should be used as follows:

•1st cycle: 1/2 teaspoon (twice daily) on arising and at bedtime. The contents of one two-ounce jar should last one month.

•2nd cycle onwards: 1/4 teaspoon (twice daily). Contents of one two-ounce jar should last two months.

The cream should be gently massaged into soft tissue areas such as the chest, breast, under arms, inner arms and wrist area, abdomen, or inner thighs. Apply to a different area each day to avoid saturating fat cells.

However, for women with only slight bone loss, low hormone levels of progesterone or for prevention, the following schedule should be followed:

•Days 1 to 14 of cycle: no application

•Days 15 to 28: 1/8 to 1/4 teaspoon once daily.

Progesterone is one of the female body's most important hormones and has benefits far beyond its role in menstrual cycles and pregnancy, says Dr. Lee. The menopausal decrease in progesterone production can be correlated not only with accelerated bone mass loss but also with many functions associated with what is commonly interpreted as aging. Proper supplementation with natural progesterone prevents and can even reverse these supposed aging phenomena. Natural progesterone should never be confused with the synthetic progestins promoted by the pharmaceutical industry and so often prescribed by physicians as progesterone substitutes. These synthetic substitutes do not duplicate natural progesterone's full spectrum of benefits, and all carry multiple potential undesirable side effects The many benefits from natural progesterone include blood sugar normalization, more efficient utilization of fat for energy, bone formation, protection against cancer, enhancement of thyroid hormone, anti-depressant activity, and blockage of estrogen side effects.

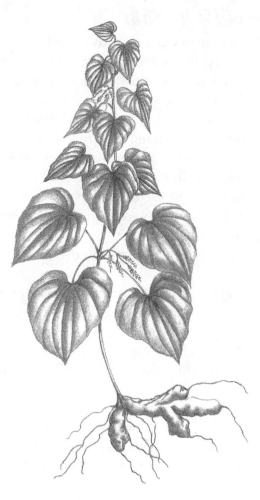

(Dioscorea villosa) Wild Yam

Says Lee: "After menopause, estrogen supplementation will retard osteoporosis but it will not correct the bone loss that has occurred. Bone formation is the function of progesterone. In most menopausal women, the loss of progesterone and the consequent loss of bone building is the major cause of osteoporosis. In my clinical experience, osteoporosis can be reversed in many women simply by restoring adequate progesterone. Synthetic progestins vary in their ability to activate osteoblast function and none are as good as natural progesterone."

There are many other anti-aging benefits of natural progesterone, notes Dr. Lee. As women approach menopause, they find themselves losing energy, retaining fluids, fighting fat, developing wrinkles and facial hairs, prone to headaches and depression, and less interested in sex. Common wisdom assigns these symptoms to simply aging. They see their doctors, take their diuretics and, occasionally, thyroid medication, and face their future with fading enthusiasm. They seek out cosmeticians for their wrinkles, see their beauticians more often for their thinning hair, and take more calcium for their thinning bones. What they are unaware of is the importance of proper hormonal balance, particularly the lack of this singularly important hormone, progesterone.

How does progesterone work? Progesterone is a primary precursor in the biosynthesis of the adrenal corticosteroids, says Dr. Lee. Without adequate progesterone, synthesis of cortisone is impaired and the body turns to an alternative pathway via dihydroandrosterone and androstendeione. This alternative pathway has androgenic (i.e., masculinizing) side effects which cause the long facial hairs of elderly postmenopausal women and thinning of their scalp hair. When progesterone is supplemented, it is quite common to witness the clearing of facial hair and the return of healthy scalp hair in these women. Furthermore, impaired cortisone synthesis results in a decrease in one's ability to handle stress whether this stress be induced by surgery, trauma or emotional turmoil. Yet with adequate progesterone, one's ability to deal with stress improves.

Benefits of naturally derived progesterone from wild yam include:
•Protects against fibrocysts
•Maintains secretory endometrium
•Natural diuretic
•Helps use fat for energy
•Natural anti-depressant
•Helps thyroid hormone action
•Normalizes blood clotting
•Restores libido
•Normalizes blood sugar levels
•Normalizes zinc and copper levels
•Restores proper cell oxygen levels
•Prevents endometrial cancer
•Helps prevent breast cancer
•Stimulates osteoblast bone building
•Necessary for survival of embryo
•Precursor of cortisone synthesis

Natural progesterone is available without a prescription in a variety of forms—skin cremes, drops, and capsules. Progesterone is well absorbed transdermally into the fatty layer under the skin. *Skin areas to which progesterone creme has been applied will be seen to become less dry and more youthful in texture.* Skin aging is prevented more effectively with progesterone than with estrogen cremes. With continued use, the progesterone is distributed throughout the body via the blood stream. Thus, full benefits may not become apparent until after several weeks or even several cycles of use, depending on the difference in body fat content and the relative progesterone deficiency status of the patient.

Progesterone is quickly absorbed through the mucosa of the mouth. Thus, oral drops retained in the buccal areas or under the tongue are quickly absorbed into the blood stream. Notes Dr. Lee, "For prompt response, as needed in migraine headaches or hot flushes for example, oral drops are superior. Taken orally, progesterone, like vitamin A, is fat-soluble and much is acquired by the liver where it is secreted and thus, in bile. Oral doses must be 5-10 times greater than transdermal doses to achieve equivalent effects."

A Final Note

The best combination for many post-menstrual women will be to use a plant-based estrogen formula along with a dietary osteoporosis formula as discussed in *Chapter 17.* They will work together to provide the absolute best guarantee of a smooth transition, helping alleviate the hot flashes, vaginal discomfort and other symptoms of emerging menopause and—equally important—offer you needed protection against the onset of osteoporosis.

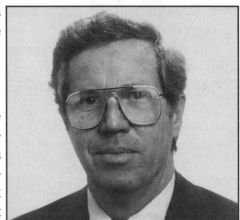

John Lee, M.D., is one of the leading experts on the use of wild yam for prevention of osteoporosis. He recommends that women use wild yam-derived progesterone as a cream or oral supplement whether they are pre-menopausal, menopausal or past menopause.

19. Smart Skin Sense

Skin. It is the body's largest organ and one of its most important. The skin's functions include protection, tempera-ture regulation, vitamin D synthesis, and sensation. Ideally, for reasons of both health and appearance, the skin should always remain soft and supple.

The earliest skin care treatments known by archaeologists date back to the ancient Egyptians. Early skin cremes were made from bees wax, almond oil, and herbs. As skin care became popular in the Mediterranean countries, the herbs lavender and chamomile were used for dry skin, sage was combined with aloe for sunburn, and elm leaves were used for oily skin needs. Depending on the type of treatment desired, the herbs were heated with almond oil until thick with their scent. Bees wax was then added and the mixture was beaten into a creme. Lemon, rosemary or parsley were also added to help bleach out skin blotches or freckles. Fascination with skin care has been shared throughout history and many of these age old remedies are still being used today.

Cleopatra reportedly spent hours soaking in buttermilk to bleach her skin. The Romans packed themselves in a nutrient rich clay mud called *fango* to keep their skin firm and youthful looking. Later, they discovered an indigenous seaweed called *iridea* and applied it to rid themselves of unwanted wrinkles and stretch marks. The Aztec and Mayan peoples used natural papaya as a skin moisturizer.

Victorian women used honey as a facial mask and steeped fresh violets in warm milk overnight to use as a solution for oily skin. To this day, women make facial masks out of mashed avocados, sliced cucumbers, oatmeal, and egg whites, not to mention spending millions of dollars on commercial skin care products in hopes of keeping their skin supple, smooth, and wrinkle-free.

Recent research, however, is beginning to support the theory that healthy, radiant skin comes from within. Specially formulated topical creams and oils combined with nutritional support can slow down the skin's aging process.

Skin Facts

Rapid skin deterioration usually begins by the age of 30. Oil gland functions slow down, hormonal changes occur, and the body gradually begins to lose its moisture. However, according to biochemists, most of the skin's wear and tear occurs in the connective tissue, of which collagen and elastin are the principal components. Both are complicated protein fibers which are the skin's underlying support system. When these protein structures deteriorate, the skin becomes rigid and inelastic. The skin's thickness may decrease by 50 to 75 percent by the age of 75. As the skin's tissue changes, the water binding proteins, vitamins, and minerals which ensure regeneration eventually deteriorate.

Photoaging

Most dermatologists agree that the least expensive and the longest lasting way to ensure a youthful appearance is to protect your skin from an early age. They also agree that the single most destructive force to human skin is the sun. Sunlight accounts for most of the visible signs we associate with the aging process. Science calls sun damage "photoaging." Ultraviolet light breaks down the skin's collagen and elastin fibers, producing brown "age spots," deep wrinkles, and giving the skin a leathery texture. Studies point out that the sun depletes vitamin C levels in the skin. Vitamin C is one of the major stimulants of collagen production. UV light can promote the generation of free radicals in the skin, which in turn, decreases antioxidant enzymes and vitamin E. Wrinkles, many believe, may largely be due to the release of free radicals in the body. Richard Passwater, Ph.D., a supporter of the free radical theory of aging, refers to them as "chemical terrorists." Free radicals are oxygen-based compounds which, when released by the body, damage cellular membranes, as well as the proteins that make-up the skin. More and more doctors are now subscribing to the free radical theory, especially as it relates to disease and aging. Roy Walford, M.D., another long-time subscriber, believes "that many of the substances that cause or promote cancer may do so by stimulating cells to produce free radicals which then damage or alter the blueprint until the cell becomes cancerous."

Ozone

Sun damage and skin cancer statistics are on the rise. Now more than ever, skin protection is essential. In 1978, the government acknowledged sunlight to be a prime factor in premature aging and skin cancer. In the 1980s the American Cancer Society (ACS) reported that a newborn's chance of developing melanoma (skin cancer) is 1 in 105 during his or her lifetime. The ACS warned that by the year 2000 the risk will be increased to one in 75. In 1988, the Environmental Protection Agency (EPA) estimated that every one percent decrease in the ozone layer contributes a 4 to 6 percent increase in skin cancers. Some 3.2 million deaths from skin cancer are possible from ozone depletion alone by the year 2075, reports EPA. By 1991, the EPA updated its study and found larger ozone holes over the United States, bringing the estimated total of projected skin cancer cases up to 42 million by the year 2040. This year, the ACS believes that of the 32,000 new cases of melanoma reported, 25 percent of them will occur in persons 39 years or younger!

Smoking

From observing facial changes in persons puffing on a cigarette, it is easy to detect expression lines of where the mouth puckers and the eyes squint. In 1991, *The Annals of Internal Medicine* and the *Journal of the American Medical Association* both stated, "Cigarette smoking is an independent risk factor for the development of premature wrinkling. Heavy smokers were 4.7 times more likely to be prematurely wrinkled than nonsmokers." Smokers have been found to have a much lower concentration of ascorbic acid (vitamin C) than non-smokers. Lower levels of vitamin C contribute to the break down of the skin's connective tissue. As the skin's elasticity wears thin, the skin develops a dryer texture that creates more wrinkles and less flexibility.

Alcohol

The effects of alcohol on the skin are similar to those of cigarette smoking. Alcohol dehydrates the body and restricts the blood flow to the skin's cells. When consuming alcohol, the skin's cells lose essential nutrients that are needed to replenish the body. Malabsorption may result in abnormal dryness of the skin due to the lack of essential vitamins, namely vitamin A. Vitamin A is needed to maintain healthy skin, nails, and hair. Furthermore, studies indicate that vitamin A may help to reduce the effects of skin aging. A high intake of food sources rich in vitamin A and vitamin A's precursor beta carotene (dark leafy green vegetables, squash, carrots, swordfish, halibut, salmon, whitefish, and crab) and vitamin C appears to act as a protective against certain types of photoaging and skin diseases. Science is just beginning to tap into the skin healing properties of vitamin A's complex structure of retinoids. The restorative properties of beta carotene-rich foods and supplements appear to be unlimited. Vitamin A may also be useful during the body's hormonal changes. Vitamin A, suggests *The American Journal of Epidemiology,* reacts positively to menopausal estrogens.

Diet and Stress

Stress, diet, and environmental conditions all take their toll on the skin. Daily wear and tear are inevitable. All three conditions combined, however, may inhibit the body from receiving the natural nutrients it needs. Diet obviously plays a huge role in the achievement of radiant and healthy skin. Eating a vitamin-rich diet, low in fats and alcohol, plus plenty of exercise, and sleep are all major contributors to good skin care.

Environmental conditions and stress may lead to a lack of zinc and calcium in the body. About zinc, longevity expert Dr. Hans Kugler notes, "the American diet is often deficient in this mineral. Men, particularly, are prone to this deficiency." Zinc is proving to be helpful in acting as an anti-inflammatory agent on skin lesions. Calcium is an essential element being used to help ease the symptoms of stress and anxiety. Diets that lack calcium may suffer from anxiety disorders. Psychosocial stress has been found to affect the skin and in some cases is directly linked to psoriasis. Scaling skin may also find a relief from an essential trace element known as silica, reports the *Journal of Investigative Dermatology.* Silica is needed by the body to help form connective tissue. Collagen contains silica. Silica promotes firmness and strength in the skin's tissues.

Working from the Inside Out

Recent research indicates that by ingesting marine protein fractions (fish and other aquatic-based proteins) and polysaccharides (complex carbohydrates found in whole grains), positive structural and anti-aging improvement of the skin will become visible over time. This suggests what science has been trying to prove for quite some time, that changes in the skin occur gradually and from within. When marine proteins and polysaccharides are taken over a period of time (3 to 6 months) they work internally to eliminate cellulite, diminish stretch marks, soften the skin's texture, erase wrinkles, and acne scars. The more damaged the skin, the more dramatic the results. Yellowish tones, due to over exposure to the sun, can also be normalized. Combined with proper nutrients such as ascorbic acid (vitamin C), vitamin A, zinc, calcium, silica, and cysteine, the skin's elasticity begins to regain its original thickness. More collagen and moisture are supplied. Cysteine has been found to aid in the detoxification of toxic chemicals that enter the body due to cigarette smoking and other pollutants. The combined and synergistic action created by all of these ingredients allows the skin's cells to once again retain their nutrients and thus replenish themselves. Reversing the signs of the aging process is is no longer a mere possibility, where skin aging is concerned. Within several months it has been witnessed that the skin can blossom into its natural state of overall radiance and health. The age old wives' tale "beauty comes from within" is proving to be true in the up and coming world of skin care research.

Vitamin C & Selenium Skin and Sun Repair

One of the growing areas of nutrition is with cosmeceuticals—products that are delivered topically through the skin yet contain dietary nutrients. In the following material, I will discuss sunscreens with the caveat that they are regulated as OTC products by the Food and Drug Administration and thus subject to different criteria. It may be that ultimately, if we like the idea, we will have to promote our product not as a sunscreen but as a product fulfilling a different function.

Presently, the most popular sunscreens are topical agents in the form of solutions, gels, creams, or ointments. The central ingredient is generally a vitamin, para-aminobenzoic acid (PABA) and its derivatives. But, unfortunately, there's increasing evidence that these common and conventional sunscreens may interfere with vitamin D synthesis. In other words, the situation is one where our greatest protection against the sun is made possbily by means of a vitamin (PABA) which, in turn, interferes with the synthesis of still another vitamin (D). So the question becomes whether it is possible to provide the sunscreen effect by other means? It now looks like still another vitamin (C) may be the answer.

John Murray and his Duke University colleagues have shown significant UV protection to pig skin by topical applications of the ascorbates.

It logically followed to test this out in humans. To do this, 10 volunteers were pretreated with a 10% l-ascorbic acid solution or an indistinguisable placebo, then irradiated with UV. At 24 hours, both arms were photographed using color slide film. The slides were then analyzed for erythema (redness) effect. By careful measurement, only the sites treated with topical vitamin C showed a 22% significant reduction of redness. Even simple inspection confirmed the protective effect of the ascorbates.

Another report: "A 10% ascorbic acid solution was topically applied to the skin of domestic pigs who were exposed to ultraviolet radiation. Results showed that skin levels of vitamin C rose 4- to 40-fold or more following following multiple treatment with the vitamin. The topical vitamin C applied 15 to 30 minutes before UV exposure also protected porcine skin from UVB and UVA damage. A single application provided significant protection; mutiple applications, however, produced even better results."

Since the vitamin C does not produce a "sunscreen" effect, the researchers conclude that the reduced skin damaged is caused by biological, not physicial effects. However, since vitamin C levels were significantly reduced as a result of exposure to ultraviolet light, the researchers speculate that normal skin concentrations of vitamin C are probably severely depleted during exposure to sunlight, and

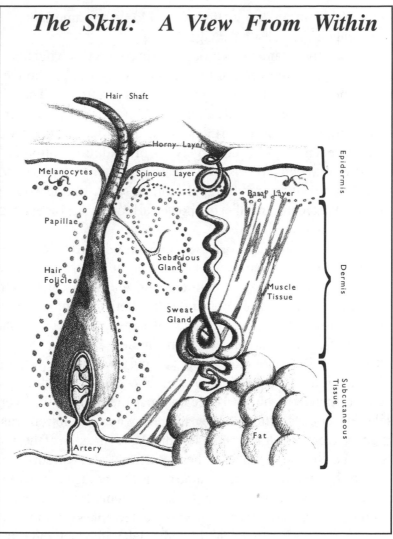

The Skin: A View From Within

Human skin has three layers of tissue—the epidermis, the dermis, and subcutaneous tissue. The epidermis consists of four layers of cells—horny, granular, spinous, and basal. The skin also has hair and two kinds of glands, sebaceous and sweat.

"replenishment of skin vitamin C would be an important pharmacological intervention against sun damage."

Frequently, vitamin C is brought up in context with the free radical theory. It is probably well to emphasize the story once again. Simple sunburn is an excellent example of the ravages of oxidative damage. The ascorbates in the form of an ointment provide a superb illustration of the protective effects of a powerful antioxidant. Up to this point in its medical history, the use of ascrobic acid has been emphasized largely by oral administration and parenterally (mostly intravenously). Now we learn that vitamin C can serve a potentially useful purpose by inunction (applied to the skin). Its effect does not seem to be that of a sunscreen, but rather of a powerful biochemical agent that mitigates free radical damage.

Selenium in the form of L-selenomethionine (SeMet) also appears to be helpful. Recently a study was conducted to determine oral and/or topical selenium protects against pigmentation and skin cancer induced by UV irradiation. This study demonstrated that both oral and topical SeMet supplementation can reduce the incidence of acute and chronic damage to the skin (i.e., sunburn and tanning or pigmentation and skin cancer) induced by ultraviolet (UV) irradiation without giving any signs of symptoms of toxicity. The selenium concentrations of skin and liver showed that both means of delivery increased the level of selenium in the skin and the liver, with the skin selenium concentrations higher in areas where the lotion was applied. UV irradiation caused significantly less damage to the skin of the mice treated with selenium. No animals given either topical or oral selenium developed Scoring of skin pigmentation demonstrated reduced tanning (a measure of free radical damage to the skin) in the selenium-supplemented mice. Furthermore, weekly counts of the total number of clinically detectable skin tumors desmonstrated that mice treated with selenium had a delayed onset and a markedly lesser incidence of skin cancer induced by the UV irradiation. Notes Dr. Karen E. Burke, M.D., Ph.D., attending physician at the Cabrini Medical Center, New York, NY: "If mouse tumorigenesis, with its short latent period, can be inhibited effectively with topical or oral SeMet as the experiments presented demonstrate, a similar effect might be expected for humans with their long latent period. Therefore, the protection that might be provided by either topically or orally administered SeMet may be of great significance to individual health.

This is of special importance, especially today, when because of the decrease in the protective filtering of UV-irradiation by the ozone layer and increased outdoor leisure, the number of skin cancers has increased more than any other form of cancer."

Getting Older Isn't What it Used to Be

Getting older today isn't what it used to be. Americans are living longer. Trend setters have even coined a new word for Americans' longer life expectancy—it's called "down-aging." Thirty million people are now over the age of 65, compared to 17 million just 25 years ago says the National Institute on Aging (NIA). Indeed, NIA scientists are validating that to a certain extent people are able to control their own rate of aging. How? Through their lifestyle. No one is immune to the ravages of time or gravity, but developing a well-rounded lifestyle seems to be one of the major factors in downaging. A healthy lifestyle that includes protection from the sun is recognized as an absolute factor in helping to slow down or inhibit the skin's premature aging process. One of the most obvious ways in which to appear more youthful is to develop and maintain healthy and radiant skin. By making positive choices in diet and lifestyle, it is possible to keep the skin smooth and healthy well into your golden years, thereby improving not only the appearance, but the overall health of the body. Eating sensibly, limiting sun exposure, as well as supplementing the diet with vitamins A and C, minerals such as zinc and calcium, and marine proteins are all important factors in keeping the skin healthy.

Smart Skin Sense

Once again, here's what you need to do
for more beautiful, youthful skin:
• Create a healthy lifestyle
• Exercise regularly
• Limit exposure to the sun
• Dry brush the skin
• Use a sunscreen
• Get plenty of sleep
• Limit alcohol intake
• Quit smoking
• Drink plenty of water
• Moisturize

Where to Find the Formula

Editor's Note: Although finding each of the ingredients discussed in this report will prove difficult at most supermarkets, drug stores and health food shops, we recently learned of an American company, Gero Vita International, that has put together a formula, called Dermatein, that combines marine polysaccharide fractions with other proven agents such as selenomethionine, for reversing wrinkling and helping prevent sun damage including skin cancer. In fact, the formula recently was tested on a group of women, by several physicians, and proven to actually reverse wrinkling and smoothen skin. Apparently, it works quite well, based on this study, which will soon be published in a major international nutritional journal, and it may soon become an American classic. Order Dermatein now, while supplies are available, by calling (800) 825-8482.

20. Sexual Potency

In a Los Angeles suburb a husband came home with a new nutritional supplement that contained quebracho bark which is cultivated from plants in the Andean region of Argentina and Chile. He and his wife each ingested a single pill. Soon after ingesting the supplement, they began acting like two insatiable sexual animals.

Good health equals good sex! Few people would disagree with the idea that sex is basic to human existence. It is not only a tremendous source of pleasure but also a key element of both male and female identity. It involves far more than mere instinct or physical drive, bringing into play a wide range of emotional and sensory impulses that enable us to build self-esteem, experience joy and love, and cope with the demands and stresses of everyday life. Sexuality energizes virtually every part of the human body, with the brain being the most potent sensory organ of all. The most universal of all desires and pursuits, sex is in some ways the essence of the person; it is vital to our physical and mental well-being, whatever our age, gender, ethnicity, or social background.

Optimum sexuality requires a thriving lifestyle that in turn depends upon our full physical and mental strength. We can be sexually active well beyond our youth, into our seventies, even eighties and beyond, so long as we possess the necessary libido and capacity.

It was an amazing newspaper report. The happiest men and women in America are married couples who have sex frequently after age 60, says a report by the Rev. Andrew M. Greeley, the sociologist-priest-novelist who is a sociology professor at the University of Chicago and the University of Arizona and a research associate at the former's National Opinion Research Center.

According to the Greeley report which involved a total of 5,738 subjects interviewed between 1988 and 1991: 37 percent of married people over 60 make love once a week or more, and 16 percent make love several times a week. Furthermore, men and women who engage in frequent sex after 60 report the happiest marriages and are more likely to report that they are living exciting lives, the report said.

In fact, 38 percent of those in their sixties and 12 percent of those in their 70s said they experience ecstasy during lovemaking, according to the Greeley report. And 55 percent of those over 60 said their spouses are skilled lovers. "Also, older men and women did not confine passion to the bedroom: one-third swam nude together; one-third showered together; one-half enjoyed extended sexual play; and two-thirds experimented sexually," reported the San Francisco *Chronicle-Examiner* newspapers.

However, many people experience a sharp decline in sexual interest and performance beginning in their thirties and even sooner. Some lose their sexual powers altogether. Sex researchers estimate that in the U.S. about one in four persons suffers from some kind of sexual dysfunction—and the situation appears to be worsening. The atrophy of sexual functioning has many causes: poor nutrition, stress, exposure to toxic substances, alcohol and drugs, bad sleeping habits, lack of exercise, and more. The aging process too can take its toll on the orgasmic potential of both men and women, on the ability of men to get and sustain erections, and on the overall sex drive for both genders.

Four specific areas are closely associated with sexual functioning:

•*Sex Hormones.* The most basic and commonly understood fact is that the sex hormones are responsible for sexual functioning. If a man comes to a doctor's office and complains about a decreasing sex life, a prescription for testosterone is often given if a physical doesn't show any abnormalities. However, prescription drugs often have undesirable side-effects and therefore should be last on the list of things to do.

•*Health and special nutrients for the sex glands.* Your sex glands must be in optimal health. For example, a man came to Hans Kugler, Ph.D., for general health counseling. "In the process of our discussion," recalls Dr. Kugler, "he expressed worries about his sex life. He was able to reach an erection, but had great difficulties to ejaculate. The man was referred to a doctor for a prostate examination and was found to have a mild chronic prostate infection. When it was cured, he was able to ejaculate easily." The prostate must always be in optimal health for maximum sexual potency. The key nutrient in preventing prostate trouble is the mineral zinc; a zinc deficiency can lead to prostate atrophy. Ninety percent of Americans consume zinc-deficient diets, according to Dr. Harman. (See Chapter 16 on prostate health.)

•*Muscular and physical strength.* Physical strength and virility are closely connected: more muscular men usually have higher testosterone levels. Biochemical feedback mechanisms also affect testosterone levels: a man who starts a strong exercise program that includes muscle-building will also increase his blood testosterone levels. Strong exercise stimulates not only the sex glands, it also causes the pituitary to release growth hormones. Substances that have an effect on athletic strength and performance are closely related to male sex hormones. The anabolic effect of these substances is to shift body chemistry more towards muscle formation.

•*Activators.* Natural, hormone-like substances that have an effect on sexual functi oning usually work both anabolically (increasing muscle strength) and hormonally. In many plants we find a number of compounds known as *steroles* that have similar but less dangerous properties than synthetic steroids.

Throughout history both men and women have sought so-called aphrodisiacs, or love potions, with the aim of sharpening and extending their sexual pleasure. All societies, from the ancient Greeks and Romans to modern-day industrial societies in Europe and North America, have discovered in nature or in laboratories what they believe to be the ultimate sex remedies and stimulants.

"Is there any quest more universal than the pursuit of sexual vigor?" writes Kirk Johnson in *East West* magazine. "Our lust for sex is a passion matched only, perhaps, by the eternal pursuit of youth. The two are fittingly intertwined. When we are young, there is no reason to even consider increasing a raging sex drive that, if I may speak from experience, drives us to distraction and frequently clear to the other side. But in every era and in every culture, the unrelenting tick of the biological clock has brought such a loss of sexual vitality, or fear of it, that people have employed an imaginative array of remedies—from rare plants and herbs to precious bones and desiccated animal parts—to restore it."

The search for the one "true" aphrodisiac has been never-ending. Teas of tarot root, ginseng, rice wine, live snakes, ground deer horn and crushed rhino tusks have all been said to improve sexual desire and performance. Similar claims have been made for Spanish fly, cocaine, oysters, asparagus, marijuana and even alcohol and caffeine. There is a ceaseless fascination with oils, leaves, roots, berries, seeds, juices, and sprouts. As Johnson reports, "One Arabian manual suggests a daily dish of asparagus to heighten sexual prowess. In the Amazon of central Brazil, men of the Mehinaku tribe rub needlefish against their penises in the hope that their organs will become similarly long and hard . . . . In Johannesburg, Bantu men are fond of bagalala, a wild plant found in the hills of South Africa."

"I have long believed that sex plays a major role in health," notes Cynthia Watson, M.D., author of *Love Potions*. "The basic medical questionnaire I ask my patients to complete has always included the question, 'Are you having any problems with sex?' The patient's answer, or non-answer, has enabled me to broach this delicate subject and offer whatever help I could.

"I have also long realized that the Western medical approach to this issue is far too limited. That is why I have devoted a great deal of study to herbal tonics and love potions; in the long history of aphrodisia I found many of the answers I sought.

"Aphrodisiacs have taken the shape of food or drink, herb or spice, charm or ritual, drug, homeopathic remedy, flower essence, or aroma. Although they varied in form, aphrodisiacs were among the ancient cultures' great common denominators: Remedies promising similar results have been found in the traditions of China, Egypt, Mesopotamia, India, Europe, Africa, South America, Polynesia.

For example, from ancient Egypt to the present day, honey has been served at wedding feasts. This is no coincidence or mindless ritual: Honey contains B-complex vitamins and certain minerals that promote sexual health in men and women as well as providing the easily absorbed sugar needed to replenish semen.

Sea horses, used by the Chinese for centuries in the treatment of male infertility, recently have been shown to contain vital proteins and amino acids that can increase semen production. Early American colonists who recommended dandelion weed for impotence were unaware that the plant's leaves contain an astronomically high amount of vitamin A, essential to the production of sex hormones in both men and women. The time-honored notion that special plant and animal substances have an affinity with the human reproductive system persists even today.

But researchers, highly trained in scientific protocols and the value of rigorous occidental scientific methods, would be appalled that few of these substances have undergone the kinds of controlled, double-blind studies that modern medicine demands. The effects of sexual stimulants have, until recently, remained in the sphere of folklore and myth; they have no real scientific validity—even if they are truly effective, and that has hurt the reputation of botanical aphrodisiacs. At the same time, Western practitioners have generally treated poor sexual performance by means of counseling and drugs, including sex and thyroid hormones. They have not tested natural substances long regarded as aphrodisiacs, so we have little more than anecdotal evidence to support their benefits and claims of effectiveness. "The more we doctors learn about the sexual physiology of the human body, the better we understand the underlying truth of so many ancient remedies, a truth that is largely a matter of chemistry," says Dr. Watson.

Plant-based natural aphrodisiacs have nonetheless gained increased respect in health and medical circles.

Quebracho Bark

In Argentina quebracho has long been considered an aphrodisiac (Lewis 1977). Quebracho bark comes from a South American plant known technically as *Aspidosperma quebracho-blanco*. Recent reports have centered on its ability to stimulate sexual interest in users through an overall increase in the intensity of sensation. There is a strong reason for this effect. One of its active ingredients, known as *quebrachine*, is chemically equivalent to yohimbine and we know a lot about this botanical.

Extensive research has been done on the African herb extract that contains the yohimbine compounds. This herb, like quebracho, is also taken from the bark of a tree—the *Corynanthe yohimbe* from Cameroon.

Tests conducted by Dr. Julian Davidson and others at Stanford University suggest that yohimbine has highly positive effects on the libido, often leading to "erotic" feelings and dramatic improvement in sexual performance. The Stanford researchers reported in the August 1984 issue of *Science* that when impotent male rats were given yohimbine they went wild and mounted female animals as much as 45 times in less than 15 minutes. Yohimbine has been subsequently used to treat penile erectile dysfunctions in the U.S. and elsewhere.

In 1987 Dr. Alvaro Morales, a urologist, reported "modest effectiveness" for the use of yohimbine on 100 organically impotent men. In August 1987, Reid and colleagues reported in *The Lancet* that yohimbine is a safe treatment for sexual impotence, one that *"seems to be as effective as sex and marital therapy for restoring sexual functioning."* Similar results were reported by Susset and colleagues in the June 1989 issue of *Urology* where more than one-third of 82 men, suffering organic sexual impotence, demonstrated positive improvement after one month of

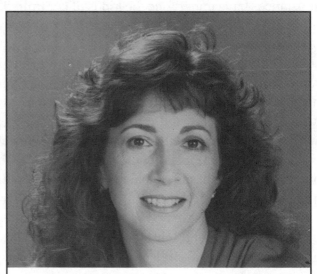

Cynthia Watson, M.D., is an expert on aphrodisiacs and sexual stimulants. Her book *Love Potions: A Doctor's Guide to Aphrodisiacs and Sexual Pleasures* (Jeremy Tarcher, 1993) is available at book stores throughout the nation. Dr. Watson is a regular contributor to the cutting edge *Journal of Longevity Research.* In her practice, she uses many of the botanicalsand supplements described in this chapter—and reports fantastic treatment with yohimbine.

Here's an anecdotal story that holds true, owing to the objective nature of the person who related it. A friend gave his wife a supplement containing quebracho, knowing nothing at the time of the potential sexually stimulating properties in quebracho bark. He later reported that within an hour of her use of this supplement that his wife was experiencing strong sexual urges and that she literally threw him on their bed, ripped off his clothing and made passionate love for hours! The friend reports that this pattern has continued following use of the quebracho-containing supplement.

Avena Sativa & Nettle

A number of studies published worldwide have documented the accidental findings of a Chinese farmer, Lee Zhang. Lee raised carp both for profit and as a main source of food for his family. But carp are notoriously lazy breeders.

One day, Zhang asked his son to take on a new chore which consisted of feeding the carp each morning before leaving for school. Mistakenly, the farmer's young son fed the fish green oats (*Avena sativa*). It was not until his father discovered this mistake and confronted his son that they both realized the boy had been feeding the carp the wrong food for months. Rushing to the pond to check on his precious commodity, the farmer was astounded by what he discovered. Hundreds of baby fish were swarming in the pond, and he had to admit that his older carp appeared much healthier too.

This 'mistake' led to a number of efforts by Chinese scientists to isolate physiological changes in the carp, as well as the active ingredients in the green oats that resulted in the farmer's most fortuitous discovery. Researchers were especially interested in the increased hormone levels found in the fish, which were nearly one third higher than normal. Eventually international researchers turned their attention to the human potential of *Avena sativa* to help the approximately 15 million men and 35 million women in America alone who suffer from a lack of sexual desire and diminished performance (Institute for Advanced Study of Human Sexuality 1990).

Even greater strides have been made in documenting the aphrodisiac effects of the natural botanicals *Avena sativa* (green oats) and *Urtica dioica* (nettle) on

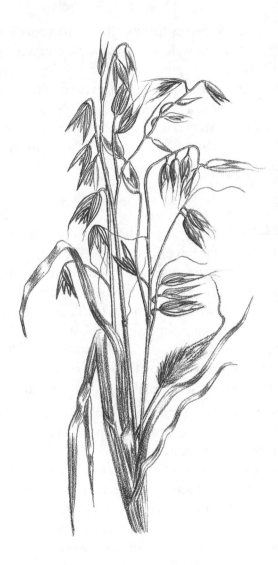

Avena Sativa

both men and women. The sex-stimulating qualities of *Avena sativa* were first noted two centuries ago in the German Pharmacopoeia, and have been referred to in many books and articles since.

Historically, the term "feeling your oats" suggested a person filled with energy and ready to experience life. Oats have been used to treat problems of digestion and circulation as well as allergies, depression, insomnia, and eczema. But it is the powerful impact of *Avena sativa* on sexual desire and performance that has most intrigued the health and scientific communities.

Nettle, obtained from the stinging nettle plant found in every part of the world, has long been used as a remedy for urinary tract disorders and prostate ailments. Rich in minerals including iron, vitamins, lipids, and chlorophyll, nettle, also known as *Urtica dioica*, is one of the most potent medicinal plants known. It has been used to treat anemia, food poisoning, hypoglycemia, and a host of other health problems.

The combination of oats and nettle has been shown to exert a powerful effect on human sexuality. Dr. Robert Frankl of Budapest University in Hungary

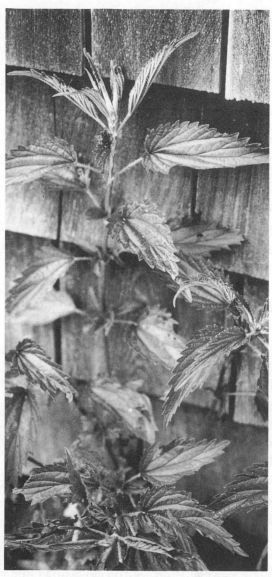

Urtica Dioica

found a vast increase in aerobic power, muscle strength, and sexual vitality among 12 males using a combination of nettle and oats. Additionally their testosterone levels increased remarkably. Dr. Frankl reported in 1984 that oats and nettle increase the libido in men by freeing the bio-availability of testosterone. The promise that this compound will help millions of people in this country suffering from low sexual interest or dysfunction is unlimited.

Meanwhile researchers from Northwestern Ohio University's College of Medicine, in Akron, demonstrated that the use of *Avena sativa* improved erectile ability and sexual functioning in men experiencing erectile dysfunction. Additionally, male blood hormone levels increased by approximately 30 percent.

The Institute for the Advanced Study of Human Sexuality in San Francisco, California, is dedicated to building upon this research with the goal of helping men and women with sexual problems recover their desire and vitality. They highly recommend the use of *Avena sativa* for some of the problems associated with sexual dysfunction. Why? Because the Institute has proven that *Avena sativa* works! After a six-week pilot program using *Avena sativa* on 40 men and women, Dr. Loretta Haroian of the Institute found that 90 percent of the men tested had greater sexual desire, performance, and sensation. One man who hadn't had an erection in six years was now able to have fulfilling sex three or four times a week. Most men reported firmer erections and more intense orgasm. One woman said that *Avena sativa* saved her marriage.

Encouraged by these results, researchers at the Institute moved to a cross-over, double blind study of over 120 men and women and achieved even more phenomenal results. Following an eight week program, men of all ages reported significant enhancement of sexual energy and performance, with testosterone increases of up to 185 percent after one month (IASHSRD 1990). This is very significant. As the researchers concluded, "Given that testosterone is the hormonal determinant of the attributes of manhood, sufficient bio-available levels should prolong the feelings and abilities associated with post-pubescent masculinity. It may very well be that many aspects of aging are due in part to low levels of free testosterone and that by supporting the integrity of bio-available testosterone, more men can retain youthful vitality including sexual interest and capacity as they age" (IASHSRD 1990).

According to Dr. Haroian, the active ingredient in *Avena sativa* isn't concentrated in the grain of the plants. She says that a "special extraction process that is quite different from the harvesting and processing of the grain" is required to isolate the active enzymes. Until recently, she noted, "No one had the special processing equipment necessary to extract the pure living oat enzymes." Some 24 enzymes have been isolated in the extract of *Avena sativa* alone but scientists have found that one particular substance, *Avena orientalis*, has a natural affinity for bonding with human testosterone, which in turn helps the male body produce more numerous healthy sperm.

The long search for sexual rejuvenation through natural remedies and stimulants seems to have finally achieved the scientific stamp of approval. Products incorporating quebracho bark and a mixture of *Avena sativa* and *Urtica dioica* have long been popular in Europe. Both hold promise for helping men and women fulfill their natural and healthy sexual urges and as restorers and preservers of sexual power. The basic message here is that "feeling your oats" is indeed sexy.

Television talk show host Geraldo Rivera recently interviewed a participant in the sexuality studies, 68-year-old Ray McIlvenna, introducing him as a "lack of desire victim." Rivera should have described him more accurately as a former victim!

After McIlvenna told about how his use of *Avena sativa* made him feel and perform "the way I was in my 30s and 40s"—Rivera's reply was short and sweet: "Well, God bless!"

Wild Yam

The last place you would expect to find some of the world's leading experts in the field of sexual performance would be in some muddy south-of-the-border yam field! But that's exactly where medical researchers have been focusing their attention, investigating the connection between orange-fleshed sweet potato and man's most pleasurable pastime—making love. And if preliminary indications hold true after the completion of more strict laboratory and clinical studies, there may well be a grain of truth to the myth of the hot-blooded Latin lover.

Scientists have discovered an amazing fact about the lowly wild yam (*Dioscorea villosa*). It seems that this edible starchy tuberous root used for centuries as a staple food throughout the tropical regions of the world is mother nature's number one source of pure, unadulterated steroids. That's right, steroids, the same stuff that you've been reading about in the newspapers during each Olympiad. Steroids are what help the power lifter lift greater amounts of weight, speed the sprinter to record times never before possible, and help professional football players fight off a double-team block. And the steroids in wild yam can dramatically improve your sex life. Completely safe from any of the side effects common to custom-tailored, laboratory-designed steroids which athletes use, this natural extract, taken in pill form, can have an amazing effect on the human male's performance in the bedroom. Many men, no matter how old they are, report a new-found vigor and rejuvenation of their ability and interest to make love.

Why is this? One of these natural sterols found in yams is a precursor to a hormone found in the human body called DHEA (dehydroepiandrosterone). This compound, and other sex-hormone-like substances are found in large amounts in yams, and therefore men in Mexico and South America countries have been taking preparations made from this plant to enhance their sexual potency. As one research noted, "Frankly we were caught by surprise. The isolation of the active ingredient we extracted from the Mexican yam proved to be far more powerful than originally thought."

Data, published in *The Proceedings of the New York Academy of Sciences,* explains why DHEA can have great benefits to human health and functioning. DHEA decreases in the body as we get older. In animal tests it has been shown that giving older animals DHEA supplements increases their immune function. Dr. Roger Loria of the Medical College of Virginia in Richmond has demonstrated that DHEA supplements can increase immune function to provide excellent protection against viral infections, from the common cold to herpes. How does this connect to sexual functioning? Simple. The immunologic theory on aging states that decreases in bodily functions are due to decreasing immune functions. Being able to increase immune functions means a slowing down of the aging process and a revitalization of bodily functions.

But there is more to the DHEA-sexual functioning story! Several doctors presented research findings at preventive medicine meetings that have shown a connection between blood sugar disorders and decreased sexual functioning. In summary: low blood sugar means bad sex. In several studies DHEA has been shown to be very effective in normalizing blood sugar levels, which was even found to be beneficial for diabetics.

DHEA acts like a buffer hormone to help maintain normal body composition. It has demonstrated potential to be effective in both weight-loss and weight-gain. How much of these substances should a man take? Recommended amounts are usually listed on the packages. However, the effectiveness is often increased if such formulations are taken in cycles; larger amounts for a few weeks, interrupted by taking nothing for one or two weeks (and then starting the cycle again) is often more effective than taking a small amount at all times. So be sure to take your wild yam supplements!

Ginkgo

A tree native to China and Japan, *Ginkgo* is cultivated and revered in temple gardens. *Ginkgo* has been known to aid the flow of blood and oxygen to the brain, thus increasing memory and awareness. This powerful and versatile herb also contains chemicals that prevent damage from free radicals. Because it improves circulation, it can help in cases where a man has circulation-related difficulties in getting an erection.

Sarsaparilla

Sarsaparilla is an herb found in Mexico, the Caribbean and the Orient that has been shown to affect testosterone levels in men. Testosterone-like substances in the herb cause this effect.

Licentious Goat Wort (Horny Goat Weed)

Funny name aside, this extract works! "The essential active element in this remarkable herb has natural affinities for the suprarenal glands and for the circulatory system," says Daniel Reid, author of *Chinese Herbal Medicine.* "Recent studies have shown that sperm count and semen density increase substantially in men during the first few hours after ingestion of this herb. Besides stimulating hormone production in the suprarenal glands, which in turn stimulates other related glands, this drug has a salutory effect on circulation of blood. When it enters blood vessels, especially the finer capillaries, its presence there causes them to dilate, thereby greatly enhancing circulation in tissues fed mainly by small capillaries, such as a man's penis. It also facilitates delivery of the extra hormones secreted into the bloodstream by the same drug. And, since it expands blood vessels, it causes a proportional decrease in blood pressure, making the herb safe for those who need it most."

Speaking to Women

The key to increasing sexual libido in both men *and women* is a gentle but subtle increase in their body's levels of testosterone. When this startling announcement was made by a world famous medical researcher at a recent scientific convention in Colorado, the eyes of both men and women lighted up with anticipation: finally the medical world had discovered a key sexual aphrodisiac!

Increasing testosterone in women is an important sexual enhancer, according to Julian Whitaker. M.D., editor of *Health & Healing,* the largest circulation medical newsletter in the world. "Testosterone enhances libido in both men and women," Dr. Whitaker reported at the proceedings of the American College of Advancement in Medicine at its annual meeting in Colorado Springs in November 1992. "Women with higher testosterone levels have more sex, increased libido, more orgasms and tighter bonds with their mates. It is a potent sexual enhancer."

Dr. Whitaker said that one patient whom he put on a testosterone-increasing program "has such a radiance of sensuality. She is a siren—thanks to increased testosterone." Her experience is typical of many women, he added. He noted that increasing testosterone in males also acts as a potent sexual potentiator.

So what can women do who want to empower themselves with an even stronger and more radiant sexuality? Clearly, a small increase in body testosterone is important. And the safest way of gently stimulating the body's own natural production of testosterone is through the use of *Avena sativa*.

Researchers at The Institute for Advanced Study of Human Sexuality who have studied the sexy benefits of *Avena sativa* note, "It is generally accepted that testosterone is the basis of libido in women" (1990). *Avena sativa,* they note, was instrumental in elevating testosterone levels in women and men. "It seems there is much work to be done if we are to understand the potential of *Avena Sativa* to enhance, restore and protect sexuality," say the researchers. "It is an exciting challenge, not only because the results are so welcome, *but because there are no harmful side effects.*"

The Institute for Advanced Study of Human Sexuality Research Department published in 1990 results from a crossover double blind study which looked at the sex enhancing effects of *Avena sativa* on women, "Some individual women reported significant improvement on one or more parameters," the report said.

Among the findings:

•A 28-year old female, using 300 milligrams of *Avena sativa* daily, reported that she, "felt better, more intense orgasms, more sexual dreams." She said she wanted "to keep taking [*Avena sativa*] and would like to try larger doses for special occasions."

•A 39-year old female reported that she liked her "more aggressive feelings about sex." She noted that *Avena sativa* "should be used by couples."

•A 25-year-old female ingested as much as 1,800 milligrams of *Avena sativa* prior to sexual encounters and reported increased tactile sensitivity and prolonged sexual desire with a focus on the physical and no need or desire for fantasy. "You are supersensitive to touch, sexual and nonsexual, especially in your mouth," she told researchers. "You just want to be all tangled up and real intense . . . You can go forever."

"For men, there is no doubt that *Avena sativa* is an effective enhancer of sexual desire, performance and activity," note the researchers.

"[Men] describe vigor and urgency reminiscent of their youth . . . The overall effect for the men who reported improvement can be summarized as a generalized sense of well-being with increased ability to function sexually . . . [with] a calm, confident capacity to initiate, perform and enjoy sexual activity."

A Final Word

The essential requirements—the foundation—for good sexual functioning consist of:

•*Physical Activity.* Exercise is the most effective way to stimulate endocrine functions. An exercised body is a body capable of doing physical things, and sex is certainly a physical thing.

•*Normal Weight.* Being overweight—especially in combination with eating the average high-fat diet—makes the blood cells in your body clot together, and reduces oxygen supply to the various organs. Instead of being ready-to-go, you become tired and ready to fall asleep. In addition, overweight people have lower sex hormone levels than people with normal weight.

•*Handling Stress.* If you are under stress and your mind is on something else that worries you, this is not conducive to a relaxed evening of good sex. Take care of the distress in your life first. This is often easier said than done, but it is something that you must take into consideration.

•*Smoking Cigarettes.* Several publications regarding cigarette smoking show a connection between number of years smoked, daily number of cigarettes smoked, and a decrease in sex hormones. The athlete or tough guy often represented in cigarette advertising is—in reality—not such a hot item. Athletic performance, sex and smoking just don't go together.

"Like all herbal therapy, aphrodisiacs must be taken over an extended period of time in order to have the desired effects," explains Reid. "Since they employ no synthetic chemicals or other artificial ingredients, they must work naturally with the body's circulatory and endocrine systems, and this takes time. Count on two or three months of daily doses for noticeable enhancement of sexual potency to become apparent."

Many health professionals believe that when taken regularly such tonics can increase hormone production, build overall strength, increase resistance to illness, and promote longevity—along with their sexually revitalizing powers. When supplements containing these botanical substances are used over weeks and months, they appear to work naturally with the body's endocrine and circulatory systems to perk up the libido, stimulate glandular secretions, enhance circulation, and flush the organs with heat and energy creating a build-up of erotic impulses.

Dr. Watson's Herbal Pharmacy
of Sexual Stimulants and Sexy Energizers

The following herbs are discussed by Dr. Watson in her fantastic new book *Love Potions*, available now in bookstores to provide you with a storehouse of information on how to make your sex life sizzling. These are just a few of the herbal stimulants recommended. They can be used in one of two ways: taken daily to boost overall vitality in the long term or more specifically as aphrodisiacs to strengthen sexual organs and ignite passion in preparation for lovemaking.

Suma. Suma (*Pfaffia paniculata*) is also known as Brazilian ginseng. Probably it acquired the nickname because like ginseng it is adaptogenic and can be taken to stimulate the immune system and vitality in general. Suma can be taken as a tonic daily for energy and stamina to fortify hormones and stabilize blood sugar. It has even been reported to help reduce tumors and cancers. Doses of at least 9 grams daily are recommended.

Guarana. Guarana (*Paullinia cupana*) is indigenous to Brazil. Natives of South America make a powdered substance from the dry bark of this jungle vine and mix it with water as a pick-me-up. It is remarkable for relieving mental exhaustion, as a remendy for a hang-over headache, and as an appetite suppressant (not surprising, as guarana contains three times more caffeine than coffee).

Panax Ginseng. Ginseng is perhaps the best known of the so-called aphrodisiac herbs.

Animal research indicates that despite its reputation, while it does not have a specific effect on the sexual organs, the plant has gained its reputation because of its ability to increase all-around well-being, stamina, and endurance.

Ancient Vedic texts from India claim that ginseng "bestows the power of a bull on men both young and old." In Japan and China, ginseng is used ritually to increase longevity and prevent senility.

The most frequently used sexual stimulant preparation is made from the ginseng plant and it apparently works best on the male hormone system. Quality control is an important point with ginseng preparations, and they are only effective if taken in minimum amounts. Ginseng usually has a potentiating effect on other preparations; that means that it can be taken together with other natural preparations and to increase effectiveness.

Glycyrrhiza Glabra. A plant that has been used worldwide for centuries for medicinal and aphrodisiac purposes, the ancient Egyptians, Chinese, and Indians used it in various forms to increase longevity and to improve erotic arousal and stamina.

Glycyrrhiza Glabra contains traces of phytoestrogen sterols similar to those produced by the adrenal glands.

Bee Pollen. A compact package of nutrients, pollen contains B vitamins, vitamin C, trace minerals, unsaturated fatty acids, proteins, antibacterial and immune-boosting properties, and—you guessed it!—substances that stimulate the sex glands and hormone production. No more than a couple of teaspoons of bee pollen granules a day will yield powerful results.

Where to Find the Formula

Editor's Note: Fortunately, for men and women who wish to take advantage of the powerful herbs *Avena sativa* and *Urtica dioica*, there is now a formula that combines them in a synergistic base of zinc and boron. This formula is called Sexativa. It is based on the same formula proven to work by the Institute for Advanced Study of Human Sexuality. Sexativa, with *Avena sativa* and *Urtica dioica*, can be ordered by calling (800) 825-8482. Another great formula with quebracho bark and L-arginine that readers might be interested in is called Mood Elevator and it can also be ordered from the same company. L-arginine is especially important for men suffering common forms of impotency, since its presence in the body stimulates formation of nitric oxide which is necessary for erections. The combination of quebracho bark and L-arginine appears to work synergistically for both men and women.

21. *Increased Energy*

How would you like to go all day and into the night, calm, directed and with a quiet, steady driving flow of energy? How would you like to avoid the lethargy associated with transient depression or sluggishness? How would you like to have the calmness of mind to let the little things, that really don't matter, slide? Would you like to feel that you have the mental power to handle any problem? By using the powerful nutrients in your growing phyto-pharmacy, you can enjoy day long serenity and a kind of energy that burns like the even flame of a candle in a still room. We're going to tell you about several plant substances that can convey those powers.

"We have all at some point in our life experienced anxiety," says David Hoffmann, author of *The New Holistic Herbal* (1990). "Normally the feeling lasts only for a short time and is caused by some relevant external problem." However, when we experience anxiety habitually, he says, our thoughts and behavior are unduly influenced by anxiety; he says we perceive the world filtered through our attitude of anxiety and we act accordingly. "We enter a vicious circle where anxiety produces more anxiety."

When anxiety, hyperactivity and depression become all too powerful in your life, that's when you will find nervous system relaxants, derived from botanical extracts and amino acids, helpful. They provide a buffer from the anxiety cycle. "In addition to the nervine relaxants," Hoffmann says, "the anti-spasmodic herbs are useful, as often in cases of anxiety there is also muscle tension, the relief of which helps the whole being to move to a state of ease and well-being, the perfect inner state within which to bring about healing."

Getting from here to there, creating energy flow, the calmness of mind and steady driving force necessary to productive days is all that much easier when you know which phytochemicals and nutrients are are your special allies.

Symphytum

The key energy compound in the human body is called adenosine triphosphate (ATP). One of the key stimulators of ATP production in the body is allantoin. Typically, people with sufficient allantoin in their systems are bright, alert and feel naturally spirited.

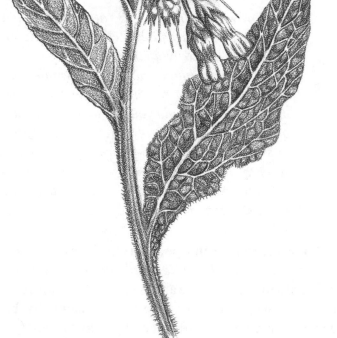

Symphytum

What happens when we don't have enough ATP to sustain optimal body function? Cellular reproduction slows, the body begins feeling sluggish, and our vital organs start to wear.

Unfortunately many people have diets with low quantities of allantoin partly because processing foods—especially grains—destroys allantoin. How can we ingest enough allantoin to ease depression?

We must go to nature's storehouse: *Symphytum,* more commonly known as comfrey—one of the most valuable herbs known to botanical pharmaceutical experts. Comfrey is a rich source of allantoin which stimulates the cells to increase their production of ATP. This herb with its beautiful purple-white flowers and large fuzzy leaves is nature's allantoin warehouse. Ancient herbalists and healers used comfrey for hundreds of ailments including anemia, arthritis, boils, bruises, burns, diarrhea, emphysema, eczema, gangrene, gout, hay fever, pleurisy. "The impressive wound-healing properties of comfrey are partially due to the presence of allantoin," notes David Hoffmann. "This chemical stimulates cell proliferation and so augments wound-healing both inside and out."

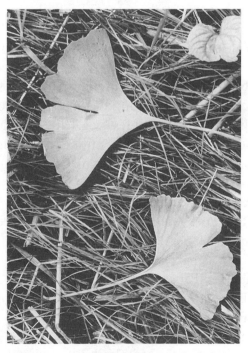

In addition to containing allantoin, comfrey is loaded with vitamins A and C, calcium, potassium, phosphorous, protein, iron, magnesium, sulfur, copper, zinc, and 18 amino acids.

Ginkgo Biloba

Yet another safe herbal remedy designed to battle depression that can result from the stress and tension of modern living comes from the oldest tree in the world. This

Ginkgo Biloba

amazing tree, part of the family known as *Ginkgoaceae,* can be traced back 200 million years. Although little known or used in the United States, physicians worldwide wrote in 1989 more than 10 million prescriptions for this tree's extract, known as *Ginkgo biloba.* Indeed, annual sales are estimated at $500 million, and one European phytopharmaceutical company has established a twelve-hundred-tree plantation in South Carolina (Pelton 1989).

We can thank the dedicated environmentalists of ancient China for its survival. Ross Pelton, Ph.D., explains: "The ginkgo tree nearly became extinct during the last Ice Age. Two thousand years ago it was nearly driven to extinction by the advance of civilization in China. It was saved by Chinese monks who considered it a sacred tree and grew it inside their temples. In addition to its beauty, the ginkgo tree has another unique characteristic. At high temperatures it secretes a sap that acts as a fire retardant. It is thought that this protective quality is one reason why ginkgo trees surround many Buddhist temples throughout China and Japan . . . . Ginkgo trees now line the streets in many cities around the world. Powerful antioxidant compounds in the ginkgo tree are thought to be responsible for the tree's hardiness and ability to thrive in polluted city environments."

The leaves of the tree possess a number of compounds that have therapeutic benefits. In addition to being prescribed to counter depression, *Ginkgo biloba* has been used for cardiovascular problems, senility, and impotence. Some 34 major studies concerning the healing powers of *Ginkgo* extracts have been published over the last few years and worldwide interest in this ancient tree's powers continues to grow stronger. In March 1988, *The New York Times* reported laboratory synthesis of the compound ginkgolide B eventually could lead to its widespread use in treating asthma, toxic shock, Alzheimer's disease, and various circulatory disorders.

How does *Ginkgo biloba* work? As Pelton (1989) explains its actions include:

•Increasing circulation to the brain by increasing blood flow through capillaries that are farthest from the heart.

•Preventing oxygen free radical damage to the brain.

•Protecting nerve tissue from damage due to decreased blood flow and oxygen deficit.

•Enhancing the brain's ability to metabolize the energy fuel, glucose.

•Increasing nerve transmission.

•Repairing lesions in cell membranes caused by oxygen free radical damage.

Ginkgo biloba is an especially important nutrient for people as they age and their heart grows weaker and blood doesn't move as fast. This condition is known as vascular insufficiency. In one study, *Ginkgo biloba* was given to 166 senior citizens suffering from vascular insufficiency. *Ginkgo biloba* created a statistically significant improvement in cerebral vascular circulation and mental functioning (Pelton 1989). Perhaps most intriguing is *Ginkgo biloba's* effects on mental alertness. Pelton (1989) reports that: *"Ginkgo* affects mental alertness by actually changing the frequency of brain waves. A double-blind study, in which EEG monitors were used on the subjects, showed that *Ginkgo* extract increases brain alpha rhythms. These are the brain wave frequencies associated with mental alertness. The monitors also indicated a decrease in brain theta rhythms, which are the slower brain frequencies associated with a lack of attention and an 'unfocused' state of mind."

The way that *Ginkgo* is used is important. Its half-life in the body is only about three hours which means that at that time only about half of what was ingested will remain active with the rest having been metabolized or excreted (Pelton 1989). Furthermore, although high doses have led to short-term memory improvement, *Ginkgo biloba* acts slowly, its effects building over time. Experts recommend a disciplined use of ginkgo, three times daily, to maintain therapeutic blood levels (Pelton 1989). Stay with ginkgo. Sometimes three to six months are needed for improvement to become evident.

Valerian Root

When Friar Lawrence gave Juliet a potion to make her sleep in William Shakespeare's *Romeo and Juliet* its main ingredient was valerian root.

Valeriana officinalis has some 170 varieties spread throughout North America, Europe and Asia. More than 50 tons of valerian root are sold each year in France where it is a popular over-the-counter sedative. Even though valerian has been used as a medication for as long as historical information has been available, it has only recently been the object of scientific scrutiny. Mowrey (1986) reports that: "In a remarkable series of animal experiments that followed, the herb was proven to be sedative, to improve coordination, and to antagonize the hypnotic effects of alcohol. Meanwhile, clinical evidence obtained by careful testing by trained medical practitioners was accumulating. This evidence showed that in humans, Valerian root was strongly sedative. It also had a marked tendency to increase concentration ability, as well as energy level . . . . Valmane, a German drug containing pure substances from Valerian root, has been frequently studied. It has been shown to suppress and regulate the autonomic nervous system in patients with control disorders, to be mildly sedative, to help regulate psychosomatic disorders, and relieve tension and restlessness. In another study, hypertensive men were given a glass of water containing extract of Valerian root. After

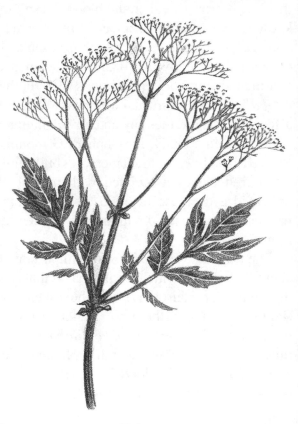

Valerian

a given period of time an examination revealed a general tranquilizing effect and EEG readings that indicated an elective neurotropic action on higher brain centers, thereby fulfilling criterion for being labeled a tranquilizer."

One-hundred-sixty-six volunteers took part in a Swiss test designed to prove once and for all whether Valerian root can improve sleep. Using the double-blind format, half the subjects were given capsules containing valerian extract. Every one of the subjects reported great improvement in both the quality and quantity of their sleep. That test also revealed several curious results. Smokers reported that they slept better with the valerian extract. Likewise, the usual morning hangover connected with other sleeping formulations did not occur. This suggests that sleep induced by Valerian—instead of by some narcotic drug—allows the endocrine system to function more fully and leaves one feeling refreshed in the morning.

Valerian, unlike prescribed sedatives, can safely be used with alcohol. This is due to the apparent lack of synergism between valerian and alcohol. Unlike pharmaceutical sedatives, valerian is non-addictive. In 1981, improved reaction times in patients given a preparation of valerian and hops were noted in a German test measuring stress reduction. More recently, Swedish researchers conducted a double-blind study in 1988 on 27 subjects, 21 of whom said Valerian was better than the control. Forty-four percent reported perfect sleep while eighty-nine percent reported improved sleep, all without side effects.

Other tests have proved that Valerian is also effective against stress reactions like headaches, fatigue, irritability, and that it can coax the body's natural restorative powers into action. Recent tests have shown that valerian, when ingested in combination with other natural herbs, combines the best of both worlds. Valerian helps the body sleep naturally, while the other herbs go to work helping the body restore itself. For example Valerian works well with comfrey and amino acids. As opposed to many narcotic sleeping agents which neutralize certain amino acids, Valerian is a good neighbor to all the amino acids. Valerian is a safe and effective sleeping aid, says Andrew Weil, M.D., author of *Natural Health, Natural Medicine*. For these and other reasons, it deserves serious consideration for use in this country as a mild sedative. It is a safe, herbal remedy that really works and deserves a place in the home.

Scutellaria Laterifolia

Mowrey (1986) calls *Scutellaria laterifolia,* also known as skullcap, a good tonic for excitability, restlessness and other nervous complaints. Most research, he says, has been carried out in Russia. "Some major Russian medical books discuss the scientific findings in great detail. Therein, experiments are reviewed which have proven Skullcap to be a tonic [and] sedative." In the U.S., our knowledge of skullcap dates to at least 1861 when physician J.D. Gunn, author of the *New Domestic Physician or Home Book of Health*, noted that, "Skullcap is a valuable tonic nervine and antispasmodic. It is especially useful in . . . neuralgia, convulsions, delirium tremens . . . nervous excitability, restlessness, and inability to sleep, and indeed in all nervous affections." Says Mowrey (1986), "From that time to the present, natural health experts have recognized the value of Skullcap for these kinds of problems." Hoffmann (1990) recommends the use of Skullcap along with Valerian root.

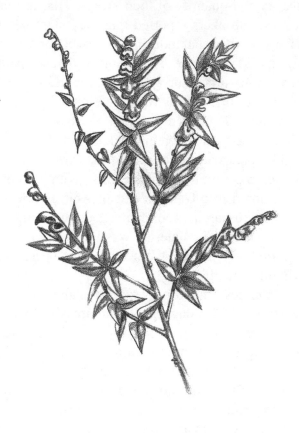

Scutellaria Laterifolia

Paullinia Cupana

Centuries ago, the Indians of Brazil discovered the seeds of a fruit similar in appearance to grapes were natural stimulants that increased energy while at the same time decreasing appetite. The natives called the plant guarana. Botanists who later studied the plant named it *Paullinia Cupana*. It belongs to the *Sapindaceae* family of plants which are indigenous to the rain forest.

In part its stimulatory effect is derived from the caffeine and tannin contained in the fruit. Not surprisingly, *Paullinia Cupana* is a major ingredient in three of the major soft drinks in Brazil.

The first recorded mention of this plant occurred in the late 1550s, following the Portuguese discovery of the Amazon (Waters 1989). The journals and log books that these explorers kept contain reports of sampling a bitter tea created from an unusual plant that had a smooth, erect stem and an ovoid fruit the size of a grape.

This tea, they learned, was used by the natives for a wide range of physical and mental problems—headaches, neuralgia, menstrual difficulties and disorders and bowel complications.

In October and November, as the fruit ripened, it was harvested and the fruits were spread in the sun to dry. When dry, the shells were cracked open and the white seeds in the center were removed. Next, the natives ground these seeds with a stone mortar in a deep dish of hard sandstone. When it was ground, they wet the powder to form a paste. Then they would add a certain amount of whole and broken seeds. Next, they molded the dough into loaves measuring five to eight inches in length, weighing 12 to 16 ounces, drying them over slow heat. After several days, when the white loaves had turned dark brown, the natives would shave off a piece, boil it in water, sit back and enjoy its medicinal qualities.

The most impressive effect this tea had on the first European explorers was that when they drank it, they experienced a feeling of pep, vitality, and alertness. The natives explained that they, too, often drank this tea when they were feeling fatigued and listless.

The explorers returned to Portugal with samples of the plant and soon it became widely used in Europe. Today, Brazilians look upon *Paullinia Cupana* as having all the exhilarating effects of other stimulants without the side effects. The herb is a staple in preparations designed to increase mental alertness, combat fatigue, and decrease hunger. It is sold throughout South America and Europe in a liquid form.

Several years ago, a botanist named Grieve wrote a now-classic reference manual called *A Modern Herbal* which explains that *Paullinia Cupana* contains several active ingredients besides caffeine and tannin. He says it's a gentle excitant and serviceable when the brain is irritated or depressed by mental exertion, fatigue or exertion from hot weather.

One reason modern Europeans and Brazilians like to buy and use *Paullinia Cupana* is the way it works in weight loss. The appetite-suppressing nature of this natural fruit, combined with its ability to give the body a feeling of a natural high, helps reduce the anxiety of a diet. One of the best things said about *Paullinia* is that people use it as a natural stimulant to reduce fatigue and hunger, so that one is encouraged to stay on a healthy, well-balanced diet.

The FDA has adopted a wait-and-see position regarding *Paullinia Cupana*, but even the agency can't deny that the tablets are being consumed by health-conscious Americans even faster than the Brazilian rain forest is being consumed by fire. We know one user who says, "It gives me a definite zap of energy. I feel mellow and laid back but I seem to have extra energy all day." Most users agree, that even though the stimulation is notable, there are no disagreeable side-effects, no heavy let down sometimes associated with other stimulants. As a matter of fact, research on *Paullinia Cupana* is now centering around just exactly how the seeds of this plant release energy in the body. One hopes that those secrets will be revealed before the plant is completely destroyed in Brazil. Because of its rapid destruction, you may well want to try the gentle stimulatory effects of *Paullinia Cupana . . . now.*

Royal Jelly

Royal Jelly is produced by worker bees and fed to a chosen ordinary female bee when in the larvae stage. The royal jelly causes the female to grow to nearly twice her normal size; she becomes incredibly fertile, laying over twice her weight in eggs in a single period. She ends up living more than five years compared to the life span of only a few weeks for other bees. Her diet is exclusively royal jelly.

In Japan, royal jelly is the most popular of all nutritional supplements but it is also extraordinarily popular in other parts of the world—perhaps because beekeepers are considered to be among the most long-lived people in the world. Not surprisingly, bee keepers will tell you that the most prized gift from their hives is royal jelly.

Royal jelly is one of the richest natural sources of pantothenic acid and is rich in many other B vitamins as well as 18 amino acids and all eight of the essential amino acids. It also contains minerals such as iron, potassium and silicon.

For several thousand years, Chinese and Japanese natives have consumed

daily doses of royal bee jelly. In these two countries royal bee jelly has been used for:
   •Helping convalescents gain weight
   •Regulating constipation and diarrhea
   •Producing energy
   •Tranquilizing effects
   •Boosting blood volume
   •Increasing the amounts of hemoglobin in the blood
   •Cleansing blood, flushing pollutants from the capillaries
   •Oxygenating the body, allowing more oxygen to reach the body's organs and brain cells

Athletes have known about the energizing effects of bee pollen for years. After the 1972 Munich Olympics, Lasse Viren, the Finnish winner of the 5,000 and 10,000 meter events, admitted that he had been eating honeybee pollen for years. Royal bee jelly is a wonderful tonic. Try some.

Tyrosine

Dr. Mindell (1980) notes that tyrosine, "is a natural amino acid that holds promise of being a major aid in the treatment of emotional or mental depression." An amino acid, tyrosine is found in complete protein foods such as meat, fish, eggs, dairy products, seeds, nuts, and some whole grains.

How does tyrosine work? Mindell (1980) explains that tyrosine "releases a substance called catecholamine which, in turn, increases the rate at which brain neurons (nerve cells with conducting fibers) produce dopamine and norepinephrine. The reaction seems to act against emotional depression."

The compounds—epinephrine and norepinephrine—have wide ranging activities that affect brain and nerve cells. Their most important quality is their ability to create a non- narcotic sensation of calmness. Both compounds are produced in nerve cells, as well as in the adrenal medulla where they can be stored. A third compound produced from tyrosine is dopamine, which affects nerve tracts in the brain. Among the studies showing tyrosine's tranquilizing power is one published in the *American Journal of Psychiatry* by Dr. Alan J. Gelenberg of the Harvard Medical School. Dr. Gelenberg's patients all responded positively to oral doses of tyrosine. In another study, three of five patients experienced at least a 50 percent reduction in depression scale scoring after four weeks of supplementation with tyrosine compared with one of four controls receiving placebo. The reduction in depression rating score was positively correlated with the increase in levels of tyrosine in blood plasma, suggesting that an adequate tyrosine level was necessary for improvement. In a small study looking at two amphetamine-dependent patients, one was able to eliminate dependency on the stimulant entirely and the other to reduce dependency by two-thirds after using tyrosine. The recommended dosage for tyrosine is 100 milligrams to two grams three times daily.

Biotin

Deficiencies in biotin may cause depression. In one case report a patient was experiencing depression along with nausea and vomiting, insomnia, paresthesias, headaches, and lethargy. Within five days after being supplemented with biotin at 300 micrograms daily, significant improvement was noted and he quickly returned to a normal non-depressed state (Levenson 1983). In an experimental study four normal subjects received a diet deficient only in biotin. After 10 weeks they were depressed, fatigued, sleepy and complained of nausea, anorexia and muscular pains. All signs and symptoms were alleviated by biotin supplementation (Sydenstricker 1940).

BH4-Biopterin

A brain chemical, BH4-biopterin has been shown to be deficient in people suffering from stress. Research in Austria has shown that a relative lack of BH4-biopterin in the brain may lead to clinical stress. That same study showed that by using BH4-biopterin supplementation, patients reported a general feeling of well-being and were more relaxed.

Depression is a cause of decreased life span. The elderly tend to become more easily depressed. That is why supplements that fight depression naturally are so important. By using the nutrients discussed in this chapter, you can give yourself a mental edge all day.

22. *Exercise*

Take care of your body. After all, it's only human!

"**We can make a 95-year-old as strong as a 50-year-old person and a** 65-year-old as physically fit as a healthy 30-year-old, and, if there are no underlying disorders, mental sharpness is retained," Dr. William Evans, chief of the Tufts University Health Science Center's human physiology laboratory, told reporters (Kotulak 1991). "Many of the biological markers of aging are not valid at all. Rather, they are markers of inactivity and poor nutrition."

The gangster Bugsy Siegel had a favorite saying—at least as portrayed by Warren Beatty in the 1992 Academy Award winning film *Bugsy*. Now, Bugsy Siegel was no role model and we wouldn't pretend that he was anything more than a low down gangster. But Bugsy had a favorite saying, short and to the point:

"Everybody deserves a fresh start."

Certainly, the best avenue for a fresh start can begin at any time—morning, afternoon or evening—when you punctuate your day with a robust aerobic exercise program. That is because exercise is the great renewer.

Exercise is one of the keys to youth. When we're young we use our bodies.

We bend, stretch, run, leap, and jump. Joy emanates from our being because of bodily movement. We just naturally twist and turn like a New York pretzel. But as we age and become consumed with wage earning, paying the mortgage, our kids' college tuition and working we begin to neglect our bodies, and we no longer exercise as much as when we were carefree children. And presto! We feel old. We lose our childlike enthusiasm and joy!

If you're feeling tired or depressed it is often not your mind that is feeling so but your body.

Fortunately, no matter how neglected your body has been, it will respond to an exercise program!

We all want a fresh start. By combining optimal nutrition with exercise that second chance will be yours.

Today's new breed of scientists and health professionals are involved in a quest for the proper combination of nutrition and exercise that can bring us to the edge of eternity.

At the Human Nutrition Research Center on Aging at Tufts University, elderly people who are in their nineties are taking up weight lifting and their muscle function is being increased by 200 to 300 percent (Kotulak 1991).

It used to be that when we thought ahead about retiring that we thought of "taking it easy," settling down in front of the TV or on a chair on the porch. Indeed physicians were part of the problem. Doctors would see a patient with white hair and say: "Well, you need to take it easy and you're not supposed to be playing tennis anyway." But we have recently learned that exercise is an absolutely essential part of any program designed to achieve maximum life span.

Indeed, health professionals today, advocate an energetic, nutritionally optimal and active lifestyle upon retirement.

"We know that nutrition and exercise can make a big difference," Dr. Evans told reporters. "The real challenge is to convince people to do it" (Kotulak 1991).

The qualities of people most of us simply call "aging" are part of a diseased state caused by "taking it easy." Loss of hair pigment, shakiness of the limbs, slow movement, deafness and even reduced lung and heart function—all of these qualities and many others are indicators of biological, not physical, age, reports Dr. James Fozard, director of the National Institute on Aging's Baltimore aging study.

The bottom line, say researchers, is that aging is intertwined with good or poor dietary habits, lifestyle factors such as lack of exercise, smoking and boozing and your outlook on life—positive or negative thinking.

"Fifteen years ago we saw aging as a disease to which every older person succumbed," says Dr. Gene D. Cohen, acting director of the National Institute on Aging, in Bethesda, MD (Kotulak 1991). "People now can have a glimpse of what could be. They see that they can live longer, and that's influencing their behavior. It changes their thinking about cigarettes, drinking, food, lack of exercise and high-risk behaviors."

"You only get one machine, and you have to take care of it," Dr. Pantel Vokonas, director of the Normative Aging Study at Boston's Veterans Administration Medical Center, told reporters. Volunteers who practice what the scientists preach live an average of 10 years longer than today's average life span of approximately 74 for men (Kotulak 1991).

Indeed, Dr. Evans says that exercise is a key to longevity and good health. He points out that his studies have shown this to be true particularly in the case of halting bone loss in postmenopausal women. Dr. Evans discovered that human subjects who did no more than walk four days a week for slightly under an hour were able to stop the onset of osteoporosis. In essence, they stopped losing bone mass. Not just a little but a lot! Dr. Everett Smith, Professor of Preventive Medicine at the University of Wisconsin in Madison, has found that women who engaged in exercise programs had a four to five percent increase in bone mass of the spine and hips after four to five years.

Another classic example: Dr. Maria Fiatarone of the Harvard Medical School took a group of aged and decrepit seniors, nursing home refugees, who were about to be confined to their beds until death. She led them through a weight-training session three times a week. That impetus got their bodies juiced up and excited like young colts, and they began walking and exercising as if 20 years of rust and disuse had been shed! Her work totally destroyed preconceptions by doctors that once muscle tone is lost it cannot be regained especially in the aged.

She told reporters that the results were all the more revealing because of the poor physical condition that these people were in when they began to exercise. Her study showed that anybody can get in shape at any age, and that if you don't use your body, you do lose its natural vitality—but not forever.

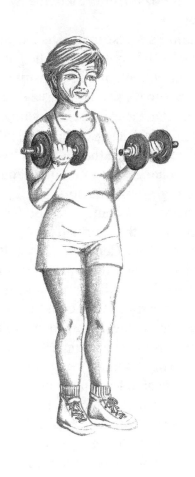

How important are optimal nutrition habits when combined with a sensible exercise program? "Various studies have shown that physical inactivity in adult life shortens life expectancy," notes *The Surgeon General's Report on Nutrition and Health* (1988).

The average male today in the U.S. lives to about 74 years of age. But volunteers, who are participating in the Baltimore Longitudinal Study and Boston Normative Aging study, are living to 80 or 82 on the average—the result of their superior nutritional and lifestyle habits.

A recent study by Dr. Glen E. Gresham, Chair of the Rehabilitation Medicine Department at the University of New York at Buffalo, used physical therapy on elderly patients with osteoarthritis in the knees and found that most had increased functional capacity and decreased pain.

Gresham and colleagues conducted their study on 80 older people with osteoarthritis of the knees, a condition that affects about ten percent of the elderly population. The three-month rehabilitation program strengthened the leg muscles around the knee by using a specially developed exercise bench; its purpose was to delay the progression of the condition and postpone artificial knee surgery. The pain and stiffness and decreased range of motion and muscle weakness that accompanies osteoarthritis can severely impair the ability of afflicted people to climb stairs, rise from a chair or even stand comfortably and walk. Yet of the 80 patients in Dr. Gresham's study, 72 experienced less pain; 68 had improved muscle strength; and endurance, and 76 had increased capacity.

"We're not claiming that you would completely do away with the need for a knee replacement, but it's quite conceivable now that it would postpone the day," said Dr. Gresham who suffers himself from the condition of osteoarthritis of the knees.

The Simple Art of Walking

We have so many conveniences today that we simply don't *need* to use our bodies as much. In the 1930s, the average person worked off about 2,600 calories daily beyond what was needed to keep the body warm and functioning.

Today, people burn only about 600 activity calories a day. That energy expenditure figure can be increased by doing simple things like walking.

Studies indicate that burning about 300 calories in activity each day can add years to a person's life. The simplest way to burn 300 or so calories is to walk about three miles—a time requirement of 45 to 60 minutes for most people.

Five Keys to Starting a Walking Program

Here are some tips for yoru walking program:
•Using a car odometer, drive one-half mile from home in several directions.
•Each day, pick one of your previously measured routes; walk out and then back. Don't hurry; take some time to marvel at the wondrous sights of life on Earth; after all, life is a gift!
•When each route can be comfortably walked in 15 minutes, increase your distance to two miles.
•Increase your distance to three miles when two miles can be covered in 30 minutes.
•The final goal is three miles in 45 minutes. Beginners can expect to spend eight to twelve weeks reaching this goal.

Keeping Up Your Exercise Program

Try these motivational strategies:
•Exercising with a friend or spouse is the best move that can be made when starting an exercise program. People who walk or work out with a partner are much more likely to keep at it, according to several studies. Whether it is the camraderie or the peer pressure, no one knows, but the buddy system seems to work.
•A lot of people seem to think of healthful eating and regular exercise as bandwagons they'd like to jump on. But that's a poor metaphor to use regarding exercise. Unfortunately, when people fall off a bandwagon, it continues to roll on out of reach. Rather you should think of healthful living via exercise as a bicycle. Sure, you may fall. But it's no problem to climb back on. Like bike riding, once the body learns how to live more healthfully, it will never forget it's a blast!

•Engage in a variety of fitness activities instead of the same thing over and over again. You will be less likely to suffer injuries, according to Dr. James Garrick, found and medical director of the Center for Sports Medicine at St. Francis Memorial Hospital in San Francisco.

• *"Think I'm a failure, huh?" you're saying. "I'll show you!"* That kind of thinking leads people—who haven't exercised in 10 years—to go to a gym, lift more weights than they should in the beginning, run faster then they ought to, and then give up. That kind of thinking leads people to move from one miracle exercise program to the next. Any exercise is great! The key is to start slowly, never exceed your comfort level and do it daily. You will improve steadily.

•Changing your physical shape with exercise is an achievable goal that can happen if you will it to happen. But don't use the word *want*. If you use *want* phrases such as, " I want to lose weight . . . I want to be strong . . . I want to be sexier . . ."—a funny psychological thing happens. You become weak. Don't ever use the word *want*. Rather, you should say, "I *am* going to lose weight . . . I *am* strong . . . I *am* sexy." Make yourself hungry for those results.

There are many ways that exercise can exert a positive effect on your health and appearance. The point is to start and enjoy the heck out of all kinds of exercising from good old fashioned stretching to swimming and perhaps even some jogging, and don't be afraid to start some huffing and puffing. After all, you've got this wonderful gift called the human body.

23. *Weight Loss: Simple and Easy!*

Although the Ice Age ended 10,000 years ago, our bodies remain genetically programmed as though we still lived during a time when food was scarce and fatty foods, with their high-caloric content, were absolutely essential.

Now you may want to lose weight—you may need to for medical reasons such as high blood pressure—but your body may have a darn good reason for preventing you from losing weight!

Genetic Vestiges of the Ice Age

Our genes still remember that during the Ice Age, food was scarce-- especially during the winter. As a result it was in the body's best survival interest that men and women should eat as much food as possible when it was plentiful. The added fat accumulated during the brief summer and fall meant survival during the long starving periods of winter. Extra body fat meant added energy to burn during the winter and added warmth (*Intelli-Scope* 1992).

Indeed, even at the turn of the century the heft of a man was thought of as a symbol of success. Our greatest men such as banker J.P. Morgan, presidents like Grover Cleveland, William McKinley and Theodore Roosevelt all had great paunches and heft, and in our primitive minds, we *knew* that these were successful men!

The Curse of Fat!

But no longer do we face the feast or famine days of the Ice Age. Whereas 10,000 years ago, death most often resulted from famine and scarcity, today we are the victims of over abundance. We have abundant supplies of beef, fowl, pork. Not surprisingly, many of our most common diseases today seem somehow connected with the excessive intake of fat—cancer, heart disease, diabetes.

Being Trim is Good!

Being trim is healthy. The National Institutes of Health is engaged in experimental studies on animals that invariably demonstrate that the most long-lived subjects are those whose diets are lowest in calories (Kotulak 1991). Researchers believe that people too can benefit from some form of caloric restriction, and that they can delay the premature aging effect often associated with excessive body weight. So, it is good to be thin—not just from the modern aesthetic but from our knowledge of longevity. Caloric restriction is absolutely important!

In addition, being trim is sexy, and it adds a certain lightness to your movement. Finally, being trim increases your self-esteem. When you know you look good, people are attracted to your positive attitude and want to be with you!

Some 95 percent of people who lose weight through caloric restriction alone end up gaining it back within one year (*Intelli-Scope* 1992).

"The bottom line is that, if you want to get rid of body fat, caloric restriction —not eating when you're hungry—is the ultimate unnatural act," longevity specialist Durk Pearson, author of *Life Extension* (Warner Books 1981) recently told a reporter. "Your genes are telling you you're going to die if you do this, and in fact, when people lose weight too fast with any technique, the master control center in their brain will actually alter their metabolism to make it very difficult to lose further fat, because that fat is their Ice Age life insurance policy."

Trick the Body!

There are five aspects to weight loss that you need to use in order to succeed.

1. The first thing that must be done is to restrict caloric intake. You need to be ruthlessly honest, look at your daily food consumption patterns and decide where you can cut out high-calorie indulgences. Then do it! All too many people are sneaks who are constantly snacking and then they wonder why they cannot lose weight.

2. Use natural thermogenic dietary supplements that increase the base metabolism so that you can burn more calories per day. These include botanical extracts such as *Ephedra sinica* and *Camellia sinsensis.* Both of these botanicals increase the rate at which the body burns fat. It is like turning up the gas under a pot of water. Both of these botanicals have the added bonus of suppressing appetite. Thus, the best time to use them is in the morning and afternoon, so that you do not end up overeating by snacking. *Ephedra* is a key weight loss ally. It is truly an amazing botanical.

3. You should not skip meals when dieting. Be sure to eat breakfast. A good breakfast is one rich in whole grains which will help transport food out of your body more quickly and offer some four to six hours of sound satiety.

4. Furthermore you should fool the body by substituting nonfat treats and foods for fatty foods. For example, you can now find nonfat cheeses and cold cuts that are 98 percent fat free. They will trick your body into thinking it is getting a fatty food, yet it isn't! You can consume nonfat frozen yogurt instead of ice cream. You should also eat plenty of complex carbohydrates (whole grains) and water-heavy fruits and vegetables.

The bottom line is that you should drastically cut down on sweets, fatty foods and increase high-fiber foods. Consumption of sugars actually induces hunger through low blood sugar levels and fatty foods remind your body how much it loves to eat more fatty foods. But there is no reason not to eat nonfat versions of your favorite foods! And be sure to supplement with a broad-based multivitamin and multimineral supplement like the one described in *Chapter 2.* With caloric restriction you have to be make sure that you are getting all the nutrients necessary for optimal nutrition both through judicious selection of foods and supplementation.

Exercise!

The fifth and final part of a successful weight-loss program is exercise. Any exercise. Even ten minutes a day of exercise. Just get that metabolism up! You can exercise before showering in the morning by doing sit-ups, lunges or aerobics.

The point is to make it vigorous (provided your physical condition allows you to do so). As Durk Pearson explains, "All exercises aren't created equally in terms of getting rid of fat. You may think that jogging for half an hour would be much better for getting rid of body fat than running as hard as you can for 30 seconds. Actually, it doesn't work that way" (*Intelli-Scope* 1992). The 30-second burst of exercise releases more noradrenaline into your bloodstream, which contributes to speeding up your metabolism for two to four or more hours.

A Final Word

Follow each step as we have outlined; be sure to work gradually at cutting down caloric intake especially through honest self-appraisal of your eating habits, and don't be a sneak! Envision your new, thin self!

Your chances at weight-loss are better than ever thanks to thermogenic botanicals to help to cut your calorie intake. But don't forget one other secret weapon on your side. To learn more, turn the page and read on about some amazing fats known as medium chain triglycerides.

24. *Medium Chain Triglycerides: Nature's Fat Burners*

There's a wonderfully funny movie starring Meryl Streep and Albert Brooks. It's called Defending Your Life. It's all about "life" up in heaven. One of the great scenes in the movie shows Albert Brooks indulging himself in an incredible breakfast... all his favorites, his taste buds at their pique. As he's relishing his meal, his superior walks in and informs him that he can eat all he wants without gaining weight. It's a dream come true. But then, this is heaven. Now, thanks to the diligent work of serious researchers, there may be a little bit of heaven here on earth.

Fats give food a special flavor which many people find hard to resist (Haas 1992).

Today, "kitchen scientists" are developing fatless foods that were once considered untouchables for the weight and fat conscious. You can find something down almost every aisle in the market: Fat-free cheese, fat-free cookies, fat-free salad dressings, fat-free sour cream, fat-free cakes and muffins and ice cream--each allows us to indulge our most sensuous culinary fantasies without really committing caloric sins!

And some of these foods mark great advances. Yet, still others mark only another tawdry example of misleading advertising. Have you ever examined the label of these "foods"? For many, the first ingredient is sugar. And sugar eventually converts into fat in the body. The majority of the rest of the ingredients could probably fill the cupboards of an industrial chemistry laboratory. Instead of eating these chemically laden foods to avoid the fat, there are chemicals within your body that may actually let you eat "fat foods" without gaining weight.

Triglycerides Hold the Key

Triglycerides are the main class of fat foods. Composed of fat molecules, they make up approximately 95 percent of all the fats we eat. Triglycerides are the main way we store energy for future use. They bond with proteins and exist in our circulatory system where they are "warehoused" until needed as fuel. They are a major source of energy and serve as the body's reserve for essential fatty acids.

When too much of these fat molecules are warehoused in the bloodstream trouble can develop, causing ailments that include diabetes, hypertension, and heart disease. Long chain triglycerides, so named because they are made up of 18 to 24 carbon atoms, are the storage form of fat. These LCTs not only can result in weight gain, but can elevate blood cholesterol and are associated with cancer (Whitaker 1993).

Certain LCTs, like those found in butter, cheese, red meat, coconut oil, sesame oil and corn oil should be avoided. They bypass the liver completely and enter the bloodstream at the level of the heart (Whitaker 1993). At this point, they are distributed throughout the body where they are added to fat stores. But since LCT energy is conserved, a diet high in LCT fats actually *decreases* your energy! However, don't sell triglycerides short. There's a lot more to the story of triglycerides than just LCTs.

MCTs Burn Fat Fast

Medium chain triglycerides (6 to 12 carbon chains) are fats that act more like a carbohydrate. According to Julian Whitaker, M.D., writing in the forward-thinking medical newsletter *Health and Healing*, medium chain triglycerides

(MCTs) "are absorbed rapidly from the intestinal tract into the bloodstream, then burn vigorously, providing the body with quick energy and actually increasing its metabolic rate, so you can burn calories quicker."

Another way to understand the phenomenon of MCTs versus LCTs is this: LCTs are too heavy to be easily absorbed by the liver. They are unable to be converted into useful energy and are simply stored as excess body fat. MCTs, however, are lighter. They are more easily absorbed by the liver and are converted almost instantly into energy.

If the liver is an important monitor for absorbed calories, which researchers agree it is, a diet with medium chain triglycerides would result in much less weight gain than a diet with comparable amounts of long chain triglycerides (Bray 1980).

One study compared the energy-burning effect of a high-calorie diet containing MCTs and LCTs. Researchers found that the number of calories burned six hours after the meal of MCTs was almost twice as much (120 vs. 66) as those burned after eating a meal of LCTs. The conclusion was that excess energy coming from fat in the form of MCTs would be burned and utilized instead of being stored as fat (Whitaker 1993).

Fat storage can vary from person to person. Excess fat in the body is usually stored in fat cells. All people have a set number of fat cells which are formed at specific times of growth, such as infancy and adolescence. These cells enlarge to accommodate the storage of increased amounts of triglycerides. Fat cells vary in size, with an obese person having much larger fat cells than a thin person.

For over 30 years, the special properties of medium chain triglycerides have been applied in human therapy, particularly in cases where digestion, absorption, or transport of usual dietary fats are disturbed. MCTs have been used successfully in adults, children and newborns with disorders concerning fat digestion. Additionally, studies covering high cholesterol disorders, such as hypercholesterolemia, have reported beneficial results replacing dietary LCTs with MCTs (Bach 1982).

MCTs and Proteins

Protein is the basic building block of all life. It was important for researchers to know if MCT metabolism affected the body's protein content. If so, continued investigation and development would be virtually useless.

A study was conducted at the Nutrition/Metabolism Laboratory at Harvard Medical School, however, which demonstrated that animals given diets containing MCTs demonstrated a *decrease in weight gain and fat content*, compared to the control group receiving LCTs.

Both groups had virtually similar diets, except for one difference. One group consumed food with MCTs. The MCT-fed group lost weight. And while fat deposits were also reduced, body protein was not (Ling 1986).

MCTs May Prevent Obesity

Researchers believe these properties found in MCTs have positive implications for the treatment of obesity. Separated from coconut oil through a water process known as hydrolyzation, MCTs are lighter than LCTs and dissolve easier in fluids. Further validation about MCTs and its potential for weight reduction comes from Dr. Allan Geliebter, reporting in the *Journal of Clinical Nutrition*. "MCT," Dr. Geliebter stated, "may have potential for dietary prevention of human obesity."

Live Longer with MCTs

MCTs offer a variety of other benefits. They provide a concentrated source of calories, even more efficient than protein or carbohydrates. MCTs may be of added value during exercise. Sustained physical exercise causes a depletion of body carbohydrates which is a major factor in the development of exhaustion. Since MCTs are known to be rapidly digested and oxidized, it appears that they provide a quick source of dietary energy. They are also a good food for anyone with increased energy needs. They are a major aid in settling digestive problems. And they have a very low tendency toward being deposited as body fat.

MCTs are especially beneficial where extra energy is necessary, such as after major surgery. LCTs are not capable of supplying quick energy in large quantities. MCTs are more easily and completely assimilated into the blood system. They also limit the build-up of cholesterol in all tissues. As a result, a diet rich in MCTs, rather than LCTs, may increase life span (Bach 1982).

L-Carnitine + MCTs = Optimum Energy Synergy

L-Carnitine is simply the active form of carnitine. Carnitine is a vitamin-like compound that is found in the diet and can be made by the body. It is an important amino acid, essential to one's health. Carnitine is found mainly in red meats, but may also be present in fish, poultry, milk products, wheat, and avocados. Stored primarily in our skeletal muscles and the heart, carnitine transforms fatty acids into energy for muscular activity. Carnitine also transports fatty acids into the energy factories of our cells, the mitochondria, and increases the rate at which the liver uses fats, another energy-producing process.

When you pair together MCTs and carnitine, the synergistic effect can be substantial. Both clean the blood system and transform fatty acids into energy. Both protect the cardiovascular system from disease. Both increase fat utilization and reduce cholesterol levels. Both provide faster weight loss and offer benefits for obesity. Carnitine appears to enhance muscle building and endurance. It can also raise HDL levels—your good cholesterol. And it may reduce the risk of fatty deposits in the liver associated with alcohol abuse (Haas 1992).

MCTs: A Rare Treasure

Today, even with all our scientific knowledge of foods containing MCTs, the American marketplace has made it extremely difficult for MCTs to reach the public. The majority of our processed foods are high in fat-producing LCTs. Restaurants, too, prepare foods using oils laden with LCTs.

For those interested in discovering the fat-reducing, energy-enhancing characteristics of MCTs, supplementation is the appropriate, beneficial avenue to take. Like so many important vitamins, minerals and nutrients that offer a promise of a healthier, longer life, adding MCTs to your diet is the surest way to take advantage of its many favorable qualities.

25. Hair Growth

*"I always wanted to be
like my dad.
But that didn't include
going bald."*
—Any man losing his hair

*"Give me a head of hair
Long, beautiful hair.
Gleaming, streaming
flocks of flaxen."*
—Hair

There are a lot of claims being made today for products that can reverse male pattern baldness and restore hair thickness. Too many claims, too much hype and too much money and not enough truth or science—a sorry comment on the field of natural hair restoration.

Yet whether we want to admit it or not, it is frustrating for any man or woman to watch handfuls of hair disappear down the drain each time they shower or bathe. A full head of hair says, "sexy," "vigorous," and "young."

Hair is an important adornment and manifestation of physical beauty. Although in the distant past, the hair of prehistoric man hair was thought to add a layer of needed warmth (and in fact, hair probably covered his whole body), today we know that hair may offer protection from sunlight and even blows to the head, but that for the most part our hair is there to act as a sexual turn-on and enhance our appearance.

A healthy adult head of hair contains about 120,000 hairs that grow approximately 11 millimeters per month. The cycle of growth of an individual hair may last three years or longer and allowed to grow full length an individual hair could measure 20 to 36 inches.

Each hair goes through a cycle of growth, fall and replacement. The period when the hair is growing is known as the *anagen* phase; the period of rest is the *telogen* phase. Hair growth depends upon the production of cells by a process called cell division or *mitosis* which is vitally dependent on energy cycles. One of the primary energizers for the hair is a chemical compound called glucose 6 phosphate dehydrogenase (G6PDH) (Adachi 1970). Scalp hair grows most rapidly between the ages of 15 and 30 and the rate declines sharply between 50 and 60. Our discussion of the theory of hair growth is important for understanding the dynamics of reversing baldness and thinning hair. That is because the key to reversing conditions of hair loss is to maintain a longer period of anagen hairs and a shorter period of telogen hair (Oba 1988). There are some other keys too including limiting the production of certain harmful forms of the male hormone testosterone that we will discuss. But the important thing to remember is that all of these theories can be unified in both topical and dietary formulations that can truly reverse the onset of balding and thinning hair.

The most common type of inherited hair loss—male-pattern baldness—has been the subject of research for hundreds of years. Yet in all this time, the shining domes of millions of balding men (who've tried so many expensive "miracle" products and haven't benefited) are eloquent and frustrating testimony to the fact that this research—even over hundreds of years—hasn't amounted to more than a hill of beans or, in this case, a few patches of hair going down the drain.

In the past, products have generally attempted to promote hair growth by supplying nutrients with vasodilators and stimulants for improving blood circulation; potential antagonistic action of female hormones; and nourishing the hair follicle with such nutrients as amino acids and vitamins (Oba 1988). Most work not at all, leaving the consumer feeling taken advantage of and the federal regulatory agency overseeing such products, the U.S. Food and Drug Administration, eager to suppress virtually any claim of hair growth.

In fact, only Upjohn, with its product known by the trade name Rogaine, can make claims for hair growth at this time, and the effectiveness of Rogaine, is receiving mixed reviews. Yes, it works in many cases, although it does not work superlatively.

Hey, but at least it produces some fuzz!

And where there's fuzz, there's hope!

There are other methods of thickening what hair one has and even promoting growth that are not being publicized and that you have probably never even heard of because FDA watch dogs are ready to pounce on such claims and shut down any companies making them. But these products do exist, and you're going to learn about them, what they contain, and why they work.

Now, let's go back to our discussion of the life cycle of the human hair—an endangered species upon the heads of some men! One of the most important breakthroughs in the prevention of male pattern baldness has come from our understanding that the life cycle of the human hair has both an anangen phase and telogen phase. A hair in the anagen phase has a high energy level (Oba 1988). But in advanced pattern baldness, there are a whole lot more hairs in the resting, or *telogen* phase—bad news, indeed, for men and women who're sorry to see their hair thinning.

"This clearly means that the level of energy metabolism becomes lower in the hair follicles of advanced alopecia and that the depression of the energy metabolism in the follicle is an important major factor for the process of alopecia" (Oba 1988). Indeed, researchers believe the first step in the promotion of hair growth is to find the cause of the depression of the energy producing system and a delivery system for an efficient and effective energy supply to the hair follicles.

So you guessed the next question: How do you provide an efficient energy supply to the hair follicles?

The answer that researchers were searching for came from rabbits which have an extraordinarily consistant hair cycle of a telogen and anagen phase that occurs every two months.

In their study, researchers clipped hairs from a small area on the rabbits precisely at the moment when their telogen stage began. The researchers dermally applied or injected test ingredients to see if the hair in that bare spot would grow back and at what rate and whether the telogen cycle could be shortened. They believed that if the material worked on the rabbit that it could work for both men and women in the case of balding and thinning hair caused by lowered metabolic activity. Some 300 substances, natural and synthetic, were screened.

Pentadecanoic Acid

The material with the highest potential was a compound called pentadecanoic acid (PDG), says Oba (1988). In these particular studies, PDG even outperformed Minoxidil, the active ingredient in Upjohn's product Rogaine. The levels of the key energy compound, adenosine triphosphate (ATP), were raised at the application site as well by as much as 3.5 times, providing further evidence that PDG boosted the metabolic energy.

This is an important observation because in common male-pattern baldness inhibition of energy production is induced by an androgenic hormone. This androgenic hormone adversely affects the production of phosphofructokinase, a major enzyme involved in the process of glycolysis, which decomposes glucose carried in the blood stream that ultimately provides the building blocks for the energy compound ATP (Oba 1988).

Oba then went on to test his theories with human subjects. He reports that he found "very good results" using PDG on 25 voluneteers with male pattern alopecia, aged 27 to 62. Upon completion of this initial study, he then asked 19 dermatologists at six sites to carry out a double-blind clinical test on a PDG-based solution in 253 volunteers with male-pattern baldness. The changes in the group using the PDG solution were very significant and the results should bring hope to all men and women suffering from hair loss: something can be done to help!

Oba reported that clinical findings consisted of the appearance of new hairs at first called *downy* hairs. These *downy* hairs changed to more mature *vellus* hairs and then to *terminal* hairs. Far fewer falling-out hairs were also observed. Oba concluded that, "It was proved that the new hair growing product containing PDG had a very high effectiveness for the male pattern alopecia." In addition, there were no side effects in haematology, liver function or urinalysis.

Japanese researchers applied in 1985 with the Japanese Ministry of Health and Welfare for a patent on a type of hair growing product based on PDG and in 1986 the product was launched on the market. Today in Japan, its market share is 25 to 30 percent (Oba 1988). The same product was next launched in Germany in October 1987 and gained a high degree of consumer acceptance.

There are other topical and dietary substances that have demonstrated some hair growth potential. Some, such as ginseng and orizanol, stimulate microcirculation throughout the scalp, enabling nutrients including energy producing compounds to reach the site of the hair follicle.

Ginseng

Ginseng produces *hyperaemia* which enhances circulation in the capillaries of the skin and increases the supply of nutrients to the epidermis, reports John Chang of Walgreen Laboratories, writing in the May 1977 issue of *Cosmetics and Toiletries*. "This prevents or retards premature aging of skin *and loss of hair*," he says. "Ginseng has also been reported to have a protective action on damaged hair and to give better manageability and less brittleness."

Orizanol

Also known as Orizagamma-V, orizanol is derived from rice oil, orizanol stimulates microcirculation and is an antioxidant.

Hinokitiol (b-Thujaplicin)

Hinokitol was discovered in the Formosan Hinoki tree by Dr. T. Nozoe in 1936 and was found in the refined oil of the Japanese Hiba tree. It is also found in the refined oil of the Western Red Cedar. It is a seven membered carbocyclic chemical which is very rare in nature. Japanese studies showed thicker hair growth on areas deprived of hair that were treated with a hair tonic containing Hinkitiol copper salt. A clinical study conducted at Nihon University's Department of Dermatology on 11 patients, both male and female, demonstrated the growth of downy hair would occur between seven and sixty days of use, while the growth of hand hair could begin after about 30 days of use. A clinical study conducted at Chiba University's Department of Dermatology on 10 patients with *alopecia areata* demonstrated 60 percent effectiveness in growing downy hair within two months of use. A clinical study conducted at Railway Hospital of Tokyo, Department of Dermatology, on 50 patients with *alopecia* was 68 percent effective in growing downy hair.

Swertia Extract

When growth of hair and acceleration of the dermal functions are expected, a substance that improves dermal blood flood is essential. Swertia, also known as *senburi*, is a botanical registered in the Japanese pharmacopecia that can be applied topically for stimulating hair roots to hasten growth. In China it is called *toyaku*.

Kallikrein Biofactor

Kallikrein is an enzyme that falls into a category of cosmetic ingredients known as skin "rectifiers" (Cook 1984). Rectifiers such as Kallikrein can:
　　　•Improve cell renewal
　　　•Increase the amount of protective lipids
　　　•Increase the uptake of oxygen by cells
　　　•Accelerate natural repair of cells damaged by UV light and other forms of radiation
　　　•Stimulate microcirculation.

According to its producer Canada Packers Chemicals, these properties are thought to be due to the basic ability of kallikrein to increase blood flow by vasodilation and by its ability to enhance the permeability of mammalian cells to nutrient flow.

Takanal

First discovered in Japan in 1954, this aminovinyl compound has been used in many of the most successful hair care and scalp treatment formulations sold worldwide. One clinical study demonstrated a 92 percent effectiveness rate for growing downy and eventually coarse hair. It has an excellent safety record and has been approved for use in cosmetic preparations by the Japanese Ministry of Health and Welfare. It is surprisingly effective even at very low concentrations.

Vitamin A

Vitamin A is known to have played an important role in the metabolism of epidermal tissues as well as protecting the mucous membrane and the skin, which are considered vital in hair growth. Thus, a concentration of 0.05 to 0.5 percent of Vitamin A should be used in a topical compound that will promote hair growth. Forms of vitamin A that appear to work best include aliphatic retinoids and aromatic retinoids such as retinol, retinal, retinol acetate or retinol palmitate.

A Final Word

We know that if you are losing your hair, it is a traumatic experience. We also know that the best results will come to those who begin quickly with a regrowth program upon realizing they are losing their hair.

Yes, you can regrow your hair!

The stimulating botanicals and other nutrients discussed in this chapter truly work when used in combination.

But the time to start is before you lose *all* your hair. The time to start is *now*.

Yes, You Can Grow Back Your Hair

An efficacy study conducted by AMA Laboratories of New York has proven that the ingredients discussed earlier in this chapter will grow back hair. The study, which involved more than 30 test subjects, found that the ingredients discussed in this chapter, when combined in a single formula, gradually increased numbers of hairs counted and that after six months, there was an average of 18 percent more hairs in men using the formula. Furthermore, 60 percent of subjects had increased hair density in previously balding areas. There was also far less hair loss. There were no adverse side effects.

The following before and after pictures of test subjects demonstrate conclusively that a formula, containing ingredients, discussed in this chapter will grow back hair in both men and women.

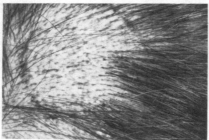 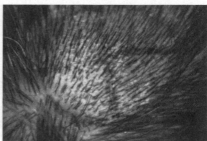

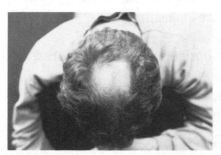 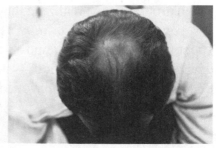

Editor's Note: Fortunately, these ingredients, proven to help regrow hair, have been combined into one formula called Trigenesis. In clinical studies, carried out by independent researchers, the Trigenesis hair restoration formula truly improves hair growth as the above photos dramatically demonstrate. Call (800) 825-8482 to order Trigenesis.

26. Heavy Metals and Oral Chelation

The man who walked in the office of Murray Susser, a physician in Santa Monica, California, was a high powered bank executive in his late thirties with prematurely graying hair. "The patient was known for his steel trap mind," says Dr. Susser, "but he started to suffer memory lapses and confusion. We talked and it came out that he was using a men's hair coloring which contained the toxic heavy metal lead acetate. It's still used in men's anti-graying products today and although we're told that the lead is not suppose to be absorbed into the body, a lot had been absorbed into his."

Dr. Susser performed first a hair analysis and then a pubic hair analysis and both samples were very high in lead. Next Dr. Susser performed a urinary provocative test, using intravenous EDTA (a chelating agent that draws lead out of the body) and he discovered that the level of lead in his patient's urine was sky high.

"So I put him on an oral chelation program using nutrients such as calcium, magnesium, vitamin A, vitamin C, cysteine, lysine, thiamin, choline and inositol and he gradually started to get better. Within one month there was a noticeable improvement again in his brain function. Within about three months he was back to normal. It was a very wonderful occurrence. It was nice to see him get back, and I don't think that the average doctor would have found out for years."

Chelation is the process of drawing harmful metals and minerals out of the body. Dr. Susser explains that minerals in the body are found in a chelated state called a lygand, which is a bond between a protein and metal molecule. Yet toxic metals such as lead and cadmium (which cause many disorders including central nervous system damage, high blood pressure, birth defects and cancer) can also form such bonds and build-up in the body. Even calcium, says Dr. Susser, becomes harmful when it becomes a soft tissue contaminant in the veins, arteries and skin. Perhaps of most concern is that lygands can accumulate in the body's vessels, preventing circulation, causing heart disease.

The only way to get rid of a metal in a lygand is to present it with another substance with a greater, more powerful bio-electrical power that will draw it out of this lygand. "Chelators," he says, "present a stronger biochemical attraction to the toxic metals and minerals to draw them out and put them in solution so that they will flow out of the kidneys."

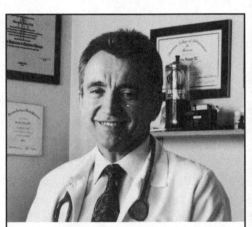

Heavy Metal Poisoning

Heavy metal poisoning is a modern disease that strikes millions of Americans and whose initial symptoms may be subclinical and not suspected by most physicians. In fact, our bodies probably carry about one-thousand times more lead today than those of

Murray Susser, M.D., is an expert in the diagnosis of heavy metal poisoning. He often recommends oral chelators to his patients. "Because metal contamination is so prevalent today in our modern society, oral chelation is an important regimen for the healthy heart, indeed, for the healthy body," he says.

our primitive ancestors (Patterson 1987). "In the polar ice pack researchers dug down to a layer that was 2,800 years old and found a relatively small concentration of lead," says Dr. Susser, referring to the landmark work performed by C.C. Patterson of the California Institute of Technology, in Pasadena, California. "But around 800 B.C., which marks the beginning of the bronze age, researchers began to find lead in the ice pack. Around 300 A.D.

they found a significantly increased lead deposition; that was when the iron age began. They found much higher concentrations of lead around 1750 with the advent of the industrial revolution. If even the remote polar ice pack can become contaminated with toxic metals, think of what's happening to our bodies today, as we go about living in busy urban areas or just about anywhere else in this heavily industrialized nation."

There is an enormous amount of research showing that millions of adults and children now contain toxic levels of lead in their bodies which is causing hypertension, diminished intelligence, birth defects, and other maladies.

But how does heavy metal poisoning affect people other than prisoners? Can anybody become contaminated with heavy metals? We are exposed to lead, sometimes in drinking water, from the exhaust fumes of cars, from paints; even serving ware with painted or glazed colors can leach lead into our food.

But our drinking water can be the most insidious cause of metal contamination.

To find out what kind of lead levels were in drinking water supplies across the nation, the Environmental Protection Agency tested water in some 660 water systems, checking homes and buildings most likely to have elevated lead levels in the water supply. The following cities are in that category, with the populations, the lead level in parts per billion and percentage of children with high lead levels.

U.S. Cities with Lead Levels Over EPA Standards

Water Supplier	Population	Lead Level	Children with High Lead Levels
Arizona			
Phoenix	907,930	19	32.3%
California			
Palo Alto	56,900	30	NA
Milpitas	NA	23	NA

Children
with High

Water Supplier	Population	Lead Level	Lead Levels
Pleasanton	NA	18	NA
San Francisco	648,000	18	55.5%
Connecticut			
Hartford	398,500	40	46.7%
District of Columbia			
Washington	1,000,000	18	51.7%
Florida			
Escambia Co.	269,545	175	NA
Pompano Beach	50,100	84	NA
Fort Myers	51,500	34	27.1%
Cocoa	171,132	32	NA
Miami Beach	96,000	27	51.2%
Daytona Beach	79,664	24	37.4%
Georgia			
Gwinnett Co.	296,281	66	NA
North Fulton	60,000	53	NA
Richmond Co.	80,000	48	NA
Clayton Co.	164,081	34	NA
Douglasville-Douglas Co.	70,070	30	NA
Cobb Co.-Marietta	425,000	22	NA
Savannah-Main	141,855	21	51.8%
Macon-Bibb Co.	143,810	17	48.8%
Guam			
Guam	61,750	25	NA
Illinois			
Oak Park	54,887	39	NA
Decatur	94,081	36	50.0%
Cicero	61,000	28	NA
Evanston	73,233	25	NA
Glenview	56,000	25	NA

Water Supplier	Population	Lead Level	Children with High Lead Levels
Illinois (cont.)			
Waukegan	69,392	20	NA
E. St. Louis	208,976	19	NA
Oak Lawn	56,182	18	NA
Bloomington	52,000	18	NA
Palatine	55,000	17	NA
Indiana			
Hammond	93,440	27	NA
Ft. Wayne	180,000	21	45.3%
Iowa			
Cedar Rapids	110,243	80	33.5%
Des Moines	196,477	21	36.1%
Maine			
Portland	132,000	70	43.9%
Maryland			
Potomac	1,000,000	39	NA
Elkridge-Howard Co.	115,000	20	NA
Massachusetts			
Newington	82,011	163	NA
Framingham	62,000	100	NA
Somerville	74,096	84	NA
Malden	51,000	71	NA
Medford	56,000	70	30.3%
Chicopee	53,325	69	48.7%
Quincy	88,000	62	NA
Brookline	59,202	62	NA
Waltham	58,350	52	NA
Lowell	100,000	51	42.5%
Boston	577,830	48	69.4%
Worcester	200,000	39	47.3%

Water Supplier	Population	Lead Level	Children with High Lead Levels
Michigan			
Royal Oak	65,410	17	NA
Minnesota			
St. Paul	385,000	54	44.9%
Minneapolis	473,073	19	44.9%
New Hampshire			
Nashua	80,000	45	29.3%
New Jersey			
Jersey City	290,618	84	NA
Southeast Morris Co.	65,000	37	NA
Wayne	52,000	29	NA
Elizabeth City	112,000	28	NA
Newark	275,221	27	NA
Milburn	183,199	25	NA
Passaic Valley	270,00	24	NA
Bayonne	61,100	18	NA
Trenton	225,00	18	59.2%
New York			
Utica	120,000	100	48.9%
Yonkers	188,082	68	NA
Mt. Vernon	67,153	62	NA
New York Aqueduct	6,552,718	55	NA
Syracuse	192,000	50	45.1%
New Rochelle	137,640	36	NA
Binghamton	55,860	20	48.1%
Elmira	62,660	20	29.7%
New York City	518,00	20	57.7%
Onondaga	198,000	20	NA
North Carolina			
Asheville	110,000	29	32.2%
Gastonia	72,000	17	40.1%
Ohio			

Water Supplier	Population	Lead Level	Children with High Lead Levels
Cleveland-Baldwin	567,680	25	64.7%
Cleveland-Nottingham	344,160	25	64.7%
Cleveland-Crown	172,000	20	64.7%
Cleveland-Morgan	156,160	20	64.7%
Oregon			
Portland	402,000	41	44.7%
Tualatin Valley	121,457	28	NA
Pennsylvania			
Westmoreland Co.			
Yough	130,000	56	NA
Williamsport	55,000	51	50.2%
Lancaster	108,000	41	52.7%
Lower Buck Co.	85,000	37	NA
Greater Johnstown	65,000	34	53.4%
Plymouth	54,288	31	NA
Bensalem	58,200	29	NA
Mill Creek	58,179	27	NA
Beaver Run	130,000	25	NA
Philadephia	1,755,000	22	62.0%
Erie	190,000	16	45.4%
Puerto Rico			
Fajardo Ceiba	56,056	60	NA
Rio Blan Vieq	135,780	29	NA
Caguas Urbano	154,948	16	NA
Metropolitan	1,510,348	16	NA
Rhode Island			
Pawtucket	105,000	29	NA
South Carolina			
Charlestown	193,276	211	38.6%
Columbia	248,650	40	40.2%

Water Supplier	Population	Lead Level	Children with High Lead Levels
South Carolina(cont.)			
Orangeburg	51,584	18	NA
Texas			
Port Arthur	60,687	28	NA
Virginia			
Chesapeake	127,980	30	NA
Portsmouth	120,000	26	47.9%
Occoquan-Woodbridge	102,440	22	NA
Richmond	209,000	16	42.6%
Washington			
Tacoma	224,600	32	37.8%
North Shore	52,000	29	NA
Alderwood	83,400	28	NA
Everett	72,480	23	39.9%
Bellingham	55,000	23	35.5%
Seattle	548,000	19	29.9%
Bellevue	100,000	19	NA
Wisconsin			
West Allis	63,240	22	NA
Racine	125,000	18	45.2%
Oshkosh	54,000	17	NA
Madison	170,616	16	29.2%

Source: Environmental Protection Agency, Environmental Defense Fund, *USA Today*

Cadmium & Aluminum

Our exposure to cadmium is equally insidious. Cadmium is used in hardening rubber tires, causing our nation's freeways and highways to be contaminated with this metal.

In addition to cadmium, some researchers assert that the need for aluminum removal is rapidly gaining increased gerontological attention because of its accumulation in the neurofibrillary tangle-bearing neurons of brains of people suffering severe Alzheimer's disease.

Furthermore, the National Academy of Sciences published a report in 1991, *Seafood Safety,* which asserted that there may well be a link between build-up of the heavy metal methylmercury in the human body and Parkinson's disease.

With this in mind it would seem that today's advocates of oral chelation may someday be shown to have been on the cutting edge of nutritional supplementation.

Perhaps most interesting and little known is the role that metals play in the onset of violent and antisocial behavior. Dr. Morton Walker (1990) tells of research conducted over the last six years by William J. Walsh and fellow analytical chemists at the Argonne National Laboratories which revealed that extremely violent people have abnormal patterns of trace metals in their hair. These patterns can be used like chemical fingerprints to identify those who are violence-prone. More than 60,000 hair samples were analyzed to establish what could be construed as normal metal content in the hair. The hairs of inmates at Stateville and Menard prisons in Illinois were compared, representing all races and socioeconomic levels. All the subjects had deliberately and repeatedly hurt other human beings (Walker 1990). The researchers found that abnormal levels of several toxic metals such as lead and cadmium could predict violent behavior.

"The world is really poisoned. It's really tragic," says Dr. Susser. "Some people tolerate pollution better than others, but we're all poisoned."

But there is something we can do about heavy metal build-up. Dr. Susser strongly urges that people use chelators because he believes that by purging the body of toxic metals, we contribute to our health and well-being. "I think people should be using oral chelators whether they are suffering visible clinical symptoms of poisoning from heavy metals or simply interested in preventing heavy metal build-up," he says.

Dr. Susser says that, "If there were more research on oral chelation, it probably could be shown that people who use such supplements live longer. One of the ingredients used in chelators is vitamin C which has already been demonstrated to increase human life expectancy by five years. Higher levels of vitamin E—another chelator—may help prevent premature death in men from heart disease. Thus you can see that the oral chelators have multiple purposes beyond chelation and almost certainly can help you decrease your chances of contracting life-threatening diseases."

Oral chelation therapy is preventive, says chelation expert Dr. Walker (1990). "So many environmental disadvantages that we can do nothing about strike all of us everyday . . . . Popping down my daily quota of oral chelates is a technique that allows me to fight for my life and health more effectively."

27. *Adaptogens*

Doctors and medical researchers who keep their finger on the pulse of medicine recognize that 21st century medicine is defined by disease prevention and anti-aging. Key components to 21st century medicine are adaptogens. Adaptogens are rare herbal roots and extracts that have the ability to bring the body back into health and balance by counteracting negative stress factors before they begin to damage the cells. Mikael Wahlstrom, author of *Adaptogens*: *Nature's Key to Well-Being* writes, "Soon over 70% of illness and disease will be conquered with the help of adaptogens." He also notes, "Nature has her own method of helping bodies withstand stress-adaptogens are stronger than stress, our rediscovered key to well-being."

Adaptogens can be traced back to Asia, specifically China and Tibet where centuries ago Tibetan monks and Chinese acupuncturists mastered the medicinal qualities and potency of these healing plants. Today medical research has begun to give credence to the highly sophisticated and intricate medical systems realized so long ago from these ancient teachings.

How Adaptogens Work

In order for the body to maintain a healthy state of well-being, it is crucial that cells are able to carry out their work and renew themselves. To do this they need to be properly nourished. Adaptogens supply the cells with energy and help the cells to optimize their use. "Adaptogens stimulate the body's own self-regeneration process and help to rebuild even under unfavorable conditions" (Wahlstrom 1987). Adaptogens are most effective when guarding the body against the consequences of environmental, physical, and emotional stress. Stress, especially long-term stress, can ravage the body by tearing down the immune system and obstructing the functions of normal, healthy cells. Adaptogens, and their active ingredients, glucosides, strengthen the cells by transforming glucose into energy. Often, when stress continues to invade the cells the use of glucose is blocked, which in turn inhibits the production of enzymes. Adaptogens help cells to shield themselves and to become more tolerant of damaging, outside stimuli.

Where Adaptogens Are Found

Adaptogens are found in rare and superior plants. According to Chinese medicine, one type of superior plant is found in every 500 to 1,000 known medicinal plants. The most widely used adaptogens are garlic powder, astragalus, *Echinacea,* Reishi mushroom, Korean ginseng, dandelion, licorice, ginger, *Schisandra* root, kelp, and *Gingko biloba.* All of these plants exhibit their own, unique adaptogen qualities.

Schisandra

As the Asians began investigating the potency of plants, one of the most sought after plants in Tibet was and is to this day *Schisandra.* It has been used for centuries as protection against liver damage. Like many adaptogens, *Schisandra* has the ability to protect the body cells against stress. *Schisandra* also is able to protect the liver, stimulate blood circulation, and increase oxygen in the cells (Wahlstrom 1987)

Perhaps the most widely acknowledged adaptogen is garlic. Garlic was coined Russian penicillin when the Russian army used it as an antibiotic during World Wars I and II. With its remarkable medicinal properties, garlic is taken quite seriously by the medical community. Some of the most impressive research on garlic and its abilities to act as an adaptogen is with lowering cholesterol levels and having an overall benefit on the heart. Apparently garlic helps to balance an improper diet, thus helping the body to "adapt." Its natural sulphur compound, allicin, has been found to lower cholesterol levels and is currently being researched for its ability to aid atherosclerosis. Six studies found that when rabbits were fed a diet high in cholesterol and garlic, blood cholesterol levels were 10 to 80 percent lower than those animals that were not fed garlic. Furthermore, atherosclerotic lesions were fewer (Mowrey 1986).

Siberian Ginseng

Another well-known adaptogen is ginseng. Used for centuries by the Chinese, ginseng has often been called a panacea and more recently a "wonder herb." Ginseng has been found to normalize the body in several ways, but perhaps the most impressive is the study at Kanazawa University in Japan. Researchers found that ginseng, "not only inhibited the growth of cancer cells, but actually converted the diseased cells in to normal cells" (Mindell 1992). Other properties known to ginseng are balancing the central nervous system (guarding the body against stress), creating a noticeable increase in mental and physical endurance, and ginseng also has the ability to regulate blood pressure (Mowrey 1986).

Ginkgo Biloba

Becoming almost as popular in the west as ginseng is *Ginkgo biloba*. The *Ginkgo* tree is thought to be over two-million years old and is considered sacred in some parts of China. Some medical researchers believe *Ginkgo's* ability to survive is an indication of its healing powers. In Europe, ginkgo, is a widely accepted herb that is sold only with a prescription. Today science has shown us that *Ginkgo* can help alleviate depression, improve mental activity, and guard against senility, including the early stages of Alzheimer's disease. Double-blind, placebo-controlled studies have shown that memory test performance was "significantly improved" after taking *Ginkgo biloba* extract. In another double-blind study, elderly patients monitored by EEG's improved their mental performance and experienced a renewed state of alertness (Voelp 1985). When *Ginkgo biloba* extract was given to 112 geriatric patients diagnosed with cerebral vascular insufficiency, the patients experienced relief from headache, ear-ringing, vertigo and short-term memory loss (VRP 1989).

Kelp

A sea-remedy that has been used as an adaptogen for centuries is kelp. Kelp is used traditionally in the Japanese diet. Slowly, kelp is making its way into American culture. Kelp is rich in iodine, calcium and potassium. It is considered a general tonic for the blood (Mowrey 1986). Researchers became intrigued with kelp's anti-neoplastic qualities when they began questioning why Japanese women have a 40% less incidence of breast cancer than American women. Laboratory studies have shown that kelp significantly inhibits the growth of mammary neoplasms (Yamamoto 1974).

An Adaptogen Formula

The University of Kansas recently studied the popular Chinese prescription that combines the adaptogens *Astragalus* with ginseng, *Angelica sinesis*, cinnamon, *Rehmannia* and licorice to isolate the mixture's active ingredients. In China, this remedy is used to nurture the body back to health after experiencing a severe illness. It is also, used to guard against anemia, fatigue, kidney, and spleen problems. Researchers isolated SQT, a potent compound found in Chinese remedies that aids in re-building the immune system after the administration of cancer therapy. SQT also has been successful in the prevention of the devastating side effects that often accompany cancer treatment therapies (Zee-Cheng 1992). This research has captured the attention of the Chinese adaptogen approach of "toning the blood and strengthening Chi (vital energy) in cancer immunotherapy."

Reishi Mushroom

In China, reishi mushroom is known as the "Mushroom of the Immortals." It is a highly regarded adaptogen and is known for its ability to defend the body against allergies, chronic fatigue syndrome, and many other immune-related diseases (McGlasson 1992). Chinese women, also drink tea made out of Reishi mushroom to give their skin a healthy glow.

Echinacea

China is not the only country rich with rare adaptogen plants. In the U.S. one of the most discussed adaptogens of the 21st century grows wild. *Echinacea,* is the purple colored, wild Native American cone flower that grows abundantly throughout the North American Plains. It was used extensively by native people as a cure-all for everything from snake- bites to the common cold. Some 80 years ago Dr. S. Foster wrote in the *Eclectic Medical Journal,* "Nature has probably destined *Echinacea* to be used as a sustainer of vitality, an organizer of the defensive powers of the immune system, to such an extent as to be justly crowned the greatest immunizing agent in the entire vegetable kingdom, as far as is known to medical science."

Nearly 100 years later modern science is still fascinated by *Echinacea's* seemingly endless healing properties. The root of *Echinacea* has been found to effectively treat viral infections, impaired immune functions and wound healing. Mild infections and cases of low immune deficiency respond to echinacea's profound immune enhancing effects. The major component of *Echinacea* is inulin. Inulin increases the body's ability to defend against, neutralize, and destroy viruses and infection-causing bacteria, creating a strong antibiotic effect.

Other studies show that *echinacea* helps to build higher resistance to infections by building the body's T-cells. T-cells are white blood cells that possess specific antigen receptors. When the body becomes invaded with foreign micro-organisms T-Cells begin their attack. Dr. Mowrey reports that, "T-cells are actually the body's main defense against acute bacterial infection; they also destroy fungi, cancerous cells, transplanted tissue, wounded cells harboring viruses and bacteria." *Echinacea* stimulates T-cell reproduction, which in turn attacks viruses and combats infection while, boosting cellular immunity.

Milk Thistle

Also found growing in North America is milk thistle. Over 200 scientific papers have been written about the liver-repairing qualities of this powerful adaptogen. Milk thistle is an important adaptogen because it helps to repair the liver. A healthy liver is vital to an overall state of well-being, since its main tasks are to break down and filter through ingested fats, making sure that the body cells receive the nutrients they need. The liver also has the job of repairing damaged blood vessels and body cells. Unfortunately, mistreated livers are often unable to carry out their tasks effectively and too often fats and toxins become stored in the liver. Studies have shown that the seed of milk thistle not only protects against liver damage, but helps to regenerate damaged liver cells (Lee 1991). Milk thistle has been shown to help detoxify alcohol-induced fat in the liver and chronic hepatitis or inflammation of the liver (AIBR Scientific Reviews 1987).

Dandelion

Lastly, the common dandelion (*Taraxacum officinale*) is one of nature's finest adaptogens. The nutrient-rich dandelion has long been used in many folk remedies. Today research science has shown that dandelions have a much greater vitamin A content than carrots (Mowrey 1986). One of the most popular ways in which dandelion root has been used is as a natural diuretic. One study found that animals who were given dandelion root "lost up to 30 percent of their weight" (Kugler 1993). Unlike over-the-counter diuretics that can often rob the body of necessary potassium, dandelion root is one of the best natural suppliers of potassium (Hoffmann 1991).

Research is only beginning to tap into these plants' vast potential. Adaptogens stimulate the immune system and block the cells against a multitude of negative stress agents. Adaptogens can be taken by anyone at any age. They help keep healthy bodies healthy and bring stressful afflictions back into balance. Dr. Wahstrom writes, "For many years modern medicine in the Western World has turned its back on the collective wisdom and learning of years of traditional medicine. Research has concentrated on the development of synthetic medicines, fast-acting and specific medicines, which are often more poisonous than medicines. Modern medicine has looked at each ailment and each organ in isolation, looking for specific cures, rather than seeing the human being as a whole. But at last scientists are taking a new look at medicine and nature, and are beginning to see how nature herself is their greatest ally in health."

28. Healing
and Preventing Ulcers

The *FDA Consumer* reports that peptic ulcers affect 1 out of 50 Americans each year and 1 out of 10 Americans will suffer from peptic ulcers during their lifetime.

According to their report, once a person develops an ulcer, the more likely they are to be susceptible to more ulcers in the future.

Recent research indicates that ulcers are related to a bacteria, *Helicobacter pylori*. *Pylori* is rarely found in people under the age of 20. Researchers believe that it "may infect more than 60 percent of Americans over 65." At high risk for ulcers are those who take nonsteroidal anti-inflammatory drugs (NSAIDs), like high-dose aspirin, ibuprofen, naproxen and piroxicam.

Recognize Symptoms

For the ulcer sufferer, discomfort is mostly felt in the middle or upper abdomen and the pain often strikes inbetween meals or in the middle of the night. Over-the-counter, synthetic antacids that are made up of aluminum, calcium, or magnesium salts are generally the most sought after non-prescription choice. However these antacids can interfere with the absorption of other medications, contribute to chronic aluminum toxicity, and because of their sodium content, they may conflict with the body's basic metabolic processes--such as kidney function and increased blood pressure (Pizzorno 1991).

Chili Peppers Heal Ulcers

Contrary to the belief that hot and spicy foods create ulcers, they may actually heal. Cultures that eat curries and, specifically spicy foods with cayenne pepper, have very low incidence of peptic ulcers. As a folk remedy, cayenne pepper has been used since 7000 B.C. Today there is growing evidence to support the theory that cayenne pepper, in the form of capsicum, has a mild stimulating, anti-inflammatory, and antibiotic effect on the stomach. Capsaicin is the compound found in capsicum that gives it its healing properties. In laboratory tests capsaicin was found to stimulate the mucosal blood flow in the stomach of rats (Limlomwongse 1979). *Gastroenterology* (Holtzer 1989) reports that when rats were given high levels of acidic aspirin, "capsaicin was found to reduce ... discernible formations of mucosal lesions." Further studies showed that capsaicin on its own "did not cause any injury to the gastric mucosa" (Holtzer 1989).

Licorice Root Strengthens Your Stomach

Ulcers may be caused by increased pepsin and hydrochloric acid release, reduced mucus production, and factors that irritate the gastrointestinal lining such as alcohol, or drugs of the aspirin group which can also act as irritants or reduce mucus production. Eventually the lining loses its ability to protect the stomach from its own digestive juices. Glycyrrhetinic acid, a compound found in licorice root (*Glycyrrhiza Glabra*), helps to strengthen the stomach's natural defenses. Licorice root has also been found to have an anti-inflammatory effect on the stomach's mucous membranes (Mowrey 1990).

Vitamin C Rejuvenates Stomach

Studies show that people suffering from peptic ulcers have deficient levels of Vitamin C (O'Connor 1989). Only one out of eighty guinea pigs that received vitamin C supplements, along with a basic diet developed a peptic ulcer. Whereas, those that were deficient in vitamin C developed peptic ulcers similar in location and appearance to those found in humans. Guinea pigs that were fed diets deficient in vitamins A, B-complex, and D, but continued to receive an adequate supply of C did not develop ulcers (Smith 1933). All studies concluded that an abundance of vitamin C would help prevent and heal lesions caused by peptic ulcers.

Ginger

Originating in southeast Asia, ginger (*Zingiber officinale*) has numerous health benefits, including its anti-inflammatory action and soothing effects on heartburn and indigestion. Combined with licorice root, ginger has been used as a natural stomach and digestive aid in Chinese medicine for centuries. Ginger helps to stimulate the flow of saliva which then increases the flow of a digestive enzyme, amylase, found in saliva (Mowrey 1986). Modern medical research recently found that ginger inhibits gastric lesions in rats by 97.5 percent. Studies also have shown that ginger is able to prevent the occurrence of ulcers in rats caused by NSAIDs (Yamahara 1988).

Fenugreek Seeds

The mucilaginous nature of fenugreek seeds (*Trigonella foenum-graecum*) is able to soothe irritations and to ease the pain associated with peptic ulcers. Not long ago it was discovered that fenugreek seeds help to stimulate pancreatic secretion, which helps to improve digestion (Mowrey 1986).

Bromelain—Digestive Enzyme

Derived from pineapple, bromelain is a protein-digesting enzyme that has a mild anti-inflammatory effect, notes Murray (1991).

For millions of Americans with ulcers, these substances promote important healing.

29. *Understanding Your Medical Tests*

K. enters his doctor's office looking terrible. He is withdrawn and complains of general malaise.

The physician examines K. and finds a widespread bronze color on the face, arms, trunk, and legs. There is tenderness in the stomach and intestine. Also, dark pigmented spots on the mucosa lining of Kyle's mouth and lips signal illness.

K.'s doctor is concerned because she is familiar with his medical history and can see her patient is ill.

The doctor requests a standard blood test and finds elevated levels of potassium and nitrogen with decreased sodium, chloride, bicarbonate, and glucose.

There is a decrease in bicarbonate which usually means kidney insufficiency and hypotension. From this information, K.'s doctor suspects K. has Addison's disease. His blood workup also indicates hypoglycemia, which occurs in Addison's disease. The doctor runs more specific tests, confirms the illness, and is ready to begin treatment after informing K. of his situation. Thanks to his medical tests, K. will be able to take care of his illness before it advances to an untreatable stage.

If Gilda Radner had known more about the hereditary link of ovarian cancer and sought out the CA 125 lab test at an earlier time, she might be alive today. True, she would have been faced with the difficult decision to have her ovaries removed during the time when she heard her biological clock ticking. But she would have had a choice. Instead, Glida lacked knowledge of this treacherous killer slithering through the female population. And so, comedy lost one of its best players, for Gilda mirrored what was so right in our world.

How many other countless thousands have been lost because they too lacked information to make the right decisions? How many countless people suffer unspeakable pain for years because they never find an answer for their physical distress?

Because informed patients have a greater opportunity to communicate with doctors and thus be an active part of the healing or treatment process, this chapter seeks to take the mystery out of understanding basic medical tests; point out the high and low ranges of test criteria and what they mean; create awareness of potential errors and variability in medical tests; and show why patients should work with a reputable doctor in the interpretation of results.

The Diagnostic Process

As medical tests are the basic indicators of good or failing health, carefully analyzed blood, urine, hair, and stool samples are the windows to the inside our body.

Many people do not understand why physicians often take an exhaustive medical history. What patients need to know is that doctors look for trends and patterns, making a judgement call on which informational track they will pursue to arrive at the cause of a patient's problem.   Once this is accomplished, the physician then decides which medical lab tests to request towards more specific knowledge of the patient's health problem.

Understanding a Laboratory Report

After obtaining the patient's medical history, a blood scan is an analytical starting point giving doctors specific data on a patient's health.

Blood is analyzed on the basis of elevated or decreased biochemical laboratory values within established ranges of good health. When certain components of blood are higher or lower than the normal range, a competent physician is able to interpret these variations in tandem with a patient's medical history and identify illness with greater accuracy.

An informed patient is better able to understand his or her physician's goals in the healing process. Such interactive communication is bound to save the patient money and the doctor time.

The Basic Blood Test

The following is a list of major blood test factors to help the reader grow familiar with blood analysis:

GLUCOSE

Range	Elevated	Decreased
80-125 mg/dl	diabetes	excess insulin
	adrenal tumors	pancreatic disorder
	pituitary tumors	endocrine problem
	brain damage	enzymatic dysfunction
	hyperthyroidism	liver damage

UREA NITROGEN

Range	Elevated	Decreased
07-25 mg/dl	kidney disease	liver insufficiency
	heart failure	late pregnancy
	shock	low protein diet
	dehydration	excess IV fluids

CREATININE

Range	Elevated
0.7-1.4mg/dl	kidney disease
	acromegaly

CREATINE PHOSPHOKINASE (CPK)

Range	Elevated	Decreased
women 15-57u/liter	heart attack	early pregnancy
men 23-99u/liter	muscular dystrophy	drug interference
	cerebrovascular	
	underactive thyroid	

SODIUM

Range	Elevated	Decreased
135-148meq/l	dehydration	excess water
	adrenal cortex	kidney failure
	tumors	underactive adrenals
	pituitary disorders	thyroid disfunction
	cerebral damage	high fat level
	excess salt	vomiting

POTASSIUM

Range	Elevated	Decreased
3.5-5.3meq/l	diabetes	laxative abuse
	acidosis	diuretics
	kidney failure	cortisone therapy
	underactive	adrenal cortex tumors
	adrenals	cancer

CHLORIDE

Range	Elevated	Decreased
96-112meq/l	high salt intake	vomiting
	kidney failure	Addison's disease
	metabolic acidosis	inappropriate ADH
	dehydration	metabolic alkalosis
	respiratory	excess water
	alkalosis	

CALCIUM

Range	Elevated	Decreased
8.5-10.6mg/dl	hyper-parathyroidism	hypoparathyroidism
	bone metastases	pseudohypopara-thyroid
	multiple myeloma	malabsorption
	hyperthyroidism	pancreatitis
	kidney failure	low albumin
	excess vitamin D	

INORGANIC PHOSPHORUS

Range	Elevated	Decreased
2.5-4.5mg/dl	renal insufficiency	hyperparathyroidism
	hypoparathyroidism	excess IV glucose
	diabetes mellitus	liver function loss
		hypokalemia
		salicylate poisoning
		antacid overuse

TOTAL PROTEIN

Range	Elevated	Decreased
6.0-8.5g/dl	dehydration	overhydration
	hyperglobulinemia	immunoglobulin deficiency
	Waldenstrom	
	multiple myeloma	malnutrition
	malignancy	malabsorption
	liver disease	generalized dermatitis
	infection	nephrosis

TOTAL CHOLESTEROL

Range	Elevated	Decreased
less than 200mg/dl or greater	hypothyroidism	liver failure
	obstructive	inanition
	inflamed kidney	hyperthyroidism
	diabetes	malabsorption

Range	GOOD CHOLESTEROL (high density)
55 or greater mg/dl	healthy state

Range	BAD CHOLESTEROL (low density)
less than 130 mg/dl	high risk for coronary artery disease

Range	CHOLESTEROL/HDL RATIO
4.4 or less WD	optimal condition

ALBUMIN

Range	Elevated	Decreased
3.2-5.5g/dl	dehydration	overhydration
		liver insufficiency
		malnutrition
		burns
		dermatitis,
		general nephrosis

TOTAL GLOBULIN

Range	
1.5-3.8g/dl	healthy range

BILIRUBIN

Range	Elevated	Decreased
0.2-1.2mg/dl	red blood cell	anemia
	destruction	decreased albumin
	liver disease	
	obstructed jaundice	
	pulmonary infarction	
	large hematoma	
	possible cancer	
	bile duct blockage	

ALKALINE PHOSPHATASE

Range	Elevated	Decreased
20-140u/l	liver disease	underactive thyroid
	gall bladder	anemia
	disease	malnutrition
	jaundice	hypophosphatasia
	osteoblastic	oxulate anticoagulant
	lesions	
	peptic ulcer	
	Paget's disease	
	kidney infarction	
	pulmonary infarction	
	pregnancy	

LACTATE DEHYDROGENASE

Range	Elevated	Decreased
0-250u/l	cerebral damage	anticoagulant usage
	myocardial	clofibrate usage
	infarction	
	lung infarction	
	muscle necrosis	
	kidney infarction	
	sprue	
	liver disease	
	neoplastic disease	
	pernicious anemia	

ASPARTATE TRANSAMINASE (SGOT)

Range	Elevated	Decreased
0-50u/l	cerebral damage	pyridoxine deficiency
	mycardial	chronic dialysis
	viral hepatitis	pregnancy
	liver disease	beriberi
	muscle necrosis	

URIC ACID

Range	Elevated	Decreased
2.5-7.5mg/dl	leukemia	xanthinuria
	polycythemia	x-ray contrast agents
	acidosis	glyceryl guaiacolate
	psoriasis	nephropathy in cancer
	hypothyroidism	
	tissue necrosis	
	inflammation	
	gout, if nitrogen	
	is high	

TOTAL IRON

(storage estimate)

Range	Elevated	Decreased
women 80-150mcg/dl	iron overload	iron deficiency
men 70-150mcg/dl		

IRON BINDING CAPACITY

(shows how many free binding sites are available for iron)

Range	Elevated	Decreased
250-425mcg/dl	need iron	may have too much iron

(Recent data show excess iron may be associated with increased incidence of heart disease.)

IRON SATURATION

(indicates the percentage of binding sites filled with iron)

Range
12-57%

TRIGLYCERIDES

Range   (screens for excess fat or lipids in the blood)
  0-29   10-140mg/dl
 30-39   10-150mg/dl
 40-49   10-160mg/dl
 50-59   10-190mg/dl

Elevated   **Decreased**
bad fat in blood   malnutrition
coronary-artery
   disease if
   cholesterol
   is high
diabetes
bile-duct obstruction
high alcohol intake

WHITE BLOOD CELL COUNT

Range   **Elevated**   **Decreased**
4,100-10,900/ul   bacterial infection   bone-marrow
                       leukemia   depression
                       tissue death   viral infection
                                                     toxic reaction to
                                                        anti-cancer drugs
                                                     heavy metal ingestion
                                                     mononucleosis
                                                     anemia
                                                     hemodilution
                                                     hemorrhage

RED BLOOD CELL COUNT (RBC)

Range	Elevated	Decreased
women 4.2- 5.4mill/mcl men 4.5-6.2mill/mcl	hemoconcentration polycythemia	anemia hemodilution recent hemorrhage

HEMOGLOBIN

Range	Elevated	Decreased
12.0-15.6g/dl	dehydration polycythemia	fluid rentention recent bleeding

HEMATOCRIT
(% of red blood cells relative to the total volume of blood

Range	Elevated	Decreased
women 38.0-46.0% men 42-54%	hemoconcentration polycythemia	anemia hemodilution recent hemorrhage

MEAN CORPUSCULAR VOLUME (MCV)
(Ratio of hematocrit to the red-blood-cell count; helps diagnose and classify anemia)

Range
84-99u3/red cell

MEAN CORPUSCULAR HEMOGLOBIN (MCH)
(red-blood-cell-ratio)

Range
26-32pg/red

MEAN CORPUSCULAR HEMOGLOBIN CONCENTRATION (MCHC)

Range
30-36%

Elevated levels in all three indicate:
•macrocytic anemia (abnormal presence of large fragile, red blood cells) caused by inherited disorders due to faulty DNA synthesis.

•megaloblastic anemia; caused by folic-acid deficiency. May be accompanied by iron-deficiency.

•reticulocytosis (too many reticulocytes in the blood).

Decreased levels in all three indicate:
•Microcytic or hypochromic anemia caused by iron deficiency
•B-1 vitamin deficiency
•thalassemia, inherited Mediterranean anemia characterized by small red blood cells with less hemoglobin than normal.

PLATELET COUNT

Range	Decreased
130,000-370,000 cubic mm	causes spontaneous bleeding below 50,000; death below 5,000 cubic mm

NEUTROPHILS

Range	Elevated	Decreased
40-75%	bacterial infection severe stress	immune deficiency—death could result

LYMPHOCYTES
(one of several types of white blood cells which help fight infection)

Range	Elevated	Decreased
16-46%	mononucleosis multiple myeloma lymphocytic anemia	AIDS lymphocytic leukemia T-cell deficiency

EOSINOPHILS

Range	Elevated
0-7.0%	allergies
	parasites

There are more extensive blood tests, but this basic blood scan gives the physician a look inside the body and helps to narrow down the disease problem.

The Urine Test

The kidneys and bladder help filter and pass waste material and toxins from the body. Urine tests give particular data to a physician on the metabolic function of the body. Also, a routine urine analysis will show how much protein is spilling out of the kidneys and tell how much sugar is in the blood. Diabetes is usually confirmed through the urine test.

The Normal Test. When the body is healthy, urine excretion from the kidneys with will be straw color, clear, and with a slightly aromatic smell. The specific gravity will range from 1.005 to 1.020 and will range from an acidic 4.5 to an alkaline 8.0.

The following basic urinalysis gives a general overview of certain components which, if present in urine, signal a malfunction or disease. For instance, a high level of ketones, which should not be present, indicates the body may be deydrated and burning fat rather than sugar. High levels of bilirubin signal a possible blockage in the bile ducts, possible cancer, or jaundice.

Basic Urinanalysis

Substance	Presence	Elevated
protein	normally none	multiple myeloma
		Waldenstrom's
		macroglobulinemia
glucose	normally none	diabetes
ketones	normally none	diabetes out of control
bilirubin	normally none	jaundice, duct blockage
blood	normally none	infection, kidney stones

With the aid of a microscope, the presence of certain cells in a higher than normal range indicates possible infection or disease, while other cells should not be present at all. A high level of leukocytes indicates the body is at war with an invader, particularly if the nitrate level is also high.

Cells	Presence
red blood cells	0 to 3/high-powered field
white blood cells	0 to 4/high-power field
epithelial cells	few
casts	none, except for a few hyaline casts
crystals	present
yeast cells	none
parasites	none

The Abnormal Urinalysis and What It Signals

Result	Possible Problem
Nonstraw color	diet, drugs, inflammatory disease, infectious disease, increased specify gravity
"Fruity" odor	ketones in urine, burning fat
Bad smell	urinary-tract infection
Cloudy or murky	fat, germs, kidney infection, red blood cells, white blood cells
Sp. gravity <than 1.005	congestive heart failure, dehydration, diabetes, kidney damage or infection liver failure, nephrosis, shock
pH alkaline	alkalosis, dietary factors, Fanconi's syndrome, increased consumption of vegetables, citrus, dairy products urinary tract infection
pH acid	acidosis, high-protein diet, fever
Protein	kidney infection, kidney stones, multiple myeloma, polycystic kidney disease, renal failure

Sugars	Cushing's syndrome, diabetes, increased intracranial pressure
Ketones	diabetes mellitus, diarrhea, starvation state, vomiting
Cells	bleeding disorder, cystitis, kidney dis ease, genitourinary tract bleeding, hydronephrosis, infection, inflammation, lupus nephritis, malaria, obstruction, parasitic bladder infection, renal hypertension, renal tuberculosis, scurvy
Casts	Acute inflammation, acute or chronic renal failure, kidney disease, blood dyscrasias, chronic lead intoxication, collagen disease, diabetes, eclampsia, heavy-metal poisoning, lupus, malignant hypertension, nephrosis, renal tubular damage, trauma, vascular disorders
Crystals	Hypercalcemia, inborn metabolism error
Other	Parasites, prostate infections, vaginitis, urethritis, yeast cells

Specialized Urine Tests

There are several medical laboratory tests for urine which reveal more speciific information. These include:

URINE AMPHETAMINES
(tests for various drugs)

Type	Therapeutic	Toxic
amphetamine	2-3mcg/ml	greater than 30mcg/ml
dextroametamine	1-1.5mcg/ml	greater than 15mcg/ml
methamphetamine	3-5mcg/ml	greater than 40mcg/ml
phenmetrazine	5-30mcg/ml	greater than 50mcg/ml

URINE AMYLASE

(This test helps diagnose acute and chronic pancreatitis and salivary-gland disorders. Reporting methods differ from lab to lab. The Mayo Clinic lists urinary excretion of 10 to 80 amylase units/hour as normal. Please note: Certain drugs may affect test findings: bethanechol, codeine, fluorides, indomethocin, morphine, meperidine, pentazocine, thiazide diuretics. Others factors which may shift test results include alcohol, heavy bacterial contamination of the urine, and blood in the urine.)

Elevated	Decreased
actue spleen injury	alcoholism
gallbladder disease	liver cancer
mumps	chronic pancreatitis
acute pancreatitis	cirrhosis
pancrease cancer	liver abscess
perforated peptic	hepatitis
duodenal ulcers	
kidney disease with	
poor absorption	

URINE CONCENTRATION & DILUTION
(determines poor kidney function)

Normal Range

specific gravity
1.025-1.031

osmolality above
800mOsm/kg of water

Out of Normal Range

decreased kidney blood flow, loss of functional nephrons, pituitary or cardiac dysfunction tubular epithelial damage

URINE COPPER
(confirms Wilson's disease)

Normal Range

women 0.8-1.7g/24hr

Increased Level

biliary cirrhosis, urinary output, chronic active hepatitis, nephrotic syndrome, rheumatoid arthritis, liver degeneration, eye lens degeneration

URINE CREATININE
(looks at how efficiently the kidney filters and excretes creatinine)

Normal Range

women 0.8-1.7/24hrs

Decreased Level Indicates

shock, kidney stones, enlarged prostate, chronic bilateral kidney infection (which leads to loss of kidney function if not treated)

The Stool Test

Checking for blood in human waste excretion gives doctors the opportunity to learn more about the intestinal health of a patient without X-ray or surgery.

Tumors, ulcers, gastritis, colonitis, and various inflammation disorders may be characterized by small amounts of blood which will not be noticeable except by laboratory stool examination.

As more people travel aboard, immigrate to the United States, or eat sushi, stool checks for parasites have become more common. This does not mean every doctor is aware of the problem. Some continue to scoff at the idea, but you may wish to check with a specialist in this area if diarrhea, weakness, or strange stomach upsets persist beyond several months time. (Some people have had weird symptoms for a long time, only to discover their problem relates back to a trip abroad three years ago!)

Let's face it, ground water and reservoirs in the United States are no longer the pristine sources of clean drinking water they were a hundred years ago. Modern technology and urban living have added contamination. In 1993, California state health officials found wide spread amoeba contamination in city water reserves in Los Angeles, despite water purification efforts. In Milwaukee, some 400,000 residents were sickened by a microbiological pathogen.

When in doubt, have a simple stool sample checked for parasites. If symptoms persist, request a second lab report from a different laboratory.

The Hair Test

If we only knew the tales our hair can tell about the subtle contamination in our body cells from heavy metal exposure to aluminum, lead, mercury, and cadmium among other toxins.

Scientists speculate about the cause of heavy metal buildup in humans and many agree the cause points to contamination from a technological society that offers ease, speed, and convenience without adequate assurance of safety.

For instance, examine the outside box of modern cosmetics adored by women and men. A leading ingredient is aluminum in some form or another whether it be "aluminum lakes," or "aluminum powder." Cost is no protection. Just look on the labels of the most expensive cosmetic products (French included) and you will find aluminum in lipstick, eye liner, face rouge, as well as deodorant.

Hair dyes for men tend to contain high concentrations of lead and the rinses and bleaches for women often are composed of as many as four known carcinogenic substances. Yet these products continue to be sold in a profit-driven business culture.

As more and more hydrocarbon exposure enters the daily life of the modern resident from petrochemicals, plastic food packaging, pesticides, food dyes and preservatives, fixatives in cosmetics, etc., the human immune system is overloaded in its attempt to protect body organs, blood, and bones from outside poison.

Heavy metal contamination is present as well. Scientists speculate on how heavy metals enter the human body. Some believe aluminum foil and aluminum pans result in harmful contamination of the body with aluminum ions. This speculation is based on medical examinations of the brains of deceased Alzheimer victims. There is a heavy concentration of aluminum ions present in the tissue of these unfortunate patients.

The Prostate Specific Antigen Test

Massive confusion often exists when a man is told his prostate specific antigen level (PSA) is elevated beyond zero. This is frightening because it may mean his body is mobilizing soldiers to fight a cancer problem. Many times, however, when the PSA reading is low, there is some other cause for enlargement or inflammation. Identified by Dr. Richard Ablin of Stony Brook Hospital as an indication of the prostate gland's attempt to fight infection or cancer cells, PSA test results may be analyzed by one of two techniques, according to Lloyd Ney, Director and founder of the Patient Advocates for Advanced Cancer Treatments (PAACT) in Grand Rapids, Michigan. This organization is the largest prostrate information bank in the world with over two million data entries of information for interested patients, located at 1143 Parmellee NW, Grand Rapids, MI 49504, (616) 453-1477.

The confusing problem, says Ney, is that the ranges of interpretation for the two PSA analysis tests differ. Most doctors agree the best PSA score is a 0, with ranges over 3 indicating some kind of inflammation, enlargement, or benign growth. After a PSA reading of 5 and definitely over 9, a man may wish to have an exploratory biopsy done by a well respected urologist to determine the true cause for the rise in the prostate specific antigen level.

In current times, there is frustration over whether to treat prostate enlargement with immediate surgery to biopsy a mass or to try a testosterone supressing flutamide such as Eulexin, which blocks the production of male hormone at the neuroreceptors to prevent the feeding of cancer cells. Llyod Ney urges men not to undergo medical castration or radical prostatectomy without trying hormonal suppression first.

Ney should know. He developed prostate cancer in the mid 70's, was given 6 months to live, and told to forget chemotherapy. But Ney wouldn't give up.

His engineer "can do" attitude led him to Canada to the clinic of Dr. Fernand Labrie at Laval University in Quebec City and the hormone treatment which Ney says will cure most prostate cancer. Ney points out that research dating back to 1941 shows prostate enlargement and prostate cancer are basicly diseases of the endocrine system and should be treated with that in mind. Why haven't we heard this before?" "More money is spent on surgery than on hormone treatments, so doctors go with the flow," says Ney, who is indignant and sometimes outraged over the stories he hears from male prostate patients who might have been cured of their prostate cancer, but who were frightened into surgeries which limited or stopped the continuance of their male potency.

Ney's cancer had spread beyond the prostate and he had 32 tumors in his bones.

"The second day I got on the hormone therapy, the pain disappeared," says Ney. "After six months, my bone scan indicated a 60 percent reduction in tumor volume. Now 16 years later, all of Ney's 32 bone tumors have disappeared and his PSA level is zero. He did not undergo radical castration, but did stay on Eulexin for 8 years, which averaged between $180 and $250 a month.

Ney started Patient Advocates for Advanced Cancer Treatment in reaction to backward prostate cancer attitudes and treatment by U.S. doctors. His nonprofit organization has IRS clearance of its tax status, has made referrals in 85 countries around the world, and boasts of a 2,000,000 bit data bank on prostate cancer. Mr. Ney alleges that two U.S. Supreme Court Justices and Senator Robert Dole have called PAACT and used their information and referral services.

Important points for a man to remember if he receives a PSA report over 3 is: 1) the analysis and interpretation methods of PSA tests differ depending on which test was used; 2) most elevated PSA results under 7 by any test procedure is usually benign, but signals a problem which should be addressed as soon as possible; 3) there is strong indication from a variety of research and medical sources that certain herbs such as saw palmetto and *Pygemium africanium* provide effective natural blockage of testosterone at the neuro receptors, inhibiting the growth of tumor cells; and 4) researchers have found a severe zinc deficiency linked to prostate problems.

The Hybritech PSA test lists 0 to 4 as a normal antigen range in healthy men.

The Yang test shows 0 to 2.5 as the healthy range. Before you panic, find out which test has been used if the result is beyond 2.5.

PSA levels over three can be further explored with the transrectal ultrasound accompanied by a needle guided biopsy to determine the histology of any mass present in the prostate gland.

PSA levels between 3 and 9 may be just an enlargement or benign inflammation. PSA levels over 9 have a high probability of being a cancer mass. Levels over 20 indicate the cancer is not confined to the prostate and may be in the lymph glands. A PSA over 50 indicates a definite spread of prostate cancer to other areas of the body, particularly bone mass in the pelvic area.

As prostate cancer is a disease of the endocrine system, hormonal suppression at the neuro receptors should be tried before surgery pending consultation with your doctor regarding how far the disease has spread. Men over 40 years of age should get a baseline PSA level and continue checking this level every few years until 50. After that time, most doctors recommend annual testing for the prostate specific antigen. But there is a great deal of controversy over whether the PSA actually saves lives in terms of its overall, epidemiological effects. For the individual, there may be benefit.

The Thyroid Function Test

When the hypothalamus releases its thyroid-releasing hormone (TRH), this causes the anterior pituitary gland to secrete thyroid-stimulating hormone (TSH). Thyroxinc (T4) from the thyroid gland is stimulated by the TSH secretion. Thus, TSH and T4 levels are used to distinguish pituitary from thyroid dysfunctions.

A decrease in T4 level and a normal or high level of TSH can signal a thyroid disorder. A decreased T4 level with a decreased TSH level can indicate a pituitary disorder.

Aspirin, steroids, dopamine, and heparin can cause a false negative in the thyroid function test, so beware of taking these drugs prior to clinical testing.

Pitfalls in Medical Testing

There can be great variation on a number of factors among medical tests, particularly those conducted in public places. A 1990 study of public cholesterol screening programs published in the *Journal of the American Medical Association* reported only one program in four sampled was able to find consistent blood results. The other three missed the boat on accuracy.

Conducted by the Department of Health and Human Services, this survey found the staff conducting public cholesterol screening programs often had little or no training for this type of test.

Fifty percent of the people who had blood drawn at one of four mall locations indicated the staff did not put on new gloves with each patient. In the same study, 35% said those drawing blood did not wear gloves at all.

Thus, it is wise to be cautious and informed toward public testing sites. Demand that gloves be changed. Watch carefully to be certain new needles are used and beware of a fresh blood on top tables and desks.

Even doctors need to be alert to potential errors, poor interpretation technique, and the overall reputation of a medical laboratory they use for patient testing. Variation occurs because of the way samples are collected.

Glucose or blood sugar levels, for example, will show a drastic difference if taken after a food fast of 12 hours. A similar problem exists with cholesterol tests, in which fat levels may be higher if a person had a big meal right before blood was drawn. It is a good idea to fast for 12 hours before a cholesterol test for better accuracy.

Choice and Analysis of Laboratory Tests

Dr. Kenneth Blick, Associate Professor of Pathology at the University of Oklahoma Health Sciences Center, points out the importance of the choice of test. "Some tests are extremely accurate, while others may require more specific tests to confirm the initial results."

Knowing how well a laboratory analyzes its samples is often hard to judge. Most doctors go on word of mouth and reputation, but who knows what specific errors might occur which will never be detected?

A Glendale, California based physician, Dr. Anita Pepi, D.C. air mails stool samples to an out-of-state lab for parasite testing. Dr. Pepi was convinced her client had parasites from his medical history. But local testing returned a negative result. So she divided a stool sample collected from the patient. One sample went to the local lab near her office and the other to a laboratory back

East on the recommendation of another doctor. The local lab found no parasites, while the second lab not only found the presence of parasites, but was able to identify the exact type of "bug."

New Horizons in Laboratory Tests

This chapter has focused on basic lab tests ordered by a physician. New self tests conducted at home advance patient involvement with medical treatment.

One such test is the Cancer Home Screening Test. The University of Wisconsin Clinical Cancer Center reports an early detection, home test for bladder cancer and kidney disorders which allows a patient to detect infrequent, microscopic levels of blood in urine samples.

Researchers are hopeful this test will help detect early symptoms of bladder and kidney disease before tumor cells invade deep into bladder tissue. The test is done on a repeated basis.

But such self testing provides new problems as well.

Dr. Megan Shields, a family practice physician in Los Angeles,, cautions patients not to interpret medical tests alone. Dr. Shields is not an advocate of home medical testing because "someone with an illness will not be the best judge of medical test results. Doctors don't interpret their own medical tests for the same reason. It is far better to have another doctor do that when he or she is ill."

The answer to medical lab tests may reside in a combined effort on the part of the patient to understand tests more completely and for doctors to explain laboratory findings with greater care to their clients.

30. Procaine Substitutes

If you could find a nutritional supplement that could make you feel really—we mean *really*—good, help you develop a positive attitude and fight aging, would you use it? You bet you would!

Romanian cardiologist Dr. Ana Aslan, M.D., pioneered rejuvenation therapy during the 1950s with her use of the procaine-based Gerovital H3. Dr. Aslan was Romania's first female physician and cardiologist.

Procaine itself was developed in the early 1900s as a substitute for cocaine which we see in the root of the word (*pro*—instead of; *caine*—short for cocaine). Another name for procaine is Novocain.

After a year of frustration trying to help thousands of patients with age related problems, Dr. Aslan began researching the medical literature for anything that might offer a glimmer of hope that the effects of age-related disease could be staved off and at least palliated.

Dr. Aslan learned from the *Journal of Physiology* that there is an enzyme in our bodies called monoamine oxidase (MAO), which stays at about the same level until we reach age 35. Then it goes up dramatically every year as we age. MAO circulates throughout the body but its heaviest concentration is in the brain. A malfunction in the central nervous system affects every part of the body. Many doctors found that the level of MAO in the human body was much higher in people who suffered debilitating diseases such as arthritis, neuritis, arteriosclerosis, senility, and depression.

Dr. Aslan began experimenting with aged experimental animals to see whether or not various formulations would safely lower their MAO levels. After more than a year of experimentation, she found that one particular formula lowered the amount of MAO in her aged experimental animal subjects by 85 percent in two weeks.

The doctor knew she was onto something very special and continued to treat the rats with her new formula. After long years of experimentation, she was finally ready to try her formula on a human. Dr. Aslan was sure it was safe because she had given numerous experimental animals huge dosages without any ill effects.

One writer describes Dr. Aslan's initial medical application of procaine at the Imisoara Faculty of Medicine in Transylvania. "On April 15, 1949, she inquired of the staff if it had a rheumatism patient who wouldn't mind trying a new treatment. A twenty-year-old medical student, bedridden for weeks, volunteered because he was desperate: His right leg was locked stiff at the knee, totally immobile.

"She injected 10 cc of procaine . . . Almost immediately the youth burst into hysterical laughter. The pain had vanished. Moreover, he could bend his knee. Once, twice, three times. The injections continued and within days he left the hospital."

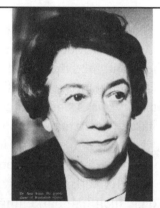

Dr. Ana Aslan, M.D., pioneered rejuvenation therapy with procaine. Her research ultimately led to the identification of the active ingredients in procaine—diethylamino-ethanol and para-amino benzoic acid—both of which are available as supplements to help develop a positive attitude and prevent free radical damage.

In the hospital where she worked, a man had arthritis so bad he couldn't even move his legs. Dr. Aslan suggested he volunteer to try her MAO-reducing formula. The bedridden, depressed man said he was willing to try anything. Within a day the man could move his legs freely. Two days later he went home, walking as if he never had arthritis. Shortly thereafter, a homeless man was brought to the hospital by the police. He was disheveled, crippled and mute, suffering depression and in a terminal stage of senility without memory. Within a year of her special therapy, the old man was alert, vigorous and mobile with his memory restored.

He was an Armenian named Parsh Margosian. Newspapers printed the story with his picture. A daughter who hadn't seen him in years recognized him as her father and brought documents to the doctor showing Parsh to be 109 years old. Rumors at the time were that Nikita Khrushchev was suffering from an unknown or secret affliction and didn't have long to live. After the news of the 109 year old man, Dr. Aslan said the KGB came to her quarters in the middle of the night and told her to pack. A month later Khrushchev appeared in public remarkably revitalized. At the same time Dr. Aslan was made the Chief Doctor and Administrator of Bucharest Geriatric Institute and soon became famous throughout the world. So did her formula which she called Gerovital H3.

Dr. Aslan kept meticulous records on 111 patients for over 15 years making sure they continued their treatment. On the average, these patients lived 29 percent longer than average life expectancy.

Clinically, Dr. Aslan worked with thousands of patients and she found that Gerovital alleviated many aging problems such as arthritis, neuritis, impotence, mental deterioration, memory loss, psoriasis, asthma, angina pectoris, ulcers, arteriosclerosis, depression, poor skin and muscle tone, diminished sexual drive, wrinkling, loss of energy, osteoporosis and hearing loss. Some patients even found their hair darkening. Elsewhere in Europe, Dr. Edith Pakesch of Vienna, Austria, reported that patients receiving treatments with Gerovital H3 all felt much better physically and it had an astonishing effect on their mental clarity and emotional stability.

Most doctors didn't believe one formula could help all these problems until 1973 when Dr. Joseph P. Hrachovac of the University of California found Gerovital did, in fact, reduce levels of MAO in the body.

Dr. David MacFarlane of the University of Southern California confirmed Dr. Hrachovac's research. Dr. Arnold Abrams of the Chicago Medical School conducted a series of carefully controlled double blind tests on GH3 with positive results. Dr. Keith Ditman, Medical Director of Vista Hill Psychiatric Foundation in San Diego, and Dr. Sidney Cohen, Professor of Psychiatry at the University of California, reported to the Gerontological Society in 1973 that 89 percent of aging patients reported less depression and an increased sense of well being after taking Gerovital H3. In describing the therapeutic benefits of Gerovital, Cohen and Ditman reported that most patients who used the supplement felt a greater sense of well-being and relaxation, slept better at night and obtained relief from depression and the discomforts of chronic inflammation and degenerative diseases. Dr. William Zung, Professor of Psychiatry at Duke University and associate professor Dr. H.S. Wang, reported at the 1975 American Geriatrics Society annual meeting that subjects in a double blind test with Gerovital H3 showed significant improvement in their mental acuity. The evidence is very strong that the ingredients in Gerovital H3 work.

Documented patient improvements included increased physical and intellectual capabilities, healthier skin, hair and nails, normalized blood pressure, increased muscular strength and joint mobility, and a delaying effect on degenerative disease. After four decades of use, Dr. Aslan (1985) reported that signs of aging in patients were not only postponed. In some cases they were reversed. Furthermore, all of these benefits were arrived at without observable side effects (Aslan 1985).

Throughout four decades, Dr. Aslan's National Geriatric Institute in Bucharest became a mecca for world leaders and celebrities who sought a scientifically proven method to slow aging.

Such notables as French president Charles De Gaulle, U.S. President John F. Kennedy, Chinese Chairman Mao Tse Tung, actors like Marlene Dietrich and Charlie Chaplin all journeyed to the Otopeni Clinic just outside the ancient city of Bucharest to partake of the rejuvenating therapy using the drug she developed, Gerovital H3. Procaine therapy via injection is now used in over 20 countries around the world.

For the average person, however, employing the institute's resources was prohibitively expensive, and the procaine-based formula was administered by injection.

It was only a matter of time before the public demanded an equally effective non-prescription formula. That need resulted in the highly successful oral version of Aslan's formula.

Historically, what exactly procaine contained that made it such a valuable longevity tool was not well understood—until recently.

The main ingredient in Dr. Aslan's original Gerovital H3 is procaine. It had to be injected daily, and few people wanted to get a shot every day. The second problem is that procaine is a drug only doctors are allowed to administer. But when Dr. Aslan discovered her procaine compound, technology was not available to follow the drug in the body to see exactly how it worked and was broken down. Today, researchers know that procaine is converted in the body to para-amino benzoic acid (PABA) and 2-Dimethyl Aminoethanol Bitartrate (DMAE). Both are substances contained in minute amounts in some foods.

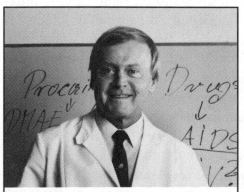

Hans Kugler, Ph.D., is one of the nation's most esteemed longevity researchers whose credentials include being president of the National Health Federation and the author of four best sellers. Dr. Kugler's ground breaking work at Roosevelt University in identifying the active ingredients of procaine is largely responsible for the availability today of an improved oral version of the Aslan formula to the general public.

Dr. Hans Kugler is probably the key figure in making this rejuvenating formula available to the widest numbers of people ultimately through his research at Roosevelt University where he learned that PABA and DMAE have virtually the same effects as procaine in the old Gerovital H3 formula. Dr. Kugler reports, "In my own longevity studies on cancer-prone mice at Roosevelt University in Chicago, we used procaine as one of the life-extending factors. In two animal studies, we compared procaine to the DMAE/PABA mixture and found literally the same positive results for the DMAE/PABA mixture as for procaine itself. If so many anti-aging effects, ranging from stimulating diuresis to recharging the formation and secretion of helpful hormones and enzymes have been traced to DMAE/PABA (which make up procaine) in the last forty years, imagine what the future might hold."

Longevity experts assert today that the multiple beneficial properties of procaine aren't solely due to the whole molecule itself but to its hydrolyzed byproducts which are quickly metabolized by the body (Kugler 1990a). The two breakdown products are diethylaminoethanol (DEAE) which is converted into dimethylaminoethanol (DMAE) and para-amino benzoic acid (PABA). Dr. Kugler (1990b) asserts that DMAE and PABA match procaine in effectiveness in enhancing brain function, cellular regeneration, and immunity.

One of the most essential and unique nutrients available to longevity seekers today is dimethylaminoethanol. Hochschild (1973) reports in *Experimental Gerontology* that cellular membrane degradation has been proposed as a prime mechanism of aging. The dimethylaminoethanol moiety is common to a number of drugs known to stabilize cellular membranes. Furthermore DMAE is the immediate precursor of choline in the biosynthesis and repair of cellular membranes. The natural presence of DMAE in living organisms has been demonstrated although concentrations are minute (Honegger 1959) presumably due to its methylation to choline. It is found most abundantly in those foods which the public tends to thinks of as "brain" foods such as anchovies and sardines.

DMAE is superior to dietary choline as a source of choline for membrane biosynthesis. Hochschild (1973) reports, "This seeming contradiction is due to the relative inability of administered choline to cross cellular membranes and to reach the site of membrane biosynthesis, in contrast to DMAE. The latter, for example, has a remarkable ability to cross the blood-brain barrier; choline does not." DMAE is superior to choline for the biosynthesis as well of acetylcholine (Hochschild 1973). Furthermore, experimental research has shown that DMAE has extended the lives of experimental animals by approximately 30 to 40 percent, according to Hochschild (1973) who concludes: "Aging is associated with an increasing biochemical imbalance. Whether this is a cause or effect of the aging process is unclear. Most likely it is both, meaning that age changes may be partly the result of cells not having optimum or correct amounts of vital substances needed for their function. Because of its essential role in membrane biosynthesis, dimethylaminoethanol is one such vital substance. The present results suggest that aging processes can be influenced by maintaining proper concentrations of dimethylaminoethanol."

DMAE also has been demonstrated to have a beneficial stimulant effect. Murphree and colleagues (1959), using double blind methods for studying DMAE under grants from Riker Laboratories, the U.S. Public Health Service Mental Health Institute and Geschickter Fund for Medical Research, report in *Clinical Pharmacology and Therapeutics* that, "Of the psychological and subjective responses, the significant findings were an increase in muscle tone, better mental concentration, and changes in sleep habits which were (1) less sleep needed, (2) sound sleep, and (3) absence of the customary period of inefficiency in the morning in the deanol (DMAE)-treated group." The exposed group generally reported favorable effects such as "improved mood," "relief of headaches," and "clearer thinking."

DMAE, reports Osvaldo (1974), has been shown to be useful in the management of learning and behavior disorders of childhood. Administration was 300 to 500 mg daily. And Pharmacist Ross Pelton reports in *Mind Food & Smart Pills* (Doubleday 1989) that, "Results from the use of DMAE have shown that it elevates mood, improves memory and learning, increases intelligence and extends life span."

Osvaldo (1974) also reports also that DMAE has been successful in treatment of Huntington's chorea probably by enhancement of cholingeric activity. He notes, "An average of 500 mg daily in children and 1,000 mg daily in adults seems to be necessary for achieving clear-cut therapeutic effects . . . . The best clinical effects have been achieved after three months of treatment in children and there seems to be a minimum period of time for best effects."

Miller (1974) reported the results of DMAE therapy in 11 Parkinsonian patients with levodopa-induced dyskinesia. At a dosage between 500 and 900 mg daily, dyskinesias were completely eliminated in eight patients and greatly improved in a ninth. The therapeutic response began 10 to 14 days after initiation of treatment. In five patients successfully treated with deanol (DMAE), placebo was substituted after four weeks and dyskinesias reappeared within three to eight days. One of the two patients who did not respond discontinued treatment because of fatigue. No other side effects were reported.

The U.S. Food and Drug Administration originally allowed DMAE to be marketed as a prescription drug by Riker Laboratories under the trade name Deaner and authorized Riker to claim it was "possibly effective" for (1) learning problems associated with underachieving and shortened attention span (2) behavior problems associated with hyperactivity and (3) combined hyperkinetic behavior and learning disorders with underachieving, reading and speech difficulties, impaired motor coordination, and impulsive/compulsive behavior, often described as asocial, antisocial, or delinquent."

Pelton reports that in 1983, however, Riker "discontinued making Deaner because the FDA asked for an efficacy study. An efficacy study would give more solid proof of the effectiveness of the drug in producing the above-listed results. Since the market was too small to make the costs of such a study worthwhile, Riker decided to drop the product."

There are other mechanisms by which DMAE probably works. The active ingredients in the original formula—and probably the offspring oral formulae—inhibit the activity of an enzyme called monoamine oxidase (MAO). Ordinarily, MAO holds in check brain neurotransmitters. But with advancing age, levels of MAO tend to increase. A number of MAO inhibitors are being marketed in the U.S. as antidepressants. Gerovital proved to be a better inhibitor of MAO than prescription drugs which produced liver damage, hypertension, chest pain and headache as side effects. Gerovital has demonstrated no such side effects.

In order to better understand his clinical successes, Ronald L. Peters, M.D., who has used amino acid therapies for a number of years, looked more carefully at the combination of nutrients in one of Dr. Aslan's offspring products which combined DMAE and PABA with amino acids. He reports, "Glutamic acid is a stimulant neurotransmitter while l-taurine is the second most plentiful amino acid in the brain, and serves a major role in ion exchange and stabilizing electrical membranes. And, of course, magnesium is essential to membrane electrical stability throughout the body and is deficient in many people with frequently associated fatigue."

PABA is also part of the Dr. Aslan-spawned products. Dr. Earl Mindell (1991) reports that, "In experiments with animals, it has worked with pantothenic acid to restore gray hair to its natural color." Other studies have demonstrated that PABA may help keep skin healthy and smooth and may help in delaying wrinkles.

Thus, the combination of PABA and DMAE appears to be a powerful aid in not only staying young but feeling young.

One of the best combinations we have found to promote an optimal positive attitude and high energy is to supplement with the following nutrients—including vitamins, minerals amino acids—in these amounts which are in ideal proportion.

Procaine-based Positive Attitude Supplement

L-Tyrosine	200 mg
Glutamine	200 mg
Dimethylaminoethanol	200 mg
Para Amino Benzoic Acid	100 mg
Choline	100 mg
L-Taurine	100 mg
Ascorbic Acid	42 mg
Vitamin B-6	30 mg
Vitamin B-12	200 mcg
Vitamin E	60 IU
Magnesium	100 mg

Where to Find the Formula

Although it can be difficult to find suppliers of oral forms GH3 in the U.S., one formula that supplies the active metabolites of procaine therapy—and that has received tremendously positive accolades from users—can be purchased by calling (800) 825-8482. It has been formulated to contain each of the essential nutrients and herbs discussed in this report, especially DMAE and PABA which are, of course, the active ingredients of procaine once metabolized in the body. It is the non-drug form of procaine therapy.

31. *Virtual Eternity*

On the Edge of Eternity

Aging and death do seem to be

What Nature has Planned for us

But what if we have other plans?

—Bernard Strehler, Biogerontologist

What will life extension be like in the Twenty-first Century? How will medical science increase maximum life span? "Maybe every newborn would get an injection," reports USA Today. *"Maybe every adult would consume a third less calories. Maybe every pharmacy would sell pills to rid old bodies of harmful compounds that build with age."*

A man lovingly had the head of his mother severed from her body. His name is Saul Kent. His organization, Life Extension, is pursuing not only longevity—but eternity—with every means available. His mother's head is

*frozen, kept in a state of suspended animation. Kent and his mother are not
alone.*

   In Riverside, Calif., in an industrial park, human heads, severed from
their bodies, are kept in a state of suspended animation in tall, thin cylinders.
They are part of a program of cryogenics—the freezing of the human body,
preserving it for later reanimation. When—and if—medical science learns to
clone bodies, the heads will be reattached to the cloned bodies. Call it a
"gambler's gamble." The process is obviously unproven. How much damage
will the cells go through in the moments following death before they are frozen
and all biological action is halted? And will tomorrow's scientists have the
power to clone bodies from the genetic scriptures within those preserved cells?
The answers are unclear. But people are willing to take the risk. One Florida
man has even willed his house to a trust, so that when he and his wife are
reanimated sometime in the next few hundred years they can return to their
lodgings. He knows it is a long shot. But if cryogenics works, he and his
beloved wife will someday be reunited; if it doesn't work, he loses nothing—
except money, which he couldn't take with him anyway!
   Yet, some scientists put the odds that cryogenics will work at no better than
a generous 10 percent. If you want to achieve longevity *now*, there are many
key supplements and dietary practices available *now*. Because later—in the near
future—breakthroughs in longevity will promise people the opportunity for
virtual eternity.

   Sound like more empty promises from the proverbial fountain of youth? Not
for long.
   Let's listen in on a ficticious conversation in the year 2300 between a man
and his "younger" wife. His name is Burton. He is 251 years old. She is a
youngster at 198. When they met, so afraid was she that he would think she was
too young at 150 that she lied about her age and told him she was actually 180
years. He knew she was lying; after all, she didn't look a day older than 140!
But he liked her. After all, Astrid had lived a varied life. She had gone to college
until she was 75 and learned seven languages before embarking upon her career
as a medical doctor. But at 105, having grown bored with the simplicity of
medicine as it was practiced then, she turned to more adventurous pursuits,

taking an advanced degree in intergalactic agriculture and living on Mars for a number of years, returning back to Earth to take a triple degree in philosophy, literature, and law. This time she stayed in school for two decades, and she was able to read every major classic written, all the philosophers and specialize in several areas of law. After all, there was no hurry. Average life expectancy was now 700 years.

She had raised her children who were now in their early 100s and after 75 years of marriage she and her first husband parted amicably. She expected this, her second marriage, to last at least 150 years. They had many plans. Then she would find somebody, perhaps take a younger lover in his early 100s. After all, marriage for eternity was no longer the standard. Who could live with another for 700 years? Two hundred years—maybe. But anything more with Burton would simply be impossible! thought Astrid as she looked affectionately at her husband.

But today she and her husband, Burton, were going shopping at the local organ exchange. Burton, at 251 and suffering a midlife crisis, wanted a new heart, knees and eyes that would allow him to pursue a career in track and field against much younger men in their early 100s. (Sometimes Burton worried about losing Astrid to one of these younger men even though among *her* friends Astrid bragged that Burton had the sexual powers of a man not a day over 90— especially when he swallowed his DHEA supplements and they added a quick spike of testosterone circulating throughout his body!) Still, Burton worried about getting old, and he wanted to prove to himself that he wasn't, and now he planned to take up a career in track and field.

"If I'm not happy with the heart and knees," he said as they entered the store that was located on Santa Monica Boulevard in Los Angeles, "I swear to you I'm going to directly to the Gene Bank and order some of Carl Harris's genetic blueprints."

"Wasn't he the fellow who ran the 90 second mile?"

"Yeah, and I want his genes! They're on special sale!"

"Well, let's see how this new heart does for you."

Burton looked over the varieties of hearts and finally selected one which promised to make him feel like he was 100 again; upon his arrival home, he unzipped his chest and implanted the new heart in a 20 minute operation, and then he had dinner.

For the next three days Burton worked out at the track and field dome and then he rested, using his muscle rejuvenators to recuperate. While he waited for his muscles to ready themselves, he read for five days. Many centuries ago, Burton read in his history books, people were in a hurry and drove in polluting gas guzzling monstrous cars that seemed to always become mired in traffic jams and people snapped at each other and never had time to *just talk, or just watch a flower bloom. How strange, he thought. How could people live their lives so much in a rush? How could they put their work ahead of the world?*

These days people had plenty of time to talk or do whatever they wanted, and it wasn't uncommon for Burton to get involved in long philosophical discussions with his wife Astrid on just about anything. Putting down his book, Burton turned to Astrid and they spoke intimately for two weeks; although she had been planning to start a new class on the ecology of Galacta, she decided it could wait. After all, what was the hurry? Instead they discussed the looming population crisis in Asia and Africa.

The problem was that the longevity ejections that had been developed by the industrialized west were now being pirated and used by even the poorer peoples of the world (who were not suppose to receive them, according to treaties signed by the major international powers, the U.S., Japan, Germany and China); but the formulae were too easy to reproduce. Unfortunately all too many nations had no national strategies to control population and morning after pills were being withheld in many of the South American nations in deference to the Natural Church which had refused to change its stance of opposition to technology for more than 1,000 years despite the mounting population problems. As a result family size had exploded from the historically small number of seven to ten in an immediate family to more than 100; yet with the proliferation of greenhouse gases and climactic change, agricultural production lagged; the once fertile lands of South America, Asia and Eastern Africa were now eroded barren deserts—largely the result of intensive chemical farming methods that stripped the soil instead of nourishing it. The rain forests that had once offered economic vitality had been destroyed by greedy corporations who logged them for their immediate profits. These lands were now deserts and food riots were spreading throughout the world; famine was a reality for the half of the world's population.

After 150 years of marriage, Burton was now in his 373rd year, and he had begun to feel some of the effects of old age, requiring new eyes, new teeth, and brain. Feeling that he was too old, he had an affair with a younger woman, an astronomer, who was only 93. Astrid accused Burton of "robbing the cradle" and left him in a huff. The fight lasted several years. Astrid had taken on another career, leading guided tours to the newly discovered planet of Xerxes. Burton soon grew tired of the astronomer; she had no life experience! He and Astrid both met somebody new, but there was no pain in their divorce: people no longer expected to marry for life. After all, who could want to live with the same person for 500 years?

"Could there ever be a time when you could be bored with life?" asked his son Edgar who was only a child at 75.

"No, Edgar, life is a gift, and we have only a short time on Earth," replied Burton.

But the real Burton had disappeared. The "Burton" speaking with his grandson Edgar actually had been engineered at the cloning/engineering clinic. The real Burton had left Earth to embark upon an exploration of the world in the Penultimate Galactic Universe #3 which had been discovered in the year 2,422. It was the first time that Earthlings learned they were not alone in the universe and the presence of other life forms had virtually destroyed religions that had posited faith in a single god, for the newer life forms could demonstrate profound powers upon Earth such as parting the seas, causing drought and pestilence and even ordaining the meeting of souls.

Not knowing when he would return from his adventure, expecting to be gone a century or longer and wishing to spare his children the trauma of growing up without a father, Burton had done the only thing he could and cloned himself.

When Burton returned 100 years later at age 463, he met Astrid at the local rejuvenation bar and they toasted, holding their hormonal cocktails, to their adventures over the last 100 years. She looked great for a woman of 411 years, remarked Burton. She had managed to retain her youthful appearance with human skin transplants. She didn't have a single wrinkle. "I think you could pass for a woman of 300," said Burton.

They spent the evening together and they decided to remarry and have more children. So they went to the cyrogenic facility and reunited egg and sperm and watched their fetus develop within its artificial placenta at the baby factory.

When they were 600, Burton and Astrid decided they wanted to experience the ultimate in life—and taste death. But when they went to the physician of death to receive their anti-longevity injections, Burton and Astrid discovered that they themselves were both clones! There would be no death, for their master geneticists had left Earth for a trip to Galaxy Number Nine and had never returned, and only the holders of master genetic codes could destroy a clone. Burton and Astrid held each other tightly upon hearing the news because now they lived in fear—the fear of endless life!

Rapid Strides

Scientists are making rapid strides that may fundamentally change the process of aging—from genetic engineering to nutrition. Researchers believe there are about 100,000 human genes in the body. They have identified 10,000 of them but expect to have them all identified by the year 2000. Progress is increasing exponentially. The limits are endless. When the genes are discovered that turn on and turn off death (there are such genes, researchers believe)—virtual eternity will have arrived!

"There's no limit, as far as we know, to doubling or tripling human life span," says biogerontologist Richard Cutler at the National Institute on Aging's Gerontology's Research Center in Baltimore. "What we really need," he says, "is to declare a war on aging . . ."

The headline in the October 16, 1992 issue of *The Wall Street Journal* was no surprise to those experts in the fields of gerontology and longevity.

Fountain of Youth May Not Be Fairy Tale, Study Finds

Nor was the newspaper's lead:

"In experiments shattering common notions about life expectancy, scientists uncovered the first evidence suggesting there may be no inborn limit to how old people can grow."

This is the present situation in which we find ourselves: Upon reaching the age of 65 American men can expect to live another 15.4 years with 13.4 years of relatively good health, two years of disability. Women age 65 have a life expectancy of 20.5 years with 16.2 years of active living and 4.3 years of disability.

But these statistics don't have to mean anything to your life. *You* can beat these odds. Each time experts predict a maximum life expectancy, says Duke University demographer Kenneth Manton, "five to 10 years later, we approach the limit and they raise it a little higher."

Ten years ago, the mere mention of living to 100 would have seemed out of reach for most people. But not today.

In the past decade, the number of Americans 100 years or older has doubled to reach an extraordinary 35,800 centenarians, reported *USA Today* in its July 23, 1992 edition. By the year 2000, the count of American centenarians will almost double again, the Census Bureau projects—and by 2050 Americans living to 100 could number in the millions.

The paper tells the story of 101-year-old widower Herald Greene who reads two newspapers, mows the lawn at the Elliott County, Ky., home where he lives with daughters—he has five children ages 59 to 71—fishes and plays the coronet.

He was a boy, *USA Today* reports, when tuberculosis killed his mother; a teen-ager when pneumonia killed his two-year-old half-brother; a young man when the 1918 flu epidemic killed 500,000 in the U.S. By 1900, when he was only a boy, the average American's life span was only 47 years. Today, it is about 75 years. "The doctors are doing wonderful things," Green says.

After a life of hard work on a farm and in a soda factory, Greene told *USA Today:* "I'm very fortunate. I have a good memory . . . . I have no major ailments. I'm just hanging on, hanging on. I want to hang on a long while if I can."

Then there is Wilk Peters who at 91 still drives, keeps a 151-foot hedge trimmed and takes French, reports *USA Today.*

More than ever before in the history of humankind, we have the greatest opportunity to live to the age of 100-years-old and beyond! And we're talking about life free from illness, mental and physical debility, and disease.

"What drives most of this research is not the desire to be immortal," says biologist Richard Sprott of the National Institute on Aging. "It's the desire not to die in a nursing home.

"I think most of us would trade dying at age 85 rather than 105 if we knew we could be healthy up to 85 and that we could have one last cigar or bourbon and kick off."

One of the most promising areas of longevity research is the study of the internally controlled processes that control aging within each animal--from fruit fly to *homo sapien*. "Mounting evidence points to a multitude of parallel and often interacting processes, many of them genetically controlled, that combine to ensure eventual decrepitude," reports *Scientific American* in its December 1992 issue. The key is that these processes appear to be genetically controlled.

Researchers today are learning more about influencing the effects of genes on living organisms.

The facts tell the story:

•Evolutionary biologist Michael R. Rose, at the University of California at Irvine, has been able to breed a strain of fruit fly that is able to live almost twice as long as ordinary fruit flies. Not only do they live longer, these super flies are far more robust than the ordinary ones. The reason for their longevity seems to be linked with their genetic superiority; the super flies are producing an even more effective form of the cellular antioxidant superoxide dismutase. "The work on Drosophila is trial-run stuff for doing the same thing in mice," he told *Scientific American* (Rusting 1992). "If we can create long-lived mice, specific genes, enzymes and cell processes involved in longevity should be revealed."

•European scientists have discovered the human gene responsible for asthma and say that asthma can be wiped out within five years.

•In one experiment, reported in *The Chicago Tribune*, research Michael West, a molecular biologist at the University of Texas Southwestern Medical Center in Dallas, found that two mortality genes, known as M-1 and M-2, can speed aging or reverse aging whether they are turned "on" or "off." Aging cells have these genes in the "on" position. When West turned "off" the M-1 gene, the cells not only became younger in overall functioning, they increased the number of times they could divide. By turning "off" the second, M-2 gene, the cells appeared to go on agelessly, dividing indefinitely. Turning "on" the M-1 gene results in the aging process. By controlling these genes, West speculates, life can be extended to 200, 400 or even 500 years. *The Chicago Tribune* reports that West has started his own biotechnology company in Dallas, called Geron, devoted to developing those genetic tools that hold potential to reverse aging. "There's no turning back," West told reporters for the *Tribune*. "For the first time in history we have the power to manipulate aging on a very profound level."

•In another related experiment, biologist Thomas Johnson of the Institute for Behavioral Genetics at the University of Colorado in Boulder recently found that the life span of soil-dwelling roundworms can be doubled by altering only one gene. This marks the first time an animal's life span has been significantly increased by genetic controls. "Strikingly, the mutant worms produce elevated levels of antioxidants (both cytoplasmic superoxide dismutase and an enzyme called catalase) and are more resistant to the toxic effects of paraquat, a herbicide that leads to generation of the superoxide radical," notes *Scientific American* (Rusting 1992). Johnson is now searching through the human gene pool to uncover similar genes. Will he find them? Johnson looks to German philosopher Friedrich Nietzsche's book *Thus Spoke Zarathustra* for inspiration: "You have made your way from worm to man, and much in you is still worm." When he finds such a gene, he predicts, human life span will be doubled from 115 years to 230 years.

•The life span of skin cells is doubled by switching off a gene that controls production of the protein called interleukin 1, based on research by molecular biologist Thomas Maciag of the American Red Cross's Jerome Holland Laboratory for the Biosciences in Rockville, Maryland (Kotulak 1991). The technique employed by Maciag is called antisense, which is already used to create ageless tomatoes that stay ripe indefinitely.

"For the first time, after years of evolution, we are on the verge of influencing our fate. Nothing, nothing is impossible," exulted Dr. John Shepherd, a biophysicist at the University of Sussex, Brighton, England, in a recent interview with *Life* magazine.

Other theories are interwoven with the genetic theory of aging. For example, some experts believe that the body's imperfect ability to cope with oxidative stress causes aging (*i.e.*, the free radical theory of aging). The daily wear and tear on our bodies caused by oxidative processes, pollution and other environmental stresses ultimately produces cumulative damage.

The genetic theory and the free radical theory are not mutually exclusive. Perhaps the most long-lived persons today are those whose genes have an unique ability to stimulate highly active, ample supplies of antioxidants.

You can already dramatically cut your risk of dying prematurely from cancer, heart disease, Alzheimer's or other leading killers of Americans today. But soon there will be additional potent anti-aging tools available--pending approval by the U.S. Food and Drug Administration.

Some of the most promising include:

•*Centrophenoxine.* Approved for use throughout Europe although not in the U.S., centrophenoxine can block accumulation of age-related celluar garbage (lipofuscin).

•*Deprenyl.* Already approved for the treatment of Parkinson's disease, deprenyl has been shown to slow the onset of Alzheimer's disease and has shown promise as a life extender.

•*DHEA (dehydroepiandrosterone).* An all-around rejuvenator, DHEA can enhance the immune system, prevent cancer and has far-ranging beneficial influences throughout the human body.

•*Growth Hormone Releasing Hormone.* Not yet FDA approved, it stimulates production of human growth hormone.

•*Human Growth Hormone.* Although approved for the treatment of dwarfism, HGH has shown promise for rebuilding muscle mass in the aged. However, many experts believe its benefits to the aged human body are far more wide ranging and rejuvenating.

•*Insulin-like Growth Factor.* Not yet FDA approved, it stimulates HGH production.

•*Isoprinosine.* Not yet FDA approved, isoprinosine is an immune booster.

•*Nerve Growth Factor.* Although not yet FDA approved, nerve growth factor has shown strong promise as a mind rejuvenator capable of restoring memory to even people severely afflicted with Alzheimer's disease.

•*PBN (alphaphenyltertiarybutylnitrone).* This promising compound, based on exciting animal studies, can block free radicals as well as extend life and improve memory.

•*Thymosins.* One of the keys to understanding the aging process is the thymus gland, which appears to play a pivotal role in immune function, as well as in the endocrine system. Not yet approved, thymosins are immune boosters. They are a group of hormones taken from the thymus gland. Our body's immune cells go to the thymus gland before they are mature; there, they are provided with their instructions for fulfilling their specialized functions. By the time people are aged, their thymus gland is a shrunken vestige of its once vital self. The goal of biochemists is to use thymosins for the rejuvenation of the immune system by remultiplying the body's T-cell count. One of the leading advocates for the thymosins is Dr. Allan Goldstein, chairman of the biochemistry department at George Washington University, Washington, D.C. Dr. Goldstein believes that the thymus gland may have a potentially greater role in aging than in its mastery over the body's immune system. He notes that there is a feedback pathway between the brain and the thymus gland. When the brain secretes the body's flight-or-fight hormone, ACTH, the thymus becomes smaller and reduces the secretion of ACTH. However thymosins also seem to stimulate the brain's release of other hormones and neurotransmitters. Thus, if the thymus shrinks, apparently the brain's production of these other important chemicals also declines. Yet thymosins can reinvigorate the brain to produce more of these other important chemicals. Within the very near future, people will probably be taking thymosin supplements which could help push average life span up to 80 or 90, simply through their stimulation of immune function and the production of important brain chemicals.

Blazing the Trail of Gene Therapy

You just learned the good news. You're going to be a parent. However, you have a history of Alzheimer's disease in your family. In the early embryonic stage of your baby's growth, science has discovered a way to let you know if your baby will suffer from the disease. Do you go ahead with the test? What do you do if it comes up positive? Do you abort? Do you have the baby, knowing it will surely suffer from Alzheimer's as an adult?

The gene for Huntington's disease, the frightening neuro-degenerative illness that killed folk singer Woody Guthrie, has been identified. Through DNA testing, you could find out if you are carrying it. Do you want to know, knowing there is nothing you can do if you have it?

These aren't scenarios to ponder for future generations. Such life and death ethical dilemmas are confronting more and more individuals as you read this. Genetic engineering, or what some may call genetic tinkering, is a scientific reality.

The purpose of this book is to help you live a longer, healthier, happier life.

Within each cell of our body are 23 pairs of chromosomes. Together, these chromosomes contain as many as 100,000 genes. These genes makeup who we are. Upon each gene is "imprinted" a specific genetic code, the instructions that make that particular gene unique. These instructions are our DNA. When the genetic code for that gene is printed incorrectly, the gene receives the wrong information and diseases can occur ranging from Alzheimer's to cancer. What if, locked away in these genes, is the time and nature of your own death. Would you want to know?

Gene doctors are cracking the code of many diseases. Their microscopes are trained on a wide range of such serious ailments as prostate cancer, heart disease, AIDS, multiple sclerosis, and sterility. Human trials, in which patients are having better genes implanted in their cells, have already begun. These include several types of cancer, cystic fibrosis, rare forms of immunodeficiency and high cholesterol. Twenty years ago genetic scientists could identify only 15 genes. Today, that number has shot up to 2,972.

Gene Hunters

Trying to find one small mistake, a wrong letter or two in the genetic code that breaks the normal pattern, is the colossal task researchers must face when trying to identify a mutant gene. Gene hunters use tiny probes, called *markers*, designed to recognize the genetic error. Hunting for the bad gene starts by first finding the marker.

In the spring of 1993, scientists at Boston Massachusetts General Hospital and a dozen other collaborating institutions discovered the mutant gene for a form of Lou Gehrig's disease. Now a person may be able to discover if they have the disease before symptoms arise. By drawing blood and testing the DNA, the mutant gene will show up. As far as diagnostic technology goes, it's really a very simple test. The hard part is developing a workable gene therapy to get rid of the disease. Scientists would have to implant an unmutated copy of the Lou Gehrig's gene, or cap off the faulty gene, in the specific cells that are malfunctioning. It requires getting the exact one-billionth-of-a-millimeter-sized part inside millions of cells into some of the most heavily sealed, hard-to-reach recesses of the human body.

One way is using a virus to transport the DNA. Such a technique is being used with patients suffering from cholesterol problems. Extracted liver cells are infected with a virus containing a gene important to the elimination of cholesterol, then reintroduced back into the patients' cells.

For now, however, discovery of a gene can lead to new therapy. Scientists have learned that Lou Gehrig's disease is caused by a defect in the body's antioxidant system and are planning trials with antioxidant medications such as vitamin E (Maugh 1993).

Gene fixers envision a day when they will have a whole fleet of gene vehicles at their disposal. Some may be viruses, parts of viruses and other microorganisms. Each would be specially designed to zip through the bloodstream and home in on a specific spot.

Being able to find a gene means that diseases can be predicted, or even better, prevented, before they strike.

First Genetic Testing

Finding the right gene is like searching through a jigsaw puzzle of 100,000 pieces. But as more and more pieces are uncovered, the search becomes easier. Huntington's disease was the first major adult condition for which there has been gene testing in this country. A genetic *marker* was discovered in the mid 1980's. Then, in March of 1993, the actual *gene* was identified. Soon, scientists hope to be able to predict the onset of the disease. Thus, a person will not only know that he carries the disease, but when it will become active whether it be in 20 months or 20 years.

Most diseases, however, are far more complicated to track down. The vast majority of common human illnesses are caused by multiple genes working together with multiple environmental factors. Looking for a specific gene without genetic markers is more difficult than looking for a needle in a haystack. And finding one, or even a few, of the genes involved only determines the person's susceptibility to getting sick.

A Family Affair

Identifying defective genes requires studying a family with a history of the particular disease being researched. The bigger the family, the better. The key in using families is to locate genetic markers that are inherited by those who have the disease, not by healthy family members. When such inheritance occurs, it means that a marker exists that lies close to the defective gene. As researchers discover other markers in the same region, it enables them to home in on the defective gene until it is identified.

Hitting the Mark

The closer the marker to the actual gene, the higher the percentage of success in predicting whether or not an individual will develop the disease. Alzheimer's researchers are confident they will find a genetic marker determining susceptibility for the most common forms of the disease within the next couple of years. The discovery of still more markers may be on the near horizon for heart disease, high blood pressure, common forms of cancer, Parkinson's disease, manic depression and schizophrenia.

Such insight into our future health needn't force us to live in fear of what might be. A positive test for skin cancer will let you know to stay out of the sun. Testing positive for prostate cancer simply means adhering to a routine of rigorous check-ups to make sure things remain alright. Early detection may be the key to successful treatment. And in genetic testing, early means early.

In one such case, an infant was tested for cystic fibrosis when he was only eight cells big. Both parents were carriers of the disease. Since it's a "recessive" genetic trait, the offspring needs to get a "bad" copy of the gene from each parent in order to get the disease. By drawing a single cell from the embryo in a petri dish and running a genetic test on the DNA for the cystic fibrosis gene, doctors were able to tell whether or not this embryo would carry both bad genes and get the disease. In this instance, the cell was healthy and the embryo was implanted in the woman's uterus.

Outdated Miracles

Soon, even this miraculous procedure will be outdated. A test using high-tech chip technology will scan a person's DNA with synthetic mutant genes and markers attached to it. Wherever the real, human DNA finds a mutation matching its own, a fluorescent speck will light up. This way, many conditions could be screened for in less time than it takes to do one test now. Someday, Americans may carry computerized cards describing their "carrier" status for the 20 most common inherited ailments. Human embryos and fetuses may be routinely put through a genetic checklist of as many as 50 traits. Ethical questions and value judgments will be challenged like never before. What about selective breeding?

As life gets better, the issues get tougher.

From a purely technological point of view, gene therapy on embryos would have tremendous advantages. Early embryonic cells have the ability to pass on their DNA to future generations. A disease-carrying couple would undergo preimplantation gene therapy, replacing bad genes with good ones. Their child, and their child's children and grandchildren would never have to worry about the ailment again.

Cancer: A Disease of Our Genes

A gene that tells a cell when to divide and when to stop is the cause of all cancers. Some cancers are passed on to the next generation as a result of inherited diseases. These are the cancers we are born with. Others occur in our body on their own. All react to the same sort of error. They are mutations in critical control genes. These mutations can strike completely out of the blue. Or they may be caused by smoking, pollution, diet, or chemicals in our food or environment.

According to Bob Weinberg, a biologist at the Whitehead Institute in Cambridge, Massachusetts, the information which makes a cell cancerous is carried in the DNA of certain kind of gene.

Knowledge about cancer genetics has skyrocketed in the last several years. Treatment of cancer will be radically different as a result of this knowledge. Dennis Slaymin of the University of California at Los Angeles has developed an antibody to fight breast cancer. Pat Stieg of the National Institutes of Health has discovered a single gene that could be responsible for blocking the metastasis of breast tumors. And the day may be near where we can custom design a treatment for the molecular characteristics of the tumor in a woman with breast cancer.

Science is working to discover what gene plays a role in triggering certain cancers. Gene transplantation could be one route in preventing metastasis. Genetic researchers have already discovered the chromosome responsible for inherited breast cancer. Now all they have to do is find the one exact gene, among thousands, that is responsible for this breast cancer in order to cure it.

Very early diagnosis, detection when there are only a few cells, would enable doctors to remove the altered cells. The site would be too small to be felt or seen on a mammogram. Doctors could just "reach in" and pluck out the cells that have gone bad.

A Futuristic Tour

What was unimaginable yesterday is a clear reality today. We have begun putting new genes into defective cells. Embryos are being checked for imperfect genes. Soon we will be able to put new genes directly into embryos and correct genetic problems before a baby grows. Close to 100 gene therapy projects are approved or under way around the world (Maugh 1993).

As we continue on this fantastic voyage there is much to think about. According to Leroy Hood, biologist at the University of Washington, we will have the capability, within the next 20 to 40 years, to virtually wipe out the major diseases that plague mankind. Will genetic engineering, or what might be thought of as "genetic domineering", lead us to genetic conformity? Diversity is nature's key to survival. But will we soon live in a society where choosing our own genes becomes fashionably irresistible?

Today, we are taking into our own hands the machinery that has made us human. We can't afford to make mistakes.

But there's so much more to come, says Hans Kugler, Ph.D who provided his ideas on life extension breakthroughs between today and the year 2030. "We will be able to virtually eliminate many diseases, from Alzheimer's and birth defects to osteoporosis, within the next two decades," predicts Dr. Kugler. For example, says Dr. Kugler, "By 1995, I predict that routine blood testing will be available to test for cystic fibrosis carriers. Treatments will be developed using alpha-hydroxy acids for wrinkled skin that will have far fewer side effects than Retin-A. And the first really effective drugs for Alzheimer's disease will become available that could help 50 percent of all those afflicted. We'll see leukotriene antagonists used to really help doctors relieve asthmatics of their symptoms. In the area of preventive medicine, each person's risk of cancer and heart disease will be determined through routine blood screens for levels of antioxidants. In the area of gene research, we will learn that lung cancer and alcoholism both have genetic links which can make people susceptible to these diseases, and we will be able to determine colon cancer at much earlier stages with genetic screening exams that determine whether there are mutations in the p53 gene. And for men and women concerned about thinning hairlines, new drugs which are much more effective than Rogaine will become available. They will work by inhibiting 5-alpha-reductase. The widespread availability of Taxol will be possible through laboratory synthesis, benefiting millions of people with ovarian and other cancers. Foods will be designed to include specific disease-fighting nutrients and food labeling laws will be liberalized to allow companies to make disease-fighting claims. Fetal tissue transplants will relieve the suffering of Parkinson's sufferers. And that's all within the next two or three years!"

Dr. Kugler says that by the year 2000:

•Nerve growth factor drugs will be able to cure 80 percent of Alzheimer's sufferers, bringing back floods of memories

•The first AIDS vaccine will be approved.

•Vitamins and other nutrients will be routinely prescribed by physicians for the prevention of cancer and heart disease.

•Powerful anti-rejection drugs will be developed to allow the widespread use of organ transplantation, extending life for millions of Americans. Meanwhile, donor laws will be liberalized, allowing the use of organs from deceased individuals--unless they specifically deny their use prior to death.

•Consumers will be able to order blood tests directly without the need of physician's prescriptions.

•Dentures will be replaced by permanent implants made from titanium.

•Eyeglasses will be replaced by laser cornea sculpting.

•The first anti-aging hormone therapies will be available using safe genetically engineered versions of human growth hormone and and DHEA.

Soon to follow will be the use of nerve growth factor for maintenance of our brain and its memory and learning functions.

•Women will be able to give birth at any age! Their eggs will be fertilized in advance when they are younger, frozen in storage and implanted at a later date!

•On the other hand, birth control vaccinations will be available that last an entire year, using anti-human chorionic gonadotropin.

•The first sub-two hour marathon will be through super nutrition and training methods.

•Skin cancer will be prevented with topical and oral DNA repair enzymes.

•Breast cancer will be treated with laser therapy.

•Victims of stroke will be restored to complete normalcy through rejuvenating drugs known as lazaroids (named after Lazarus who rose from death), and the use of deprenyl and glutamate blockers (since

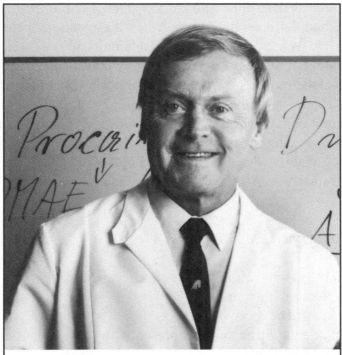

Hans Kugler, Ph. D., predicts that the future life span of people will be well in excess of 150 years. Cures will be found for the major killers today including cancer, diabetes, Alzheimer's, AIDS and stroke. "The age of bionic men and women, who trade in worn body parts for new ones, is not long off," he says.

Dr. Kugler's newest book *Tripping the Aging Clock* is now available through Health Quest Publications.

large amounts of glutamate are released following stroke, causing largescale damage).

•Antioxidant therapy will be used routinely to prevent cataracts.

•Prostate cancer will be treated without cancer; meanwhile other drugs will prevent its and other cancers' spread through the body (*i.e.*, anti-metastasis medications).

•Laparoscopic surgery will be used for removing gallstones, negating the use of surgery; new drugs will become available to prevent the build-up of gallstones from accumulated cholesterol and other substances.

•The RDAs for vitamins C, E, and beta carotene will finally be revised upward to reflect the needs for optimal nutrition! Additional nutrients will be added and new vitamins will be discovered!

•Melatonin will become widely used in supplement form to slow down the body's aging clock.

By 2010:

•The previously deadly disease cystic fibrosis will become treatable with the addition of missing genes that people will inhaler through aerosols.

•Skin transplantation, once reserved for burn victims, will become commonly used for cosmetic purposes for treating wrinkling.

•Cures for AIDS will reduce fatality from this once deadly disease by 80 percent!

•Dramatic decreases in lung cancer will be recorded through continual campaigns aimed at stopping smoking and earlier diagnosis.

•Laser treatment of formerly deadly pancreatic cancer will become a reality. It will also be used for the treatment of breast cancer.

•Artificial hearts will Artificial hearts will replace human hearts in transplant operations. Other artificial organs such as livers, kidneys and pancreases will be available. Does this sound too fantastic to be true? There is already a spare organ company that has begun fabricating human blood vessels, skin and other body parts. It is located in Cambridge, Massachusetts and called Organogenesis. On the other hand, society has been taking advantage of spare parts for the body for a long time. We've gone from wooden peg legs to hooks on the arm (a la Captain Hook) to the ivory dentures of George Washington. Millions of people today are taking advantage of artificial hips, knees, arms, ears and legs. But one day such body parts will be generated from human tissues and become a truly organic part of the body, helping once again extend human life span.

•Deafness will be largely eliminated through bionic implants.
•Creativity genes will be discovered.
•Average life expectancy will increase to 95 years.

By 2020:

•Artificial limbs will be widely available that use bionics and nerve transplants to function as effectively as human limbs. Artificial eyes and ears will also become available.
•Reproduction will now take place, if desired, completely outside the human body.
•Major killing diseases—such as cancer of the prostate and lung, heart disease, Alzheimer's and stroke—will be reduced by 70 to 95 percent.
•Worn out body parts will be cloned through genetic engineering and replaced with new ones.
•Average life span will be 130 to 150 years.

To be sure, our use of such life extenders must be predicated upon their ultimate effectiveness and safety from unwanted side effects. And human kind's manipulation of the human genome and environment will pose new questions of morality and responsibility.   But by keeping yourself healthy today, you will be able to take advantage of these and other key life extenders tomorrow when they do become available.

Live a Healthy Lifestyle

Dr. Hans J. Kugler, Ph.D., reports that good health habits can increase average life span by up to 12 years. Furthermore Hardin Jones of the University of California, Berkeley, showed that the difference in average life spans between people with poor health habits living in a polluted environment in this country, compared to Scandinavian people with good health habits and living in a clean environment, can be as high as 35 to 40 years.

The good health habits that Dr. Kugler believes most people would benefit from include: (1) Good nutrition (2) Exercise (3) Normal weight (4) No smoking (5) Seven to eight hours sleep per day (6) Being able to handle distress and (7) Moderate alcohol consumption.

This is what is available now. But to stay abreast of the cutting edge innovations in life extension, be sure to read the *Longevity Upate* newsletter, which has been called the nation's "leading source" of information on breaking news in the area of longevity research; it will arrive to you every month. (You will find an order form, including several bonus booklets which will be available when you order *now*, at the back of this book.)

Are You Ready?

Our longer life spans mean that we as Americans must give up our preconceived notions of aging. Whereas older people were once pitied and viewed as frail and sick, today we know that it need not be this way. But will you be ready? What will you do with 40 extra years beyond retirement? Will you grow wiser? Will you enter upon a new career? Will you be financially prepared? How about three sets of hard-played tennis at age 120? *The possibilities are endless.* "Let your mind run wild," says Robert Butler of Mt. Sinai Hospital in New York whose book *Why Survive? Growing Old in America* won the Pulitzer Prize (Kotulak 1991).

Well, you've read the book. Now it's up to you. But before you start, remember these last few points. Understanding how your body works and its basic needs is one large step towards a longer and better quality life on this earth. Common sense is another. Eat properly, include five servings daily of fresh fruits and vegetables, include lots of whole grains in your meals, cut down on the fat and be sure to take your dietary supplements; exercise regularly and get plenty of good sleep and you will be amazed at the difference. We've told you in these pages how to extend the number of healthy years you spend enjoying life. We've also told you how to ensure those extra years are happy and healthful ones. Chances are you want to live to be 100, to see your grandchildren, or even great grandchildren grow up and get married. Do something about it now and you could quite possibly live to be 100-years-old and, with a little luck, much more!

Now is the time for action!

APPENDIXES

Glossary

Ascorbic Acid: Also known as vitamin C.

Alkaline Phosphatase: An enzyme with an optimal pH of 8.6.

Aluminum: One of the most common toxic metals in nature. Believed to play a role in Alzheimer's disease; researchers are not sure whether aluminum is a cause of this disease or exacerbates the condition once established in the afflicted person.

Alzheimer's Disease: A central nervous system disease marked by mental deterioration. First identified in the early part of the Twentieth century, Alzheimer's is a progressive malady that results in dementia. One of the leading killers in modern society.

Amanita toxin: A type of poisonous fungus.

Amino Acid Chelates: One of the best mineral delivery systems to ensure that the nutrient is efficiently absorbed. A mineral which is chelated with an amino acid parallels what occurs in the body's digestive tract when the mineral is surrounded by an amino acid for absorption into the blood stream.

Amino Acids: Organic compounds that make up various proteins. There are 22 known amino acids and nine which are essential to human life.

Androgenic Hormone: Hormone that produces a masculinizing effect. Among such hormones is testosterone, one of the most potent.

Anemia: A condition in which the number of red blood cells is below normal, causing skin pallor, fatigue, and dizziness.

Aneurysm: Dilatation of a blood vessel wall caused by the pressure of blood flowing through a weakened area.

Antigen: A substance such as a foreign protein that can stimulate an immune response.

Antioxidant: Substance that protects other substances from oxidation resulting from exposure to oxygen free radicals.

Anxiety: Abnormal sense of fear and apprehension, marked by sweating and an increase in pulse.

Arthritis: Disease characterized by inflammation of the joints.

Atherosclerosis: Condition marked by fatty deposits in the arteries. When severe, it can lead to heart attack, strokes, and chest pain.

Bacteria, Gram-Negative: Organisms that stain pink on the Gram method of staining. (Gram-Positive stains purple-black.)

Beta Carotene: An antioxidant. The naturally occurring precursor of vitamin A, found in plant foods such as carrots and papayas. Unlike vitamin A derived from animal sources such as shark liver, beta carotene is nontoxic; therefore upper dosage limits are virtually impossible to exceed.

Bilirubin: A red-yellow pigment, found in bile, urine, gallstones and blood.

Bioflavonoids: Naturally occurring substances, often taken from orange and lemon rinds, they are necessary for healthy capillary walls. Also known as vitamin P complex.

BUN: Short for blood-urea-nitrogen; the concentration of nitrogen in the form of urea (urine) found in the blood.

Botanicals: Plant substances such as herbs, botanicals are used as dietary supplements for their healing and preventive properties.

Calcium: Essential element from the Earth's crust, responsible for bone formation.

Cancer: Any of several diseases in which cells grow abnormally or unrestricted, resulting in malignant tumors. The uncontrolled growth of a single "immortal" cell, often caused by exposure to environmental influences including tobacco smoke, sunlight and other human sources of radiation, toxic chemicals (*i.e.*, benzene, formaldehyde, viruses and naturally occurring dietary factors.

Candida Sensitivity: Susceptibility to Candida, a kind of parasitic fungi that resembles yeast.

Carcinogen: A cancer-causing substance.

Cataracts: A loss of transparency of the lens of the eye.

Cellular Branch of the Immune System: Branch in which cellular immunity dominates; immunity is cell-mediated and the small lymphocytes play a key role in resisting certain infectious diseases, autoimmune diseases (such as lupus) and some allergies.

Chelation: The process of drawing toxic forms of minerals and heavy metals from the body by converting them into an easily digestible form.

Choline: A vitamin in the B complex, essential for proper liver function.

Chromium Picolinate: The most bioavailable form of chromium; believed beneficial to lower blood pressure, among other advantages.

Chronic Fatigue Syndrome: A condition marked by fatigue sometimes so great that activities of daily living cannot be performed. Also called chronic fatigue immune dysfunction syndrome or CFIDS. The condition often begins with an intense bout of flu but the exhaustion can last for years, making simple movement like turning over feel too difficult to do.

Collagen: A fibrous protein; the major organic constituent of bone, cartilage, and connective tissue, including skin.

Dandruff: Common condition in which dead skin is shed from the scalp and white flakes land on the collar and shoulders.

Degenerative Diseases: Condition which worsens (such as hardening of the arteries) and is marked by deterioration of a tissue or organ in which vitality is impaired.

Deoxyribonucleic Acid: The component of chromosomes and of many viruses that is responsible for the duplication of characteristics *i.e.,* the repository of heredity for each living thing.

Dessicated: The process of removing moisture from a naturally occurring nutrient (*i.e.,* dessicated liver and other glandulars).

Diabetes: Usually refers to diabetes mellitus, a condition in which there is inadequate secretion or use of insulin, excessive urine output, excessive sugar levels in the blood and urine and by excessive thirst and hunger.

Diabetic: Person with diabetes.

Dipeptide: A peptide (important constituent of proteins) which yields two amino acids when broken down.

Down's Syndrome: A chromosomal abnormality in which cells have 47 rather than 46 chromosomes. The condition is marked by mental retardation and a physical appearance in which the eyes slope upward at the outside and facial features are small.

Ellagic Acid: A compound with the ability to check bleeding by shortening the clotting time.

Emphysema: A lung disease in which the tiny air sacs become damaged. Cigarette smoking is the usual cause.

Endocrine System: Glands that secrete hormones and enzymes internally that are carried throughout the body by the blood system.

Endotoxins: A toxin arising internally.

EPA: Environmental Protection Agency, the federal agency charged with the protection and enhancement of the environment, both today and for future generations.

Enzyme: A protein secreted by cells that acts as a catalyst to induce chemical changes in other substances.

Epstein-Barr virus: A type of virus that causes infectious mononucleosis. Condition is marked by extreme fatigue so severe it is often accompanied by inability to work or complete other tasks of normal living.

Flavonoids: Compounds found in high concentrations in some foods and red wines that might help prevent heart disease by preventing oxidation of low-density lipoproteins, the so-called "bad" cholesterol.

Folic Acid: A vitamin in the B family, needed to produce red blood cells. Used in the treatment of nutritional anemia.

Food and Drug Administration (FDA): Responsible for regulating prescription and over-the-counter drugs, as well as foods, animal feeds, medical devices and other consumer goods such as cosmetics, the FDA also regulates nutritional supplements. Under the leadership of its most recent commissioner, Dr. David Kessler, and California Congressman Henry Waxman, the FDA has taken a decidedly anticonsumer stance in trying to take many supplements off the retail market including amino acids, optimal doses of vitamins and minerals and other botanicals—despite the fact that evidence indicates they are largely safer than some of the prescription drugs such as the contraceptive depo provera, as well as the drugs Halcion and Prozac, that have been allowed to stay on the market.

Free Radical Theory of Aging: A unified view of the aging process, whose founder is Dr. Denham Harman, professor emeritus of medicine and biochemistry at the University of Nebraska. Aging, so the theory goes, is the end result of the effects of oxygen-based compounds (*i.e.*, free radicals within our bodies.

Galactosamine: An amino derivative of galactose that occurs in cartilage.

Gallstones: Lumps found in the gallbladder, the tiny sac that stores bile.

Gene: The functional unit of heredity, capable of reproducing itself perfectly every time, directing enzyme and protein formation. Each gene occupies a specific place on a chromosome.

Gerontology: The scientific study of the processes and problems of aging.

Gland: A secreting organ; the secretion may be poured out upon the surface or into a cavity or may be at once taken into the blood without appearing externally.

Glandulars: Extracts of glands such as the pineal, liver, or pituitary. In nutrition, it is believed that "like attracts like," and that nutrients contained in glandular extracts will naturally be able to more likely help that particular organ. For example, some high quality supplements contain bovine eye retina which has been demonstrated to efficiently deliver needed bioflavonoids to the human eye.

Glucarates, Glycosinates: Phytochemicals believed important to boost immune system function and to serve as antioxidants.

Glucose: Blood sugar; major energy sources for the body, derived from ingestion of carbohydrates.

Glutamine: Along with glucose, an amino acid that nourishes the nervous system.

Glycogen: The body's chief storage carbohydrate, primarily n the liver.

Hang-Over: Unpleasant side-effects after excessive drinking of alcoholic beverages, marked by nausea, vertigo, and headache.

Hepatitis: Inflammation of the liver.

Hepatocyte: Liver cells that secrete bile, a yellow or greenish fluid secreted by the liver.

Hesperidin: A bioflavonoid and crucial member of the vitamin C family.

High Blood Pressure: Abnormally high blood pressure; also known as hypertension.

High Density Lipoprotein (HDL): The good cholesterol, HDLs carry harmful substances out of the blood supply and resist oxidation caused by harmful oxygen-free radicals.

Histological: Relating to a branch of anatomy that deals with animal and plant tissue structures so tiny they can only be visualized under a microscope.

Hormone: A chemical substance formed in one organ or part of the body and carried through the blood to another organ or organs.

Human Growth Hormone: Responsible for growth including bone formation, musculature and function of many essential glands, levels of this hormone decrease as people age.

Humoral Branch of the Immune System: Branch in which humoral immunity predominates; humoral immunity is acquired and the circulating antibodies ward off invaders.

Hydrochloric Acid: The body's digestive juices.

Hydroxyl: A free radical believed to play a possible role in breast cancer.

Hyperkalemia: Abnormally high levels of potassium in the blood; sometimes called hyperpotassemia.

Hypovitaminosis: A condition of poor health caused by lack of adequate ingestion of vitamins.

Immunological Theory Of Aging: A theory of aging which posits that decreased immune function leads to increased susceptibility to infection or other aging processes. It is uncertain whether aging processes damage immune function or if immune function "naturally" diminishes over time.

The immunological theory of aging is not mutually exclusive to the free radical theory of aging; indeed, both theories dovetail quite nicely and fit into a larger conception of the aging processes. In fact, free radical reactions within the body may be the "insults" to the immune system that cause decreased function and lead to increased susceptibility to diseases.

Indoles: Compounds found in intestines and feces; decomposed products of tryptophan.

Inflammation: Cellular injury response in a tissue, marked by redness, heat, pain.

Insulin: Secreted by the pancreas, insulin is a hormone that regulates sugar metabolism in the body.

Interleukin-2: Compound produced by white blood cells that help regulate the immune system.

Iron: An essential mineral needed for formation of red blood cells' pigment and other bodily functions.

Lecithin: A kind of phospholipid found in animal tissues such as the liver; essential parts of animal and vegetable cells. One of the Vitamin B complex-related nutrients needed to produce an important brain chemical.

Leukocyte: Any of the white blood cells.

Leukotriene: Any of several substances involved in allergic responses (such as the constriction of bronchial tubes in asthma). Leukotrienes are related to prostaglandins.

Linoleic Acid: A polyunsaturated fat, partly comprising the nutrient lecithin; also known as vitamin F, it is essential to life.

Lipid: Fatty substance.

Lipofuscin: Cellular "garbage" that accumulates in cells damaged by oxygen free radical processes.

Liposterolic: Steroid that is soluble in fat.

Lipotropic Agents: Nutrients that help prevent abnormal and excessive accumulation of fat in the liver.

Lymphocytes: A type of white blood cell; also known as B-cells. Important in cell-mediated immunity.

Lysyl oxidase: Enzyme that strengthens the connective tissue, which in turn binds together various body structures.

Macroxyproteinase: A "repair" enzyme that can help undo the damage done by free radical reactions.

Megavitamin Therapy: A form of medical therapy using dosages of vitamins many times above the RDAs (*see entry*) for the treatment of illness. Vitamins may be delivered intravenously for optimal assimilation.

Memory Loss: Lack of ability to reproduce or recall what has been learned and retained.

Menopause: Permanent cessation of a woman's menstrual cycle.

2-Mercaptoethylamine: A supplement believed to be capable of increasing the lifespan; helps to prevent the damage caused by iron-based oxygen free radical compounds.

Mesothelium: A kind of tissue that makes up the covering of the heart and lines certain other body cavities.

Methuselah Genes: Genes believed to be life-extending; one so-called Methuselah gene regulates high-density lipoprotein or HDL, making it very high and presumably protecting against heart disease.

Mitochondria: The energy centers of the cell, located in the cytoplasm, containing DNA and consisting of two sets of membranes.

Mitosis: The usual division of the cells that result in the duplication of two daughter cells with exactly the same chromosome and DNA content as the original cell.

Mucin: Chief constituent of mucus; the "slime" of the mucus membranes.

National Academy of Sciences: Formed in 1863 by President Abraham Lincoln to advise the government on matters of science and technology, the NAS's Food and Nutrition Board is responsible for setting RDAs (*see entry*).

Natural Killer Cells: A kind of white blood cell, also called T-cells, that destroys invader cells such as tumor cells.

Naturopathic: Relating to a system of disease treatment that emphasizes "natural" agents such as air, water and sunshine and discourages use of drugs and surgery.

Neoplasm: Abnormal tissue that grows when cells proliferate more rapidly than normal. Literally, "new growth."

Neuralgia: Pain affecting a nerve.

Neural Tube Birth Defect: Also called neural tube disorder or NTD, a disorder in which the developing neural tube, which makes up the brain, spinal column and cord, does not close over completely. Depending on where the disorder affects the neural tube, the child can be affected moderately or severely.

Nutrient: A general term, nutrients include vitamins, minerals, proteins, oils, plant substances and many other chemicals that have a positive effect on human health.

Optimal Nutrition: The theory of nutrition that posits vitamins, minerals and other nutrients are required by the body at doses above those minimally required for survival (RDAs)—in order for the body to thrive and perform at exceptional levels of strength, intelligence, endurance, and other capacities.

Orthomolecular Medicine: The medical practice of using molecular substances such as nutrients and botanicals to cure and prevent illness. Doctors practicing this therapy are known as orthomolecular physicians.

Osteoarthritis: Joint disease; the most common of more than 100 different kinds of arthritis.

Osteoporosis: Also known as "brittle bone" disease, osteoporosis is a condition that affects bone density and strength, often leading to loss of mass and eventually fracture. Although it can effect both men and women, it is most often associated with the period of menopause in women's lives. Nutritional strategies, begun early in life, can counter osteoporosis.

Oxidation: The process in which organic substances are damaged by oxygen free radicals.

Oxygen: A gaseous element and the most abundant and widely distributed of all the chemical elements in the earth's crust.

Oxygen Free Radicals: Substances with an unpaired electron, oxygen free radicals are highly unstable and can damage cellular membranes and mitochondria. Their presence is caused by normal oxygen metabolism and by the presence of viruses, harmful bacteria, other illnesses and exposure to toxic chemicals such as pesticides and industrial chemicals.

PABA: Para-aminobenzoic acid; B-complex member.

Paralysis: Loss of movement in a muscle from injury or disease to the nerve supply.

Parkinson's Disease: A neurological disorder marked by muscle tremors, rigid movements, and droopy posture.

Pellagra: Nutritional disorder, most common in poor areas. Caused by deficiency of niacin.

Pharmacopoeia: A collection of drugs; a book describing drugs and other medicinal preparations, especially if issued by an authority.

Phospholipases: Repair enzymes.

Phytochemicals: Chemicals, other than vitamins, minerals, and proteins, derived from plant substances. Includes families such as coumarins, polyacetylenes, and phenolic acids. Neither a vitamin nor mineral but a whole class of other beneficial substances.

Plaque: Fatty build-up that affects the lining of the arteries and leads to coronary heart disease.

PMS: Short for premenstrual syndrome; a variety of symptoms experienced by some women before menstruation. Symptoms might include irritability, insomnia, fatigue, depression, headache and other complaints.

Postmenopausal: The period after menopause, during which time menstruation ends and estrogen levels decline.

Praseodymium Nitrate: Toxic chemical that can produce liver damage; a flavonol called silymarin is believed protective.

Prostacyclin: A kind of prostaglandin that prevents blood cells from sticking together; causes artery dilation. Vitamin C stimulates production of prostacyclin.

Prostaglandins: A class of active substances present in many body tissues. Prostaglandins can stimulate muscles in the intestine and the uterus.

Prostate Gland: A chestnut-shaped body that surrounds the beginning of the urethra in the male, the prostate is composed of collagen and elastic fibers and many smooth muscle bundles; its secretion is a milky fluid discharged at the time of emission of semen.

Psoriasis: A skin disorder marked by patches of inflamed skin covered by silvery scales.

Pycnogenols: Oxygen free radical scavengers, pycnogenols belong to the family of plant substances known as proanthocyanosides and are derived from the bark of trees such as the Bordeaux pine of southern France.

Radiation: The use of light, X-rays, ultraviolet rays or other types of rays for treatment or diagnosis.

Recommended Daily Allowance: Minimum daily requirements for vitamin, minerals and other nutrients as recommended by the National Academy of Sciences in order to prevent the onset of deficiency disease. The RDAs (also known as USRDA) have come under heavy attack from medical experts for being too low to promote optimal nutritional habits.

Rupture: A tear or break in an organ or other body part.

Rutin: Part of the C complex, extracted from buckwheat.

Schizophrenia: A mental disorder and the most common kind of psychosis, in which patients affected have delusions and hallucinations and withdrawal of interest from the outside world.

Scurvy: A disease that can occur when the diet lacks Vitamin C. It is accompanied by swelling and hemorrhages into the skin.

Senile Dementia: A decline in mental ability, usually progressive, that can occur after age 65.

SGPT: Short for serum glutamic pyruvic transaminase. Glutamic pyruvic transaminase is an enzyme usually present in blood and body tissues, particularly in the liver. It is released into the blood as a result of tissue injury so the levels of GPT in the blood may increase when patients' liver cells are damaged.

Steroid: A kind of chemical substance in a large family that includes progesterone, gonadal hormones, bile acids and cholesterol, among others.

Sterol: A kind of steroid with lipid-like solubility, such as cholesterol.

Stroke: Damage to part of the brain caused by leakage of blood vessels or interruption of blood supply.

Superoxidase Dismutase: The enzyme that decomposes the superoxide radical, superoxide dismutase is a valuable nutrient found in dietary supplements; its activity in the body can also be induced by supplements of copper, manganese and zinc.

Synergistic: When the effects of two or more substances are greater than additive with a force greater than either substance alone.

Systemic: An effect that spreads through the entire body.

Taxol: Derived from the Pacific yew tree, taxol is used to fight breast and cervical cancer.

T-Helper Cells: A kind of white blood cell which plays an important role ion the body's immune system, helping to defend against infection and cancer. Produced by the thymus gland, T-cells control the production of B-cells that fight off attacks by bacteria, viruses and cancer-causing agents.

Tocopherols: Obtained from vegetable oils, the tocopherols include alpha, beta, delta, epsilon, eta, gamma and zeta, and make-up vitamin E.

Triglycerides: Fatty substances in the blood.

Vitamin E: A family of eight molecules called tocopherols and tocotrienols with alpha tocopherol being the most potent. Found in highest quantity in foods such as wheat germ oil, sunflower seeds, sunflower oil, safflower oil and almonds.

Wrinkling: A natural feature of aging, brought about by reduction of collagen production and loss of elasticity.

Zinc: An essential mineral, especially important in human reproduction.

Principal Sources

Introduction

Bordia, A. & Bansal, H.C. (1973). "Essential oil of garlic in prevention of atherosclerosis." *The Lancet*, p. 1491.

Cookson, F.B., Altshcul, R. & Federoff, S. (1967). "The effects of alfalfa on serum cholesterol and in modifying or preventing cholesterol induced atherosclerosis in rabbits." *Journal of Atherosclerosis Research*, v. 7, pp. 69-81.

Cookson, F.B. & Federoff, S. (1968). "Quantitative relationships between administered cholesterol and alfalfa required to prevent hypercholesterolaemia in rabbits." *British Journal of Experimental Pathology*, v. 49, pp. 348-355.

De Froment, P. (1974). "Unsaponifiable substance from alfalfa for pharmaceuticals and cosmetic uses." French Patent 2,187,328.

Fujimoto, I., Hanai, A. & Oshima, A. (1979). "Descriptive epidemiology of cancer in Japan: current cancer incidence and survival data." *National Cancer Institute Monographs*, v. 53, pp. 5-15.

Gestetner, B., Assa, Y. Henis, Y., Birk, Y. & Bondi, A. (1971). "Lucerne saponins. IV. Relation between their chemical constitution and hemolytic and antifungal activities." *Journal of Science, Food and Agriculture*, v. 22, no. 4, pp. 168-172.

Hirayama, T. (1978). "Epidemiology of breast cancer with special reference to the role of diet." *Preventive Medicine*, v. 7, pp. 173-195.

Kagawa, T. (1978). "Impact of westernization on the Japanese. Changes in physique, cancer, longevity and centerians." *Preventive Medicine*, v. 7, pp. 205-217.

Kotulak, R. & Gorner, R. (1991). "Science begins to reset the clock: new insights guide research into living younger, longer." *Chicago Tribune,* Dec. 8.

Kritchevsky, D. (1975). "Effect of garlic oil on experimental atherosclerosis in rabbits." *Artery*, v. 1, no. 4, pp. 319-323.

Malinow, M.R., Mclaughlin, P. & Papworth, L. (1976). "Hypocholesterolemic effect of alfalfa in cholesterol-fed monkeys." *IVth International Symposium on Atherosclerosis*, Tokyo, Japan.

Malinow, M.R., Mclaughlin, P., Papworth, L. & Stafford, C. *et al.* (1977). "Effect of alfalfa saponins on intestinal cholesterol absorption in rats." *American Journal of Clinical Nutrition*, v. 30, pp. 2061-2067.

Malinow, M.R., Mclaughlin, P., & Stafford, C. *et al.* (1979). "Comparative effects of alfalfa saponins and alfalfa fiber on cholesterol absorption in rats. *American Journal of Clinical Nutrition,* v. 32, pp. 1811-1812.

Mowrey, D. (1986). *The Scientific Validation of Herbal Medicine.* New Canaan, CT: Keats Publishing.

Nomura, A., Henderson, B.E. & Lee, J. (1978). "Breast cancer and diet among the Japanese in Hawaii." *American Journal of Clinical Nutrition*, v. 31, pp. 2020-2025.

Smith-Barbaro, P., Hanson, D. & Reddy, B.S. (1981). "Carcinogen binding to various types of dietary fiber." *Journal of the National Cancer Institute*, v. 67, no. 2, pp. 495-497.

Stolberg, S. (1992). "Rewiring the mind and body." *Los Angeles Times,* Nov. 30.

Tyihak, E. & Szende, B. (1970). "Basic plant proteins with antitumor activity." Hungarian Patent 798.

Wattenberg, L. (1975). "Effects of dietary constituents on the metabolism of chemical carcinogens." *Cancer Research*, v. 35, pp. 3326-3331.

Wynder, E.L. (1979). "Dietary habits and cancer epidemiology." *Cancer*, supplement, v. 43, no. 5, pp. 155-1961.

1. The RDAs

Kotulak, R. & Gorner, R. (1991). "Science begins to reset the clock: new insights guide research into living younger, longer." *Chicago Tribune,* Dec. 8.

Miller, J.Z., Nance, W.E., Norton, J.A., Wolen, R.L., Griffith, R.S., Rose, R.J. (1977). "Therapeutic effect of vitamin C, a co-twin control study." *Journal of the American Medical Association*, v. 237, pp. 248-251.

Paganelli, G.M., Biasco, G., Brandi, G., Santucci, R., Gizzi, G., Villani, V., Cianci, M. Miglioli, M. & Barbara, L. (1992). "Effect of vitamin A, C, and E supplementation on rectal cell proliferation in patients with colorectal adenomas." *Journal of the National Cancer Institute,* v. 84, no. 1, p. 4751.

Pauling, L. (1986). *How To Live Longer and Feel Better.* New York: Avon Books.

Ramesha A., Rao N., Rao A.R., *et al.* (1990). "Chemoprevention of 7,12 dimethylbenz[a]anthracene-induced mammary carcinogensis in rat by the combined actions of selenium, magensium, ascorbic acid, and reintyl acetate." *Japanese Journal of Cancer Research*, v. 81, pp. 1239-1246.

Robertson, J., Donner, A & Trevithick, J. (1991). "A possible role for vitamins C and E in cataract prevention." *American Journal of Clinical Nutrition*, v. 53, pp. 346-351.

2. *The Free Radical Theory of Aging*

Harman, D. (1981). *Proceedings of the National Academy of Sciences*, v. 78, pp. 7123-7128.

Kotulak, R. & Gorner, R. (1991). "Science begins to reset the clock: new insights guide research into living younger, longer." *Chicago Tribune,* Dec. 8.

Lippman, R. (1980). "Chemiluminescent measurement of free radicals and antioxidant molecular-protection inside living rat mitochondria." *Experimental Gerontology*, v. 15, pp. 339-351.

Passwater, R. (1991). *The New Supernutrition.* New York: Pocket Books.

3. *Superoxide Dismutase*

Harman, D. (1981). *Proceedings of the National Academy of Sciences*, v. 78, pp. 7123-7128.

Kinsella, K.G. (992). "Changes in life expectancy 1900-1990." *American Journal of Clinical Nutrition*, v. 55, pp. 1196S-1202S.

Kotulak, R. & Gorner, R. (1991). "Science begins to reset the clock: new insights guide research into living younger, longer." *Chicago Tribune,* Dec. 8.

Maugh, T.H., II, (1992). "Scientists draw back veil on the mystery of aging: success in extending animals' lives through Methuselah genes may lead to longer human life span." *Los Angeles Times,* Feb. 8.

Passwater (1991). *The New Supernutrition.* New York: Pocket Books.

Williams, D.M., Lynch, R.E. & Cartwright, G.E. (1975). "Superoxided dismutase activity in copper-deficient swine." *Proceedings of the Society for Experimental Biology and Medicine*, v. 149, pp. 534-536.

4. ACF 223: The Patented Antioxidant Formulation

Harman, D. (1981). "The aging process." *Proceedings of the National Academy of Sciences*, v.78, no. 11, pp. 7124-7128, November.

5. Pycnogenol

Havsteen, B. (1983). "Flavonoids, a class of natural products of high pharmacological potency." *Biochemical Pharmacology*, v. 32, no. 7, pp. 1141-1148.

Masquelier, J. (1980). "Natural Products as Medicinal Agents. *Journal of Natural Products,* July.

Masquelier, J. (1987). "U.S. Patent." Patent Number 4,698,360, Oct. 6.

Maynard, G., Franch, J.P. & Dorne, P.A. (1970). "Use of tetrahydroxy flaven diol in opthamology, in particular in diabetic retinopathies (based on 40 cases)." *Lyon Medical*, no. 4, Jan. 25.

Middleton, E. (1984). "The flavonoids." *TIPS*, August 1984.

Passwater (1991). *The New Supernutrition.* New York: Pocket Books.

6. Chromium Picolinate and Life Extension

Passwater, R. (1992). *Chromium Picolinate: Breakthrough in Muscle Building, Weight Control and Heart Health.* New Canaan, CT: Keats Publishing.

7. The Immune System

Beisel, W.R. (1990). "Future role of micronutrients on immune functions." *Annals of the New York Academy of Sciences,* v. 587, pp. 267-274.

Chandra, R.K. (1987). "Nutrition and immunity: I. basic considerations. II. practical applications." *J. Dent. Child.*, v. 54, no. 3, pp. 193-197.

Daly, J.M., Dudrick, S.J. & Copeland, E.M. (1978). "Effects of protein depletion and repletion on cell-mediated immunity in experimental animals." *Ann. Surg.*, v. 188, no. 6, pp. 791-796.

Lesourd, B.M. (1990). "Immunologic aging. Effect on denutrition." *Ann. Biol. Clin.*, v. 48, no. 5, pp. 309-318.

Meydani, S.N., Furukawa, T., Meydani M. & Blumberg, J.B. (1990). "Beneficial effect of dietary antioxidants on the aging immune system." Nutritional Immunology and Toxicology Laboratory, USDA Human Nutrition Research

Center of Aging, Tufts University.

Pauling, L. (1986). *How To Live Longer and Feel Better.* New York: Avon Books.

Penn, N.D. *et al.* (1990). "The effect of dietary supplementation with vitamins A, C and E on cell-mediated immune function in elderly long-stay patients: a randomized controlled trial." *Age and Ageing* v. 20, no. 20, pp. 169-174.

Peretz, A.M., *et al.* (1990). "Enhancement of the immune response by selenium: clinical trials." *Artzl. Lab.*, v. 36, pp. 299-304.

Steinman, D. (1992). *Diet for a Poisoned Planet.* New York: Ballantine Books.

Thompson, J.S., Robbins, J. & Cooper, J.K. (1987). "Nutrition and immune function in the geriatric population." *Clinic. Geriatr. Med.*, v. 3, no. 2, pp. 309-317.

Watson, R.R., *et al.* (1991). "Effect of b-carotene on lymphocyte subpopulations in the elderly humans: evidence for a dose-response relationship." *The American Journal of Clinical Nutrition*, v 53, no. 90-4.

8. *Immuno-Stimulators*

Boeryd, B. & Hallbgren, B. (1980). "The influence of the lipid composition of the feed given to mice on the immunocompetence and tumor resistance of the progeny." *International Journal of Cancer*, v. 26, pp. 241-246.

Brohult, A., Brohult, J., Brohult, S. & Joelsson, I. (1977). "Effect of alkylglycerols on the frequency of injuries following radiation therapy for carcinoma of the uterine cervix." *Acta Obstet. Gynecol. Scane.*, v. 56, no. 4, p. 441.

Graber, C. D, Goust, M.M., Glassman, A.D., Kendall, R. & Loadholt, C.B. (1981). "Immunomodulating properties of dimethylglycine in humans." *The Journal of Infectious Diseases*, v. 143, no. 1, pp. 101105.

Mowrey, D. (1986). *The Scientific Validation of Herbal Medicine.* New Canaan, CT: Keats Publishing.

Passwater, R.A. (1987). "Coenzyme Q-10: The Nutrient of the 90's." *Whole Foods*, pp. 9-13, April.

Potter, J.F. & Beevers, D.G.(1984). "Pressor effect of alcohol in hypertension." *Lancet,* pp. 119-121.

Reap, E.A. & Lawson, J.W. (1990). "Stimulation of the immune response by dimethylglycine, a nontoxic metabolite." *J. Lab. Clin. Med.*, v. 115, pp. 481-486.

9. The Healthy Heart

Beattie, A., Campbell, B., Goldberg, A. & Moore, M. (1976). "Blood-lead and hypertension." *Lancet*, ii, pp. 1-3.

Bordia, A. & Bansal, H.C. (1973). "Essential oil of garlic in prevention of atheroslcerosis." *The Lancet,* ii, p. 1491.

"Chondroitin reduces 'coronary incidents.'" *Journal of the American Medical Association*, August 24, 1970, p. 1254.

"Coenzyme Q10" (1987). AIBR Scientific Reviews, Botanical Medical Series, no. 4.

Fisher, J.A. (1990). *The Chromium Program.* New York: Harper & Row, Publishers.

Folkers, K. Watanabe, T. & Kaji, M. (1977). "Critique of coenzume Q10 in biochemical and biochemical research and in ten years of clinical research on cardiovascular disease." *J. Mol. Med.,* v. 2, pp. 431-460.

Folkers, K. & Yamamura, Y. (eds.) (1984). *Biomedical and Clinical Aspects of Coenzyme Q,* v. 4. Amsterdam: Elsevier Science Publishers.

Formann, S., Hashell, W. Vranizan, K., *et al.,* (1983). "The association of blood pressure and dietary alcohol: difference by age, sex and estrogen use." *Am. J. Epid.,* v. 118, pp. 497-507.

Glauser, S., Bello, S. & Gauser, E. (1976). "Blood-cadmium levels in normo-tensive and untreated hypertensive humans." *Lancet,* i, pp. 717-718.

Gruchow, H.W., Sobocinski, M.S. & Barboriak, J.J. (1985). "Alcohol, nutrient intake, and hypertension in U.S. adults." *Journal of the American Medical Association*, v. 253, pp. 1567-1570.

Hodges, R. & Rebello, T. (1983). "Carbohydrates and blood pressure." *Ann. Int. Med.,* v. 98, pp. 838-841.

Hunt, G.L. (1987). "Coenzyme Q10: Miracle Nutrient?" *Omni*, p. 24, Feb.

Hvalik, R., Hubert, H., Fabsitz, R. & Feinleib, M. (1983). "Weight and hypertension." *Ann. Int. Med.* v. 98, pp. 855-859.

Hypertension Detection and Follow-Up Program Cooperative Group. (1977). "Race, education and prevalence of hypertension. *American Journal of Epidemiology*, v. 106, pp. 351-361.

1988 Joint National Committee. 1988. The 1988 report of the Joint National Committee on detection, evaluation and treatment of high blood pressure. *Archives of Internal Medicine,* v. 148, pp. 36-69.

Kamanna, V.S. & Chandrasekhara, N. (1982). "Effect of garlic on serum lipoproteins and lipprotein cholesterol levels in albino rats rendered hypercholesteremic by feeding cholesterol." *Lipids*, v. 17, no. 7, pp. 483-488.

Kaplan, N.M. (1985). "Non-drug treatment of hypertension." *Annals of Internal Medicine*, v. 102, pp. 359-373.

Kershbaum, A., Pappajohn, D., Bellet, S., (1968). "Effect of smoking and nicotine on adrenocortical secretion." *Journal of the American Medical Association*, v. 203, pp. 113-116.

Khaw, K.T. & Barrett-Connor, S. (1984). "Dietary potassium and blood pressure in a population." *Am. J. Clin. Nutr.*, v. 39, pp. 963-968.

Kotulak, R. & Gorner, R. (1991). "Science begins to reset the clock: new insights guide research into living younger, longer." *Chicago Tribune,* Dec. 8.

Lang, T., Degoulet, P., Aime, F., *et al.* (1983). "Relationship between coffee drinking and blood pressure: analysis of 6,321 subjects in the Paris region." *Am. J. Card.*, v. 52, pp. 1238-1242.

Matson, F., Grundy, S. & Crouse, J. (1982). *The American Journal of Clinical Nutrition*, v. 35, pp. 697-700.

Meneely, G. & Battarbee, H. (1976). "High sodium-low potassium environment and hypertension." *Am. J. Card.*, v. 38, pp. 768-781.

Miller, O. H. "Nutritional aspects of mucopolysaccharides" in *Applied Nutrition in Clinical Practice*, edited by Michael Waldzak and Richard P. Huenior. New York: International Medical Book Corp. 1973, pp. 69-76.

Morrison, L.M. & Enrick, N.L. "Coronary heart disease: reduction of death rate by chondroitin sulphate A." *Angiology*, 1973.

Murata, K. "Inhibitory effects of chondroitin polysulphate on lipemia and atherosclerosis in connection with its anti-cagulant activity." *Naturivissenschalten*, vol. 49, 1962, p. 1. "The therapeutic effect of chondroitin polysulphate in elderly atherosclerotic patients."

Nakazawa, K. & Murata, K. Department of Medicine and Physical Therapy, faculty of Medicine, University of Tokyo, 7-3-1, Bunkyo-ku, Tokyo, Japan.

Passwater, R.A. (1987). "Coenzyme Q-10: The Nutrient of the 90's." *Whole Foods*, pp. 9-13, April.

Passwater (1991). *The New Supernutrition*. New York: Pocket Books.

Pauling, L. (1986). *How To Live Longer and Feel Better*. New York: Avon Books.

Pelletier, O. (1968). "Smoking and vitamin C levels in humans." *Am. J. Clin. Nutr.,* v. 21, pp. 1254-1258.

Pierkle, J.L., Scwartz, J. Landis, J.R. & Harlan, W.R. (1985). "The relationship between blood lead levels and blood pressure and its cardiovascular risk implications." *Am. J. Epid.,* v. 121, pp. 246-258.

Potter, J.F. & Beevers, D.G. (1984). "Pressor effect of alcohol in hypertension." *Lancet,* pp. 119-121.

Skrabal, F. Aubock, J. & Hortnagl, H. (1981). "Low sodium/high potassium diet for prevention of hypertension: probable mechanisms of action." *Lancet,* ii., pp. 895-900.

Surgeon General's Report on Nutrition and Health (1988). Washington, D.C.: U.S. Department of Health and Human Services.

Tyroler, H.A., Heyden, S. & Hames, C.G. (1975). "Weight and hypertension: Evans County studies of blacks and whites." *Epidemiology and Control of Hypertension,* ed. O. Paul, pp. 177-205. New York: Stratton.

10. Cancer Prevention

Blondell, J.M. (1980). "The anticarcinogenic effect of magnesium." *Med. Hypotheses,* v. 6, pp. 863-871.

Goldin, B.R. & Gorbach, S.L. (1984). "The effect of milk and lactobacillus feeding on human intestinal bacterial enzyme activity." *American Journal of Clinical Nutrition,* v. 39, pp. 756-761.

Habib, F.K., *et al.* (1976). "Metal-androgen interrelationships in carcinoma and hyperplasia of the human prostate." *J. Endocrinol.,* v. 71, no. 1, pp. 133-141.

Poydock, M.E., *et al.,* (1979). "Inhibiting effect of vitamins C and B-12 on the mitotic activity of ascites tumors." *Exp. Cell. Biol.,* vol. 47, no. 3, pp. 210-217.

11. Shark Cartilage and Cancer Therapy

Bertelli, A. (1991). "New Treatment Prospects for Osteoarthrosis." *Drugs Experimental Clinical Research*; XVII(1): 1-2.

Japanese Rheumatism; 2: 453.

Lane, I.W. & Comac, I. (1992). *Sharks Don't Get Cancer: How Shark Cartilage Could Save Your Life.* Garden City, N.Y.: Avery Publishing.

Lee, A. and Langer, R. (1983). "Shark Cartilage Contains Inhibitors of Tumor Angiogenesis". *Science,* v. 221; 4616: 1185-1187.

Oikawa, T., et al. (1990). "A novel angiogenic inhibitor derived from Japanese shark cartilage (I). Extraction and estimation of inhibitory activities toward tumor and embryonic angiogenesis." *Cancer Letters*; 3: 181-186.

Pipitone, V.R. (1991). "Chondroprotection with Chondroitin Sulfate." *Drugs Experimental Clinical Research* XVII(1). pp. 3-7.

12. *Liver Protection*

Abe, N., Ebina, T. & Ishida, N. (1982). "Interferon induction by glycyrrhizin and glycyrrhetinic acid in mice." *Microbial Immunol.*, v. 26, pp. 535-539.

Abonyi, M., Kisfaludy, S. & Szalay, F. (1984) Therapeutic effect of (+)-cyanidanol-3 in toxic alcoholic liver disease and in chronic active hepatits." *Acta Physiol. Hung.*, 64, pp. 455-460

Baetgen, D. (1961). "Results of the treatment of epidemic hepatitis in children with high doses of ascorbic acid for the years 1957-1958." *Medizinische Monatschrift*, v. 15, pp. 30-36.

Baraona, E. & Lieber, C. (1979). "Effects of ethanol on lipid metabolism." *J. Lipid Res.*, v. 20, pp. 289-315.

Baur, H. & Staub, H. (1954). "Treatment of hepatitis with infusions of ascorbic acid: Comparison with other therapies." *Journal of the American Medical Association*, v. 156, p. 565.

Berengo, A. & Esposito, R. (1975) "A double-blind trail of (+)-cyanidanol-3 in viral hepatitis" *New Trends in the Therapy of Liver Diseases*, Springer-Verlag, Basel, pp. 1177-1181.

Blum, A., Doelle, W., Kortum, K., et al. (1977) "Treatment of acute viral hepatitis with (+)-cyanidanol-3" *Lancet,* ii, pp. 1153-1155.

Boari, C., Montanari, M., Galleti, G.P., et al. (1975). "Occupational toxic liver diseases. Therapeutic effects of silymarin" *Min. Med.*, 72, pp. 2679-2688.

Bombardierei, G., Minalini, A., Bernardi, L. & Rossi, L. (1985). "Effects of s-adenosyl-l-methionine (SAMe) in the treatment of Gilbert's syndrome." *Curr. Ther. Res.*, v. 37, pp. 580-585.

Branch, W.T. (1982). *Office Practice of Medicine*, pp. 679-685. Philadelphia, PA: W.B. Saunders.

Canini, F., Bartolucci, A., Cristallini, E., et al. (1985). "Use of Silymarin in the treatment of alcoholic hepatic stenosis" *Clin. Ther.*, 114, pp. 307-314.

Castleman, M. (1991). *The Healing Herbs.*

Cathcart, R.F. (1981). "The method of determining proper doses of vitamin C for the treatment of disease titrating to bowel tolerance." *J. Orthmol. Psychiat.*, v. 10, pp. 125-132.

Cavalieri, S. (1974). "A controlled clinical trial of Legalon in 40 patients." *Gazz. Med. Ital.*, v. 133, pp. 628-635.

Chang, H.M. & But, P. [eds.] (1986). *Pharmacology and applications of Chinese Materia Medica.*

Conn, H. (1981) [ed.] "International Workshop on (+)-Cyanidanol-3 in Diseases of the Liver." *Royal Society of Medicine International Symposia Series no. 47,* London: Academic Press.

Demeulenaere, F., Desmet, V., Dupont, E., et al. (1981) "Study of (+)-cyanidanol-3 in chronic active hepatitis. Results of a controlled multicenter study" in Conn, H. [ed.] "International Workshop on (+)-Cyanidanol-3 in Diseases of the Liver." *Royal Society of Medicine International Symposia Series no. 47,* London: Academic Press.

Dreisbach, R.H. *Handbook of Poisoning,* 11th edition, pp. 80-83. Los Altos, CA: Lange Medical Publications.

Duke, J.A. (1985) "Handbook of Medicinal Herbs." Boca Raton, F: CRC Press.

Faber, K. (1958) "The dandelion—*Taraxacum officinale* Weber" *Pharmazie,* 13, pp. 423-435

Frezza, M., Possato, G., Chiesa, L., *et al.* (1984). "Reversal of intrahepatic cholestasis of pregnancy in women after high dose s-adenosyl-l-methionine (SAMe) administration." *Hepatology,* v. 4, pp. 274-278.

Gilbert, A. & Carnot, P. (1896). "Note prelinair sur l'opotherapie hepatique." *Compt. Rend. Soc. Biol.,* v. 48, pp. 934-937.

Hartroft, W.S., Porta, E.A. & Suzuki, M. (1964). "Effects of choline chloride on hepatic lipids after acute ethanol intoxication." *Q. J. Stuc. Alcohol,* v. 25, pp. 427-434.

Hasegaw, T. [ed.] (1975). *Proc. First Intersectional Cong. Int. Assoc. Microbiol. Soc.,* vol 3, Tokyo University Press, pp. 432-442.

Hikino, H., Kiso, Y., Wagner, H. & Fiebig, M. (1984). "Antihepatotoxic actions of flavonolignans from *Silybum marianum* fruits" *Planta Medica,* 50, pp. 248-250

Hirayama, S., Kishikawa, h., Kume, T., & Tada, H. (1978). "Therapeutic effect of liver hydrolysate on experimental liver cirrhosis." *Nisshin Igaku,* v. 45, pp. 528-533.

Hosein, E.A. & Bexton, B. "Protective action of carinitine on liver lipid metabolism after ethanol administration to rats." *Biochem. Pharm.,* v. 24, pp. 1859-1863.

Kiso, Y., Suzuki, Y., Watanabe, N., *et al.* (1983). "Antihepatotoxic principles of *curcumba longa* rhizomes." *Planta Medica,* v. 49, pp. 185-187.

Klenner, F.R. (1971). "Observations on the dose of administration of ascorbic acid when employed beyond the range of a vitamin in human pathology." *J. Applied Nutr.*, v. 23, pp. 61-88.

Knodell, R.G., *et al.* (1981). "Vitamin C prophylaxis for post-transfusion hepatitis: lack of an effect in a controlled trial." *American Journal of Clinical Nutrition*, v. 34, p. 20.

Kuagai, A., Nanboshi, M., Asanuma, Y., *et al.* (1967). "Effects of *glycyrrhizin* on thymolytic and immunosuppressive action of cortisone." *Endocrinol Japan*, v. 145, pp. 39-42.

Leung, A.Y. (1980). *Encyclopedia of Common Natural Ingredients Used in Food, Drugs and Cosmetics.* New York NY: John Wiley & Sons.

Lucas, R.M. (1991). *Miracle Medicinal Herbs,* p. 6.

Maros, T., Racz, G., Katonaj, B. & Kovacs, V. (1966, 1968). "The effects of *cynara scolymus* extracts on the regeneration of the rat liver." Arzneim-Forsch, 1966, v. 16, pp. 127-129; 1968, v. 18, pp. 884-886.

Martin, D., Mayes, P. & Rodwell, V. (1983). *Harper's Review of Biochemistry.* Los Altos, CA: Lange.

Mitscher, L., Park, Y. & Clark, D. (1980). "Antimicrobial agents from higher plants: antimicrobial isoflavonoids from *glycyrrhiza glabra L. var. typica.*" *J. Nat. Products*, v. 43, pp. 259-269.

Montgomery, R., Dryer, R., Conway, T. & Spector, A. (1980). "Biochemistry: a case-oriented approach." St. Louis, MO: Mosby.

Montini, M., Levoni, P., Angoro, A. & Pagani, G. (1975). "Controlled trial of cynarin in the treatment of the hyperlipemic syndrome." *Arzneim-Forsch*, v. 25, pp. 1311-1314.

Mowrey, D. (1990). *Next Generation Herbal Medicine*, pp. 127-129. New Canaan, CT: Keats Publishing, Inc.

Murata, A. (1975). "Viricidal activity of vitamin C: vitamin C for prevention and treatment of viral diseases" in Hasegawa, T. [ed.], *Proc. First Intersectional Cong. Int. Assoc. Microbiol. Soc.*, v. 3, pp. 432-442. Tokyo University Press.

Nagai, K. (1970). "A study of the excretory mechanism of the liver--effect of liver hydrolysate on BSP excretion." *Jap. J. Gastroenterol.*, v. 67, pp. 633-638.

Nutrition Review (1984). "Present knowledge in nutrition." *Nutrition Foundation*, Washington D.C.

Ohbayashi, A., Akoka, T. & Tasaki, H. (1972). "A study of effects of liver hydrolysate on hepatic circulation." *J. Therapy*, v. 54, pp. 1582-1585.

Padova, C., Tritapepe, R., Padova, F. *et al.* (1984). "S-adenosyl-L-methionine antagonizes oral contraceptive-induced bile cholesterol supersaturation in healthy women: preliminary report of a controlled randomized trial." *Am. J. Gastroenterol.*, v. 79, pp. 941-944.

Par A., Horvath, T., Bero, T., et al. (1984) "Inhibition of hepatic drug metabolism by (+)-cyanidanol-3 (catergen) in chronic alcoholic liver disease" *Acta Physiol. Hung.*, v. 64, pp. 449-454.

Petersdorf, R. (1983). *Harrison's Principles of Internal Medicine.* New York, NY: McGraw-Hill.

Piazza, M., Guadagnino, V., Picciotto, J., et al. (1983). "Effect of (+)-cyanidanol-3 in acute HAV, HBV, and non-A, non-B viral hepatitus." *Hepatology*, v. 3, pp. 45-49 .

Pizzorno, J.E. & Murray, M.T. (1988). *A Textbook of Natural Medicine*, ch. IV: "Hepatoprotection." Seattle, WA: John Bastyr College Publications.

Pompeii, R., Pani, A., Flore, O., Marcialis, M. & Loddo, B. (1980) "Antiviral activity of glycyrrhizic acid." *Experientia,* v. 36, pp. 304-305.

Pristautz, H. (1975). "Cynarin in the modern treatment of hyperlipemias." *Wiener Medizinische Wocheschrift,* v. 1223, pp. 705-709.

Regenstein, L. (1982). *America the Poisoned.* Washington, D.C.: Acropolis.

Robbins, S., Cotran, R. & Kuman, V. (1984). *Pathologic Basis of Disease.* Philadelphia, PA: W.B. Saunders.

Rubenstein, E. & Federman, D.D. (1988). "Scientific American medicine." *Scientific American*, pp. 4:VII:1-6.

Sachan, D.A. & Rhew, T.H. (1983). "Lipotropic effect of carnitine on alcohol-induced hepatic stenosis." *Nutr. Rep. Int.*, v. 27, pp. 1221-1226.

Sachan, D.S., Rhew, T.H. & Ruark, R.A. (1984). "Ameliorating effects of carnitine and its precursors on alcohol-induced fatty liver." *American Journal of Clinical Nutrition*, v. 39, pp. 738-744.

Salmi, H.A. & Sarna, S. (1982). "Effects of silymarin on chemical, functional and morphological alteration of the liver. A double-bind controlled study." *Scand. J. Gastroenterol.,* 17, pp. 417-421.

Sanbe, K., Murata, T., Fujisawa, K., *et al.* (1973). "Treatment of liver disease--with particular reference to liver hydrolysates." *Jap. J. Clin. Exp. Med.*, v. 50, pp. 2665-2676.

Santillo, H. (1991). *Natural Healing with Herbs.*

Sarre, H. (1971) "Experience in the treatment of chronic hepatopathies with silymarin." *Arzeim-Forsch.*, 21, pp. 1209-1212.

Scheiber V. & Wohlzogen, F.X.(1978) "Analysis of a certain type of 2 X 3 tables, exemplified by biopsy findings in a controlled clinical trial." *Int. Clin. Pharmacol.,* v. 16, pp. 533-535.

Schomerus H., Wieman, K., Dolle, W., et al. (1984) "(+)-cyanidanol-3 in the treatment of acute viral hepatitis: a randomized controlled trial." *Hepatology,* v. 4, pp. 331-335.

Stanko, R.T., Mendelow, H., Shinozuka, H. & Adibi, S.A. (1978). "Prevention of alcohol-induced fatty liver by natural metabolites and riboflavin." *J. Lab. Clin. Med.,* v. 91, pp. 228-235.

Suzuki H., et al. (1986) "Cianidanol therapy for HBe-antigen-positive chronic hepatitis: a multicenter, double-blind study." *Liver,* v. 6, p. 35.

Theodoropoulos, G., Dinos, A., Dimitriou, P. & Archimandritis, A. (1981) "Effect of (+)-cyanidanol-3 in acute hepatitus" in Conn, H. [ed], Int. Workshop on (+)-cyanidanol-3 in Diseases of the Liver." *Royal Society of Medicine International Symposia Series,* no. 47, Academic Press, London.

Tsung and Hsu (1986). Yamada, Cyong, *et al.*

Vogel, G., Trost, W., Braatz, R., et al. (1975) "Studies on pharmacodynamics, site and mechanism of action of silymarin, the antihepatotoxic principle from *Silybum marianum* (L.) Gaert." *Arzneim-Forsch.,* 25, pp. 179-185.

Wagner, H. (1981). "Plant constituents with antihepatotoxic activity" in Beal, J.L. & Reinhard, E. [eds.]. *Natural Products as Medicinal Agents.* Stuttgart: Hippokrates-Verlag.

Wagner, H. (1986). "Antihepatotoxic flavonoids" in Cody, V., Middleton, E. & Harbourne, J.B. [eds]. *Plant Flavonoids in Biology and Medicine: Biochemical, Pharmacological, and Structure-Activity Relationships.* New York, NY: Alan R. Liss.

Weiss, R.F.(1988) "Herbal Medicine" *Ab Arcanum,* Gothenburg, Sweden, Beaconsfield Publishers LTD, Beaconsfield, England, p. 82 .

Werbach, M.R. (1987). *Nutritional Influences on Illness: A Sourcebook of Clinical Research,* pp. 211-212. Tarzana, CA: Third Line Press.

Wisniewska-Knypl, J., Sokal, J., Klimczak, J. *et al.* (1981). "Protective effect of methionine against vinyl chloride-mediated depression of non-protein sulfhydryls and cytochrome P-450." *Toxicology Letters,* v. 8, pp. 147-152.

13. Relieving Arthritis

Ehrenpreis, S., Balagot, R.C., Comaty, J.E., & Myles, S. B., (1978). "Naloxone reversible analgesia in mice produced by D-phenylalanine and hydrocinamic acid, inhibitors of carboxypep-tidase A." *Advances in Pain*

Research and Therapy, vol. 3.

Kotulak, R. & Gorner, R. (1991). "Science begins to reset the clock: new insights guide research into living younger, longer." *Chicago Tribune,* Dec. 8.

Mandell, M. (1985). *Lifetime Arthritis Relief System,* Berkeley Books.

Mindell, E. (1983) "DL-Phenylalanine (DLPA) nutritional control of chronic pain."

Pauling, L. (1986). *How To Live Longer And Feel Better.* New York: Avon Books.

Passwater, R. (1991). *The New Supernutrition.* New York: Pocket Books.

Public Information Memo Adaptation (81-23). "Statement on self-management in arthritis." Atlanta, GA: Arthritis Foundation Public Education Department.

14. *Super Vision*

Ala El Din Barradah, M. Shoukry, I. & Hegazy, M. (1967). "Difrarel 100 in the treatment of retinal vascular disorders and high myopia." *Bulletin of the Opthamological Society of Egypt,* v. 60, p. 251.

Alfieri, R.& Sole, P. (1964). "Influences des anthocyanosides admistres par voie parenterale sur l'adaptoelectroretinogramme du lapin." *C.R. Soc. Biol.*v. 158, p. 2338.

Bailliart, J.P. (1969). "Tentative d' amelioration de la vision nocturne." *Le Medicine de Reserve,* v. 121.

Bever, B. & Zahnd G.R. (1979). "Plants with oral hypoglycemic action." *Quarterly Journal of Crude Drug Research,* v, 17, pp. 139-196.

Felter, H.W. (1983). *The Eclectic Materia Medica, Pharmacology and Therapeutics.* Portland, OR: Eclectic Medical Publication (first published in 1922).

Gibbs, O.S. (1947). "On the curious pharmacology of hydrastis." *Federation of American Societies for Experimental Biology. Federation Proceedings,* v. 6, no. 1, p. 332.

Gil Del Rio , E. (1968). "Los antocianosidos del *Vaccinum myrtillus* en optalmologia." *Gaz. Med. de France,* v. 18, June 25.

Jameson, P.G. (1988). *The Herbal Handbook,* London: Brighton Press.

Jayle, G.E., Aubry, M., Gavini, M. & Braccini, G. (1965). "Etude concernant l' action sur la vision nocturne des anthocyanosides extraits de *Vaccinum myrtillus.*" *Ann. Ocul.,* v. 198, p. 556.

Kotulak, R. & Gorner, R. (1991). "Science begins to reset the clock: new insights guide research into living younger, longer." *Chicago Tribune,* Dec. 8.

Milkie, G. (1972). "Diet and its effect on the visual system," presented at the Annual Meeting of the American Academy of Optometry, New York, NY, Dec. 19.

Mowrey, D. (1986). *The Scientific Validation of Herbal Medicine.* New Canaan, CT: Keats Publishing.

Nandkarni, A.K. (1954). *Indian Materia Medica.* Popular Book Depot, Bombay-7. Dhootopapeshwar Prakashan Ltd, Panvel 1954, v. 1., 3rd ed., pp. 189-190.

Pauling, L. (1986). *How to Live Longer and Feel Better.* New York: Avon Books.

Pautler, E.L., Mega, J.A. & Tengerdy, C. "A pharmacologically potent natural product in the bovine retina."

Robertson, J., Donner, A. & Trevithick, J.(1991) "A possible role for vitamins C and E in cataract prevention." *American Journal of Clinical Nutrition*, pp. 346-351, v. 53.

Toufexis, A. (1992). "The new scoop on vitamins." *Time* magazine, pp. 54-59, April 6.

15. Memory Boosters and Smart Pills

Haas, E. (1992). *Staying Healthy with Nutrition*. Berkeley, CA.: Celestial Arts. pp.51, 131-132.

Lieberman, HR. (1986). *et. al,* "Possible dietary strategies to reduce cognitive deficits in old age." Chapter in *Progress in Brain Research,* v. 30.

Lewis, A. (1990). "DMAE an overview of its health effects and central uses."

Morgenthaler, J. (1991). *Smart Drugs and Nutrients.* Santa Cruz, CA: B&J Publications.

Owasoyo, J., *et al,* (1992). "Tyrosine and its potential use as a countermeasure to performance decrement in military sustained operations." *Aviation Space and Environmental Medicine*, May, 63 (5) pp. 364-9.

Pelton, R. (1989). *Mind Food and Smart Pills.* New York, NY: Doubleday.

Pfeiffer, C. *et al,* (1968). "A critical survey of possible biochemical stimulants." U.S. Public Health Service, v.1836, pp. 269-275.

Pfeiffer, C. (1975). *Mental and Elemental Nutrients.* New Caanan, CT: Keats Publishing.

Sved, A. *et al,* (1979). "Tyrosine administration reduces blood pressure and enhances brain norepinephrine release in spontaneously hypertensive rats." *Proceedings of the National Academy of Sciences of the United States,* Jul., 76 (7) pp. 3511-4.

Taillandier, J., et al, (1986). "Traitment des troubles vu viellissement cerebral par l'extrait de Ginkgo biloba." *La Presse Medicale*, v. 15, no. 31, p. 1524.

Wood, J.L. (1982). "Effects of consumption of choline and lecithin on neurological and cardiovascular systems." Federation Proceedings, December, 41 (14) pp. 3015-21.

16. The Healthy Prostate

Altman, L. (1992)."Prostrate drug's effects cited." *New York Times*, June 23.

Ask-Upmark (1967). "Prostatitis and its treatment." *Acta Med. Scand.*, v. 181, pp. 355-357.

Barry, M. (1990). "Epidemiology and natural history of benign prostatic hyperplasia." *Urologic Clinics of North America*, v. 17, no. 3, pp. 495-507.

Boosalis, M.G., Evans, G.W. & McClain, C.J. (1983). "Impaired handling of orally administered zinc in pancreatic insufficiency." *American Journal of Clinical Nutrition*, v. 37, pp. 268-271.

Boyd, E.M. & Berry, N.E. (1939). "Prostatic hypertrophy as part of a generalized metabolic disease. Evidence of the presence of a lipopenia." *Journal of Urology*, v. 41, pp. 406-411.

Bricklin, M. (1990). "The prostatic cancer group has switched to a low-risk one." New York, NY: Penguin Books, pp. 438-439.

Cancer Research (1979). December.

Carilla, E., Briley, M., Fauran, F., *et al.* (1984). "Binding of Permixon, a new treatment for prostatic benigh hyperplasia, to the cytosolic androgen receptor in the rat prostate." *J. Steroid Biochm.*, v. 20, pp. 251-253.

Champault, G., Patel, J.C. & Bonard, A.M. (1984). "A double-blind trial of an extract of the plant *Sereno repens* in benign prostatic hyperplasia." *Brit. J. Clin. Pharmacol.*, v. 18, pp. 461-462.

Doheny, K. (1992). "New laser approach to prostate surgery." *Los Angeles Times,* Aug. 12.

Donsbach, K.W. (1989). *The Prostate.* Rosarito Beach, Mexico: Wholistic Publications.

Evans, G.W. (1980). "Normal and abnormal zinc absorption in man and animals: the tryptophan connection." *Nutrition Reviews*, v. 38, pp. 137-141.

Evans, G.W. & Johnson, E.C. (1981). . "Effect of iron, vitamin B-6 and picolinic acid on zinc absorpption in the rat." *Journal of Nutrition*, v. 111, pp. 68-75.

Fahim, W.S., Harman, J.M. Clevenger, T. H., et. al. (1982). "Effect of panax ginseng on testosterone level and prostate in male rats." *Arch. Androl.*

Feinblatt, H.M. and Gant, J.C. (1958). "Palliative treatment of benign prostatic hypertrophy: value of glycine, alanine, glutamic acid combination." *Journal of the Maine Medical Association.*

Freudenheim, M. (1992). "Prostate treatment could be bonanza." *New York Times,* June 22.

Hoffmann, D. (1991). *The New Holistic Herbal.* Rockport, MA: Element, Inc., pp. 69-70.

Horton, R. (1984). "Benign prostatic hyperplasia: a disorder of androgen metabolism in the male." *Journal of the American Geriatric Society,* v. 32, pp. 380-385.

Judd, A.M., MacLeod, R.M. and Login, I.S. (1984). "Zinc acutely, selectively and reversibly inhibits pituitary prolactin secretion." *Brain Research.* v. 294, pp. 191-192.

Krieger, I., Cash, R. & Evans, G.W. (1984). "Picolinic acid in acrodermatitis enteropathica: evidence or a disorder of tryptophan metabolism." *Journal of Pediatric Gastroenterology and Nutrition*, v. 3, pp. 62-68.

Lahtonen, R. (1985). "Zinc and cadmium concentrations in whole tissue and in separated epithelium and stroma from human benign prostatic hypertrophic glands." *Prostate*, v. 6, pp. 177-183.

Leake, A., Chisholm, G.D. & Habib, F.K. (1984a). "The effect of zinc on the 5-alpha-reduction of testosterone by the hyperplastic human prostate gland." *J. Steroid Biochem.*, v. 20, pp. 651-655.

Leake, A., Chisholm, G.D., Busuttil, A. and Habib, F.K. (1984b). "Subcellular distribution of zinc in the benign and malignant human prostate: evidence for a direct zinc androgen interaction."*Acta Endocrinology*, v. 105, pp. 281-288.

Mindell, E. (1990). *Vitamin Bible.* New York: Warner Books.

Mowrey, D. (1986). *The Scientific Validation of Herbal Medicine.* New Canaan, CT: Keats Publishing.

Pizzorno, J.E. & Murry, M.T. (1989). *A Textbook of Natural Medicine.* Seattle, WA: J.B.C. Publications.

Scott, W.W. (1945). "The lipids of the prostatic fluid, seminal plasma and enlarged prostate gland of man." *Journal of Urology*, v. 53, pp. 712-718.

Sinquin, G., Morfin, R.F., Charles, J.F. & Floch, H.H. "Testosterone metabolism by homogenates of human prostates with benign hyperplasia: effects of zinc, cadmium, and other bivalent cations." *J. Steroid Biochem.*, v. 20, pp. 733-780.

Waldholz, M. (1992). "New prostate drug from Merck wins FDA approval." *Wall Street Journal,* June 23.

Wallae, A.M. & Grant, J.E. (1975). "Effect of zinc on adrogen metabolism in the human hyperplastic prostate." *Biochem, Soc. Trans.*, v. 3, pp. 651-655.

17. Preventing Osteoporosis

Albert-Puleo, M. (1980). "Fennel and anise as estrogenic agents." *J. Ethnopharmacology*, v. 2, pp. 337-344.

Barker, H., Frank, O., Thind, I.C., *et al.* (1979). "Vitamin profiles in elderly persons living at home or in nursing homes versus profile in healthy young subjects." *J. Am. Geriatrics Society*, v. 10, pp. 444-450.

Birchall, J.D. & Espie, A.W. (1986). "Biological implications of the itneraction of silicon with metal ions." *Ciba Foundation Symposium*, v. 121, p. 140.

Brattstrom, L.E., Hultberg, B.L. & Hardebo, J.E. (1985). "Folic acid responsive postmenopausal homocysteinemia." *Metabolism*, v. 34, pp. 1073-1077.

Carlisle, E.M. (1986). "Silicon as an essential trace element in animal nutrition." *Ciba Foundation Symposium,* v. 121, p. 123.

Cohen, L. & Litzes, R. (1981). "Infrared spectroscopy and magnesium content of bone mineral in osteoporotic women." *Isr. J. Med. Sci.*, v. 17, pp. 1123-1125.

Costello, C.H. & Lynn, E.V. (1950). "Estrogenic substances from plants: I. Glycyrrhiza." *J. Am. Pharm. Soc.*, v. 39, pp. 177-180.

Duke, J.A. (1985). *Handbook of Medicinal Herbs*, Boca Raton, FL: CRC Press.

Ellis, F., Holesch, S. & Ellis, J. (1972). "Incidence of osteoporosis in vegetarians and ominivores." *American Journal of Clinical Nutrition*, v. 25, pp. 555-558.

Francis, R.M. & Beaumont, D.M. (1987). "Involutional osteoporosis." Letter to the Editor. *New England Journal of Medicine*, v. 316, p. 216.

Grossman, M., Kirsner, J. & Gillespie, I. (1963). "Basal and histalog-stimulated gastric secretion in control subjects and in patients with peptic ulcer or gastric cancer." *Gastroenterology*, v. 45, pp. 14-26.

Holl, M.G. & Allen, L.H. (1988). "Comparative effects of meals high in protein, sucrose, or starch on human mineral metabolism and insulin secretion." *American Journal of Clinical Nutrition*, v. 48, p. 1219.

Infante-Rivard, C., Krieger, M., Gascon-Barre, M. & Rivard, G.E. (1986). "Folate deficiency among institutionalized elderly, public health impact." *J. Am. Geriatrics Society*, v. 34, pp. 211-214.

Kamen, B. (1989). *Startling New Facts About Osteoporosis.* Novato, CA: Nutrition Encounter, Inc.

Krasinski, S.D., Russell, R.M., Furie, B.C., *et al.* (1985). "The prevalence of vitamin K deficiency in chronic gastrointestinal disorders." *American Journal of Clinical Nutrition*, v. 41, pp. 639-643.

Lancet (1986). "Citrate for calcium nephro-lithiasis," p. 955.

Leung, A.Y. (1980). *Encyclopedia of Common Natural Ingredients Used in Food, Drugs, and Cosmetics.* New York, NY: John Wiley & Sons.

Lewis, N.M. (1989). "Calcium supplements and milk: effects on acid-base balance and on retention of calcium, magnesium, and phosphorous." *American Journal of Clinical Nutrition,* v. 49, p. 527.

McCaslin, F.E., Jr. & Janes, J.M. (1959). "The effect of strontium lactate in the treatment of osteoporosis." *Proc. Staff Meetings Mayo Clinic*, v. 34, p. 329.

Marsh, A., Sanchez, T. Chaffee, F., *et al.*(1983). "Bone mineral mass in adult lacto-ovo-vegetarian and omnivorous adults." *American Journal of Clinical Nutrition*, v. 37, pp. 453-456.

National Institutes of Health Consensus Conference: Osteoporosis (1984). *Journal of the American Medical Association*, v. 252, p. 799

Nicar, M.J. & Pak, C.Y.C. (1985). "Calcium bioavailability from calcium carbonate and calcium citrate." *Journal of Clinical Endocrinology and Metabolism*, v. 61, pp. 391-393.

Nielsen, F.H. (1988). "Boron—an overlooked element of potential nutrition importance." *Nutrition Today,* Jan./Feb., pp. 4-7.

Nutrition Rev. (1984). "The function of the vitamin K-dependent proteins, bone GLA protein (BGP) and kidney GLA proteins (KGP)." V. 42, pp. 230-233.

Pizzorno, J.E. & Murry, M.T. (1989). *A Textbook of Natural Medicine.* Seattle, WA: John Bastyr College Publications.

Rao, C., Rao, V. & Steinman, B. (1981). "Influence of bioflavonoids on the metabolism and crosslinking of collagen." *Ital. J. Biochem.*, v. 30, pp. 259-270.

Recker, R.R. (1985). "The effect of milk supplements on calcium metabolism and calcium balance." *American Journal of Clinical Nutrition*, v. 41, p. 254).

Thom, J., Morris, J., Bishop, A. & Blacklock, J.J. (1978). "The influence of refined carbohydrate on urinary calcium excretion." *British Journal of Urology*, v. 50, pp. 459-464.

Wical & Swope (1974). *Journal of Prosthetic Dentistry*, v. 32, p. 13.

18. Easing Menopause

Beck, M. (1992). "Menopause." *Newsweek*, May 25.

Costello, C.H. & Lynn, E.V. (1950). "Estrogenic substances from plants: *glycyrrhiza glabra*." *Journal of the American Pharmaceutical Association*, v. 39, pp. 177-180.

Mowrey, D.B. (1986). *The Scientific Validation of Herbal Medicine.* New Canaan, CT: Keats Publishing, Inc.

Murav'ev, I.A. & Kononikhina, N.F. (1972). "Estrogenic properties of *glycyrrhiza glabra*." *Rastitel'nye Resursy*, v. 8, no. 4, pp. 490-497.

Passwater, R. (1991). "Easing Menopause." *The New Supernutrition*, pp. 66-70. New York: Pocket Books.

Pointet-Guillot, U. (1958). "Contribution a l'etude chimique et pharmacologique de la reglisse." These, Paris.

Sharaf, A., Gomaa, N., El-Camal, M.H.A. (1975). "*Glycyrrhetic* acid as an active estrogenic substance separated from *glycyrrihiza glabra* (licorice)." *Egyptian Journal of Pharmaceutical Science*, v. 16, no. 2, pp. 245-251.

Werbach, M.R. (1988). *Nutritional Influences on Illness*, pp. 297-298. Tarzana, CA: Third Line Press, Inc.

Yaginuma, T., Izumi, R., Yasui, H., Arai, T. & Kawabata, M. (1982). "Effect of traditional herbal medicine on serum testosterone levels and its induction of regular ovulation in hyper-androgenic and oligomenorrhetic women." *Nippon Sanka Fujinka Gakkai Zasshi*, v. 34,, no. 7, pp. 939-944.

19. Smart Skin Sense

Cunningham, S. (1992). *The Magic In Food,* Llewellyn Publications.

Dahlgren, A. (1992). "Imedeen: at last a smart nutrient for aging, damaged skin." *Swanson's Health Shopper,* June.

Darr, D., Combs, S., Dunston, E., et al. (1992). "Topical vitamin C protects procine skin from ultraviolet radiation-induced damage." *British Journal of Dermatology*, v. 127, pp. 247-253.

Emerit, I. (1992). "Free radicals and the aging of the skin." *EXS,* v. 62, pp. 328-341.

Friedman, C. (1992). "Youth Extenders." *Working Woman,* July, pp. 64-65.

Grady, D. & Ernester V. (1992). "Does cigarette smoking make you ugly and old?" *American Journal of Epidemiology,* April 15; v. 135, n. 8, pp. 839-842.

Kadunce, D.P., Burr R., Gress R., Kanner R., Lyon J.L. & Zone J.J. (1991). "Cigarette smoking: risk factor for premature facial wrinkling." *Annals of Internal Medicine,* May 15, v. 114, n. 10, pp. 840-844.

Kune G.A., Bannerman S., & Field B. (1992). "Diet, alcohol, smoking, serum beta-carotene and vitamin A in male nonmelanocytic skin cancer patient and controls." *Nutrition and Cancer,* v. 18, n. 3, pp. 237-244.

Ramsey, N. (1993). "Save Your Ski.n" *Longevity,* June, pp. 34-37.

Telesco, P. (1992). *A Victorian Grimoire.* Llewellyn Publications.

20. Sexual Potency

The Institute for Advanced Study of Human Sexuality Research Department (IASHSRD), 1990. *The* Avena sativa *Project: A Research Report on Sexual Health Care Products with Extract of* Avena sativa. San Francisco, CA: The Institute for Advanced Study of Human Sexuality.

Lewis, H.L. & Memory P.F. *Medical Botany: Plant's Affecting Man's Health,* p. 401. New York: John Wiley & Sons.

Morales, A., Condra, M., Owen, J.A., Surridge, D.H., Fenemore, J. & Harris, C. (1987). "Is yohimbine effective in the treatment of organic impotence? Results of a controlled trial." *Journal of Urology,* pp. 1168-1172, v. 137, no. 6.

Reid, K., Surridge, D.H. Morales, A., Condra, M. Harris, C., Owen, J. & Fenemore, J. (1987). "Double-blind trial of yohimbine in treatment of psychogenic impotence." *The Lancet,* v. 2, no. 8556, pp. 421-423.

Susset, J.G., Tessier, C.D., Wincze, J., Bansal, S., Malhotra, & Schwacha, M.G. (1989). "Effect of yohimbine hydrochloride on erectile impotence: a double-blind study." *Journal of Urology,* v. 141, no. 6, pp. 1360-1363.

21. Increased Energy

Hoffmann, D. (1990). *The New Holistic Herbal.* Rockport, MA: Element, Inc., pp. 69-70.

Levenson (1983). *J. Parenteral & Enteral Nutr.*, v. 7, no. 2, p. 181-183.

Mindell, E. (1980). "What about tyrosine?"

Mowrey, D. (1986). *The Scientific Validation of Herbal Medicine.* New Canaan, CT: Keats Publishing.

Pelton, R. & Pelton, T.C. (1989). *Mind Food & Smart Pills.* New York: Doubleday.

Sydenstricker, V.P., *et al.* (1940). "Observations on the 'egg white' injury in man." *Journal of the American Medical Association,* v. 118, pp. 1199-1200.

22. Exercise

Kotulak, R. & Gorner, R. (1991). "Science begins to reset the clock: new insights guide research into living younger, longer." *Chicago Tribune,* Dec. 8.

Surgeon General's Report on Nutrition and Health (1988). Washington, D.C.: U.S. Department of Health and Human Services.

23. Weight Loss: Simple and Easy!

Intelli-Scope (1992). "Natural Fat-loss," October, 1992, vol 5.

Kotulak, R. & Gorner, P. (1991). "Science begins to reset the clock; new insights guide research into living younger, longer." The Chicago Tribune, Dec. 8.

24. Medium Chain Triglycerides: Nature's Fat Burners

Bach, A. & Babayan, V. (1982). "Medium-chain triglycerides: an update." *The American Journal of Clinical Nutrition*, pp. 950-962.

Bray, G.A., Lee, M., & Bray T.L. (1980). "Weight gain of rats fed medium-chain triglycerides is less than rats fed long-chain triglycerides." *International Journal of Obesity*, 4, pp. 27-32.

Decombaz, J., et al., (1983). "Energy metabolism of medium-chain triglycerides versus carbohydrates during exercise." *European Journal of Applied Physiology* 52, pp.9-14.

Erasmus, U. (1986). *Fats And Oils*, Vancouver, British Columbia, Canada: Alive Books.

Geliebter, A., et al. (1983). "Overfeeding with medium-chain triglyceride diet results in diminished deposition of fat." *The American Journal of Clinical Nutrition*, 37, January, pp.1-4.

Haas, E. (1992). *Staying Healthy with Nutrition*, Berkeley, CA: Celestial Arts.

Ling, P., et al. (1986). "Evaluation of the protein quality of diets containing medium and long-chain triglycerides in healthy rats." *Journal of Nutrition*, 116, pp. 343-349.

Whitaker, J. (1993). "Fats that help you lose weight." *Health & Healing*, v. 3, No. 7.

25. Hair Growth

Adachi, K. & Sadai, M. (1985). "The hair growing product no. 82447." Japanese patent application.

Adachi, K. (1987). "Mechanism on hair growing effect of PDG." *Proceedings of the 17th World Congress of Dermatology.*

AMA Laboratories (1988). "Independent unpublished cross-over, double blind study conducted by AMA laboratories."

Journal of the Society of Cosmetic Chemists Japan, (1991), pp. 134-139, v. 25, no. 2.

Nishinlhon Journal of Dermatology (1986). "LKF—a research team, clinical evaluation of LKF-A on male pattern alopecia," (pp. 738-748), v. 48, no. 4.

Oba, K. (1986). "Development of hair growing product especially with a property of PDG." *Fragrance Journal* (pp. 109-114), v. 14, no. 5.

Oba, K. (1987). "Cosmetic products influencing hair growth." Presented at the *International Federation of Societies of Cosmetic Chemists,* (pp. 116-142).

Oba, K. (1988) "Cosmetic products influencing hair growth." *Cosmetics & Toiletries* (pp. 69-79), v. 103.

Sadai, M. (1987). "Effect of PDG on cultured dermal papilla cells, especially with reference to ATP production and DNA synthesis." Presented at the *17th World Congress of Dermatology.*

Watanabe, Y.(1982a). "Enzyme activity of hair follicles—especially with regard to glucose-6-phosphate dehydrogenase (G6PDH)." *Journal of the Perfume Cosmetic Society of Japan (pp. 9-414), v. 6, no. 1.*

Watanabe, Y., Adachi K.& Sadai, M. (1982b). "The activities of G6PDH in hair follicles of alopecia areata." Presented at *the 16th Congressus Internationalls Dermatologiae.*

26. *Heavy Metals and Oral Chelation*

Patterson, C.C., Shirahata, H. & Ericson, J.E. (1987). "Lead in ancient human bones and its relevance to historical developments of social problems with lead." *The Science of the Total Environment*, v. 61, pp. 167-200.

Walker, M. (1990). The Chelation Way: The Complete Book of Chelation Therapy. Garden City Park, NY; Avery Publishing Groups, Inc.

27. *Adaptogens*

Haas, E. (1992). *Staying Healthy With Nutrition.* Berkeley, CA: Celestial Arts. p. 268.

Hoffman, D. (1991). *The New Holistic Herbal.* Rockport, MA: Element Inc.

"Milk Thistle" (1987). *American Institute for Biosocial Research*, No. 18.

McGlasson, L. (1992). "Reishi: Ancient mushroom is modern hope." *Health Food Business,* v. 38, pp.47-48.

Mindell, E. (1992). *Earl Mindell's Herb Bible.* New York, NY: Simon and Schuster. pp.104-108.

Mowrey, D.B. (1986). *The Scientific Validation of Herbal Medicine.* New Canaan, CT: Keats publishing. pp.11, 20, 88.

Voelp, A., *et al.* (1985). "Study of long-term action of a *Ginkgo biloba* extract on vigilance and mental performance as determined by means of quantitative pharmaco-EEG and psychometric measurements." *American-French Drug Research,* v.9.

Wahlstrom, M. (1987). *Adaptogens, Nature's Key to Well-Being.* Utgivare.

Yamamoto, I., *et, al.* (1974). "Antitumor effect of seaweeds." Japanese Journal of Experimental Medicine, v. 44, pp. 543-546.

Zee-Chang, R.K. (1992). "SQT, A potent Chinese biological response modifier in cancer immunotherapy, potentiation and detoxification of anti cancer drugs." *Methods Find Exp Clin Pharmacology,* v.14, pp. 725-36.

28. *Healing and Preventing Ulcers*

Graham, D.Y. (1993). " Treatment of peptic ulcers caused by helicobacter pylori." *New England Journal of Medicine*, Feb. 4: 349-51.

Holtzer, P., et al. (1989). "Intragastric capsaicin protects against aspirin-induced lesion formation and bleeding in the rat gastric mucosa." *Gastroenterology,* 96: 1425-33.

Limlomwongse, L., et al. (1979). " Effect of capsaicin on gastric acid secretion and mucosal blood flow in the rats." *Journal of Nutrition*,
 109: 773-777.

Modeland, V. (1989). "Ulcers screaming or silent, watch them with care." *FDA Consumer*, June,
 pp. 14-17.

Mowrey, D.P. (1986). *Scientific Validation of Herbal Medicine,* New Canaan, CT: Keats Publishing.

Mowrey, D. P. (1990). *Next Generation Herbal Medicine*, New Canaan, CT: Keats Publishing, pp. 76, 200, 261.

Murray, M.T. (1991). *The Healing Power of*
 Herbs, Prima Publishing, pp. 181-186.

O'Connor, H.J. et al., (1989). "Vitamin C in the human stomach: relation to gastric pH gastroduodenal disease, and possible sources." *Gut*, April 30 (4): 436-442.

Pizzorno, Jr., (1991). "Changing your gut reaction." *Vegetarian Times*, November, pp. 15-19.

Podolsky, D. (1991). "Kill the bug and you kill the ulcer." *U.S. News and World Report*, May 13,
 p. 94.

Smith, D. T., et al. (1933). "Peptic ulcers (gastric, pyloric and duodenal) occurrence in guinea-pigs fed on a diet deficient in vitamin C." *Archives of Internal Medicine*.

Yamahara, J., et al. (1988). "The anti-ulcer effect
 in rats of ginger constituents." *Journal of Ethnopharmacology*, 23: 299-305.

29. *Understanding Your Medical Tests*

Griffith, M.D. & Winter, H. (1988). *Complete Guide To Medical Tests*. Tuscon, AZ: Fisher Books.

Wolf, P. (1977). *Interpretation of Biochemical Multitest Profiles: An Analysis of 100 Important Conditions*. New York: Masson Publishing.

30. *Procaine Substitutes*

Aslan, A. (1985). *Specifications Regarding the Technique and Action of Gerovital H3 Treatment After 34 Years of Usage*. Bucharest, Romania: The

National Institute of Gerontology and Geriatrics.

Hochschild, R. (1973). "Effect of dimethylaminoethanol on the life span of senile male A/J mice." *Experimental Gerontology*, v. 8, pp. 185-191.

Honegger, C. & Honegger R. (1959). "Occurrence and quantitative determination of 2-dimethylaminoethanol in animal tissue extracts." *Nature*, v. 184, pp. 550-552.

Kugler, H. (1989). "Tyrosine's effect on the depression syndrome." *Preventive Medicine Up-Date*, v. 2, no. 6.

Kugler, H. (1990a). "Procaine versus the DMAE-PABA formula." *Preventive Medicine Up-Date*, v. 4, no. 11.

Kugler, H. (1990b). "Procaine versus the DMAE-PABA formula: an evaluation and survey." *Preventive Medicine Up-Date*, v. 5, no.2.

Lewis, A. (1990) *Dimethylaminoethanol (DMAE): An Overview of its Health Effects and Potential Uses.* Belmont Chemicals, Inc.

Miller, E. (1974). "Deanol in treatment of levodopa-induced dyskinesias." *Neurology*, pp. 116-119, v. 24.

Mindell, E. (1991) *Vitamin Bible*, pp. 64-65. New York: Warner Books.

Murphree, H., Pfeiffer, C. & Backerman, I. (1959). "The stimulant effect of 2-dimethylaminoethanol (deanol) in human volunteer subjects." *Clinical Pharmacology and Therapeutics*, pp. 303-310, v. 1, n. 3.

Osvaldo, R. (1974). "2-dimethylaminoethanol (deanol): a brief review of its clinical efficacy and postulated mechanism of action." *Current Therapeutic Research*, pp. 1238-1242, v. 16, n. 11.

Pelton, R. *Mind Foods & Smart Pills.* New York: Doubleday.

Rogers, L.L. & Pelton, R.B. (1957). "Effect of glutamate on IQ scores of mentally deficient children." *Texas Reports on Biology and Children*, (pp. 84-90), v. 15, no. 1.

31. Virtual Eternity

Cohen, M. (1993). "Designer Genes." *Gentleman's Quarterly*, October, pp. 268-275.

Kotulak, R. & Gorner, R. (1991). "Science begins to reset the clock: new insights guide research into living younger, longer." *Chicago Tribune,* Dec. 8.

Maugh, T. (1993). "Unraveling the Secret of Genes." *Los Angeles Times.* Oct. 31.

Suzuki, D. (1993). *The Secret of Life*, Boston, WGEH.

Medical Professionals Specializing in Use of Nutritional Supplements

Dr. Murray Susser is the former president of the American College of Advancement in Medicine and an unabashed nutritionally oriented physician. His practice of medicine typifies the kind of physician we believe you should also seek. For example, after any tests performed on his patients, the

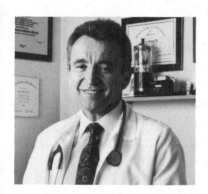

results and ensuing discussion of their meaning that occurs during sessions is taped so that the many detailed concepts and explanations can be reviewed. Dietary supplements are part of his practice. "Having treated more than 15,00 people now, I must say that the majority of my patients do much better with dietary supplements similar to those described in this book," he says. "All too many Americans suffer from what I call high calorie malnutrition, and dietary supplements play an important nutritional role." Dr. Susser supplements his daily diet with a wide array of nutri-

Murray Susser, M.D., is a former president of ACAM and nutritionally oriented physician.

ents including antioxidants and oral chelators, 40 to 50 pills daily.

Here's a sure fire way to find a physician who can help guide you to the optimal supplement program:

1) Ask your physician his/her opinion of dietary supplements.

2) Test their knowledge. Ask them about lesser known dietary aids such as pycnogenols, superoxide dismutase or DMAE.

3) Finally, use this guide as a beginning source to find the right physician. Or contact the American College of Advancement in Medicine whose physicians are more progressive and preventive oriented than those belonging to other more "mainstream" groups. Founded in the early 1970s, ACAM physicians are nutritionally oriented. ACAM has a physician referral service for the public. Their address and telephone are: 23121 Verdugo Drive, Suite 204, Laguna Hills, CA 92653 (714) 583-7666.

ALASKA

Denton, Sandra C., M.D.
Alaska Alternative
Medical Center
4115 Lake Otis Pkwy., #200
Anchorage, AK 99508
907-563-6200

Manuel, F. Russell, M.D.
4200 Lake Otis Pkwy., #304
Anchorage, AK 99508
907-562-7070

Rowen, Robert Jay, M.D.
Omni Medical Center
615 E. 82nd Ave., #300
Anchorage, AK 99518
907-344-7775

Martin, Robert E., M.D.
501 N. Knik St.
Wasilla, AK 99687
907-376-5284

ARKANSAS

Becquet, Norbert J., M.D.
115 West Sixth Street
Little Rock, AR 72201
501-375-4419

Taliaferro, Melissa, M.D.
101 Cherry St, P.O. Box 400
Leslie, AR 72645
501-447-2599

Worrell Jr., Aubrey M., M.D.
Pine Bluff Allergy Clinic
3900 Hickory Street
Pine Bluff, AR 71603
501-535-8200

ARIZONA

Armold, Lloyd D. D.O.
General Practice Assoc., P.C.
4901 W. Bell Rd., #2
Glendale, AZ 85308
602-939-8916

Ber, Abram, M.D.
20635 N. Cave Creek Road
Phoenix, AZ 85024
602-279-3795

Gordon, Garry F., M.D.
5535 S. Compass Road
Tempe, AZ 85283
602-838-2079

Friedmann, Terry Spencer, M.D.
Phoenix Health & Medical Center
7031 E. Camelback, #367
Scottsdale, AZ 85251
602-951-2605

Halcomb, William, D.O.
4323 E. Broadway Rd., #109
Mesa, AZ 85206
602-832-3014

Josephs, Gordon, M.D.
7315 E. Evans Road
Scottsdale AZ 85260-3101
602-998-9232

McGarey, Gladys Taylor, M.D.
Scottsdale Holistic Medical Group
7350 E. Stetson Dr., #128
Scottsdale, AZ 85251
602-990--1528

Meyer, Sherman W., D.O.
1713 Kofa Ave.
Suite J
Parker, AZ 85344
602-669-6618

Olsztyn, Stanley R., M.D.
3610 N. 44th Street, #210
Phoenix, AZ 85018
602-954-0811

CALIFORNIA

Abraham, Illona, M.D.
19231 Victory Blvd., #106
Reseda, CA 91335
818-345-8721

Bryce, William C., M.D.
400 N. San Gabriel Avenue
Azusa, CA 91702
818-334-1407

Belenyessy, Lazlo, M.D.
12732 Washington Blvd., Suite D
Los Angeles, CA 90066
213-822-4614

Brod, Thomas M., M.D.
12304 Santa Monica Blvd., #210
West Los Angeles, CA 90025
310-207-3337

Bryce, William C., M.D.
Competition Nutrition
16835 Aloohquin, #313
Huntington Beach, CA 92649
714-846-1901

Casanas, Robert, M.D.
P.O. 129
4979 Hwy. 140
Mariposa, CA 95338
209-742-6606

Casdorph, H.R., M.D.
Casdorph Clinic
1703 Termino Ave., Suite 201
Long Beach, CA 90804
310-597-8716

Cass, Hyla, M.D.
2730 Wilshire Blvd., #301
Santa Monica, CA 90403
310-453-4339

Cathcart, Robert F., M.D.
127 2nd Street, #4
Los Altos, CA 94022
415-949-2822

Charles, Allan S., M.D.
1414 Maria Lane
Walnut Creek, CA 94596
510-937-3331

Contreras, Victor, M.D.
247 West Harvard Blvd.
Santa Paul, CA 93060
805-525-0907

Degnan, Sean, M.D.
Preventive Medicine Clinic of
Palm Springs
2825 Tahquitz Canyon Way, #200
Palm Springs, CA 92262
619-320-4292

De Monterice, Anu, M.D.
680 East Cotati Ave.
Cotati, CA 94931
707-795-2141

Ebnother, Carl., M.D.
Creative and Natural Health
Solutions
20430 Town Center Lane, #5G
Cupertino, CA 95014
408-973-9550

Eckstein, Larry, M.D.
California Medical Group
1437 7th Street, #301
Santa Monica, CA 90401
310-458-8020

Farinella, Charles, M.D.
69730 Highway 111, #106A
Rancho Mirage, CA 92270
619-325-0734

Finkle, Eugene, M.D.
P.O. Box 309
48900 N. Highway 101
Laytonville, CA 95454
707-984-6775

Fournier, Aline, D.O.
1194 Calle Maria
San Marcos, CA 92609
619-744-6991

Freeman, David, M.D.
BioMed Health
11311 Camarillo St., #103
North Hollywood, CA 91602
818-985-1103

Gold, Robert B., D.O.
1220 Hemlock Way, #103
Santa Ana, CA 92707
714-556-4653

Gordon, Ross B., M.D.
405 Kains Avenue
Albany, CA 94706
510-526-3232

Green, Allen, M.D.
909 Electric Ave., #212
Seal Beach, CA 90740
310-493-4526

Jamangiri, M., M.D.
2156 Santa Fe
Los Angeles, CA 90058
213-587-3218

Jekot, Walter F., M.D.
Jekot Health Center
8474 W. 3rd. Street
Los Angeles, CA 90048
213-655-5900

Julian, James J., M.D.
Julian Holistic Medical Center
1654 Cahuenga Blvd.
Hollywood, CA 90028
213-467-5555

Hackethal, C.A., M.D.
Medical Alliance Associates
1766 N. Riverside Avenue
Rialto, CA 92376
714-875-8845

Hayashida, T., M.D.
1300 W. 155th Street
Gardena, CA 90247
310-323-4090

Hoegerman, H.J., M.D.
101 West Arrellaga
Santa Barbara, CA 93101
805-963-1824

Kime, Zane R., M.D..
Kime Clinic
1212 High St., #204
Auburn, CA 95603
916-823-3421

Klepp, A. Leonard, M.D.
16311 Ventura Blvd., #725
Encino, CA 91436
818-981-5511

Kwiker, Michael J., D.O.
3301 Alta Arden, #3
Sacramento, CA 95825
916-489-4400

Kunin, Richard, M.D.
2698 Pacific Ave.
San Francisco, CA 94115
415-346-2500

Langer, Stephen E., M.D.
Preventive Medicine
3031 Telegraph Avenue
Berkeley, CA 94705
510-548-7384

LeeBenner, Lord, M.D.
World Health Organization
360 San Miguel Drive, #208
Newport Beach, CA 92660
714-720-9022

Lesko, Ronald M., D.O.,
13983 Mango Drive, #102
Del Mar, CA 92014
619-259-2444

Lippman, Cathie-Ann, M.D.
8383 Wilshire Blvd., #360
Beverly Hills, CA 90211
213-653-0486

Lucidi, Edgar A., M.D.
Holistic Opthalmology
410 West Central Ave., #101
Brea, CA 92621
714-879-9500

Lynn, Paul, M.D.
San Francisco Preventive
Medical Group
345 West Portal Avenue
San Francisco, CA 94127
415-566-1000

Moharram, Mohamed, M.D.
300 W. 5th Street, #B
Oxnard, CA 93030
805-483-2355

Priestley, Joan, M.D.
7080 Hollywood Blvd., #603
Los Angeles, CA 90028

Privitera, James, M.D.
Allergy & Nutrition Clinic
105 N. Grandview Ave.
Covina, CA 91723
818-966-1618

Reiner, Donald E., M.D.
Preventive Medicine & Nutrition
1414 D South Miller St.
Santa Maria, CA 93454
805-925-0961

Resk, Joan M., D.O.
NeuroOrthopedic & Preventive
Medical Center
18821 Delaware St., #203
Huntington Beach, CA 92648
714-842-5591

Rettner, Bert, M.D.
221 Almendra Avenue
Los Gatos, CA 95030
408-354-2300

Ross, Gary S., M.D.
500 Sutter Street, #300
San Francisco, CA 94102
415-398-0555

Ross, Harvey M., M.D.
7060 Hollywood Blvd., #730
Los Angeles, CA 90028
213-466-8330

Schwartz, Barry M., M.D.
Beach Family Medical Practice
17522 Beach Blvd., #101
Huntington Beach, CA 92647
714-848-7676

Shamlin, Carol A., M.D.
Shamlin Health Group
621 E. Campbell Ave., #11A
Campbell, CA 95008
408-378-7970

Shields, Megan, M.D.
5336 Fountain
Los Angeles, CA 90029
213-467-5200

Slagle, Priscilla Anne, M.D.
12301 Wilshire Blvd., #300
Los Angeles, CA 90025
310-826-0175

Smith, Timothy J., M.D.
2635 Regent Street
Berkeley, CA 94704
510-548-8022

Steenblock, David A., D.O.
Health Restoration Clinic
22821 Lake Forest Dr., #114
El Toro, CA 92630
714-770-9616

Steiner, Pierre G., M.D.
S.D.I.C.C.
1550 Via Corona
La Jolla, CA 92037
619-488-7742

Stratford, Betty, M.D.
1501 Bollinger Canyon Road
San Ramon, CA 94583
510-837-3911

Su, Terri, M.D.
1038 Fourth St., #3
Santa Rosa, CA 95404
707-571-4424

Susser, Murray R., M.D.
2730 Wilshire Blvd., #110
Santa Monica, CA 90403
310-453-4424

Tang, David H., M.D.
Preventive Medicine Clinic of
Palm Springs
2825 Tahquitz Canyon Way, #200
Palm Springs, CA 92262
619-320-4292

Taylor, Lawrence H., M.D.
3330 3rd Avenue
San Diego, CA 92103
619-296-2952

Thomassen, Elmer, M.D.
Rancho Mediterranean Medical
Clinic
22807 Barton Road
Grand Terrace, CA 92324
714-783-2773

Tillman, Bessie Jo, M.D.
2054 Market Street
Redding, CA 96001
916-246-3022

Toth, John P., M.D.
2299 Bacon Street
Concord, CA 94520
510-682-5660

Tufft, Robert David, M.D.
Internists Medical Group
411 30th Street
Oakland, CA 94609
510-444-2155

Ullis, Karlis, M.D.
Sports Medicine/ Preventative
Medical Group
1457 Stanford ,#6
Santa Monica, CA 90404
310-829-1990

Varese, Frank, M.D.
24953 Paseo de Valencia, #7C
Laguna Hills, CA 92653

Watson, Cynthia, M.D.
530 Wilshire Blvd., #203
Santa Monica, CA 90401
310-393-0937

Wempen, Ronald, M.D.
3620 S. Bristol, #306
Santa Ana, CA 92704
714-546-4325

Wong, David Y., M.D.
3250 Lomita Blvd., #208
Torrance, CA 90505
310-326-8625

Yee, Robert Y., M.D.
3317 Chanate Road, # 2D
Santa Rosa, CA 95404
707-544-6891

COLORADO

Fish, James R., M.D.
3030 N. Hancock Ave.
Colorado Springs, CO 80907
719-471-2273

Ivker, Robert, D.O.
7580 Lost Ranger Peak
Littleton, CO 80127
303-978-1474

Juetersonke, George J., D.O.
5455 N. Union Blvd., #200
Colorado Springs, CO 80918
719-528-1960

Reed, William L., M.D.
59125 Road, #A4
Grand Junction, CO 81505
303-241-3630

Shannon, Scott, M.D.
1770 25th Avenue
Greeley, CO 80631
303-353-2000

CONNECTICUTT

Cohen, Alan R., M.D.
The Center For The Healing Arts
325 Boston Post Road
Orange, CT 06477
203-799-7733

Finnie, Jerold N., M.D.
333 Kennedy Drive L204
Torrington, CT 06790
203-489-8977

Mandell, Marshall, M.D.
Alan Mandell Center For
BioEcologic Diseases
3 Brush Street
Norwalk, CT 06850
203-838-4706

SicaCohen, Robban A., M.D.
Center For The Healing Arts
325 Boston Post Road
Orange, CT 06477
203-799-7733

DISTRICT OF COLUMBIA

Mitchell, George H., M.D.
2639 Connecticut Ave. N.W.
#C100
Washington, DC 20008
202-265-0411

FLORIDA

Barr, Ervin, D.O.
2350 W. Oakland Park Blvd.
Ft. Lauderdale, FL 33311
305-731-8080

Baxas, Sam, M.D.
Renaissance Clinic
24 West Enid Drive
Key Biscayne, FL 33149
305-361-3956

Cannon, Stanley J., M.D.
9085 SW 87th Ave.
Miami, FL 33176
305-279-3020

Caporusso, Domenico, M.D.
Center for General and
Preventative Medicine
1119 Royal Palm Beach Blvd.
Royal Palm Beach, FL 33411
407-793-7548

Carrow, Donald J., M.D.
Florida Preventive Health
Services, Inc.
3902 Henderson Blvd., Suite 206
Tampa, FL 33629
813-832-3220

Dooley, Bruce, M.D.
WellLife
1493 S.E. 17th Street
Ft. Lauderdale, FL 33316

Dayton, Martin, D.O., M.D.
18600 Collins Avenue
N. Miami Beach, FL 33160
305-931-8484

Di Mauro, Stefano, M.D.
1333 S. State Road 7
Tam O' Shanter Plaza N.
Lauderdale, FL 33162
305-940-6474

Gonzales, Carlos R., M.D.
Sugar Mill Medical Center
7991 S. Suncoast Blvd.
Homosassa, FL 32646
904-383-8282

Graves, George, D.O.
P.O. Box 2220
11512 County Road 316
Ft. McCoy, FL 32134
904-236-2525

Massam, Alfred S., M.D.
528 W. Main St.
P.O. Box 1328
Wauchula, FL 33873
813-773-6668

Melnikov, Eteri, M.D.
Manatee Family Medical
116 Manatee Ave. East
Bradenton, FL 34208
813-748-7943

Pardell, Herbert, D.O.
210 S. Federal Hwy., #302
Hollywood, FL 33020
305-989-5558

Parsons, James M., M.D.
Sunstate Preventive Medicine
Institute
2699 Lee Road, Suite 303
Winter Park, FL 32789
407-628-3399

Perlmutter, David, M.D.
Naples Neurological Associates
720 Goodlette Rd., #203
Naples, FL 33940
813-262-8971

Robinson, H.G., M.D.
4406 S. Florida Ave #30
Lakeland, FL 33813
813-646-5088

Rodgers, Robert J., M.D.
Advanced Medical Practices
2170 W. State Road 434, Suite 190
Longwood, FL 32779
407-682-5222

Schoen, Joya, M.D.
341 N. Maitland Avenue, #200
Maitland, FL 32751
407-644-1068

Slavin, Herbert R., M.D.
Institute of Advanced Medicine
7200 W. Commercial Blvd.
Suite 210
Lauderhill, Fl 33319
305-748-4991

Szabo, Imre, M.D.
17255 Davenport Road
Winter Garden, FL 34787
407-656-2780

Way, Spencer, D.O.
500 North Mills Avenue
Orlando, FL 32803
407-843-2342

Wunderlich Jr., Ray C., M.D.
666 6th Street S.
St. Petersburg, FL 337014845
813-822-3612

GEORGIA

Edelson, Stephen B., M.D.
Environmental & Preventive
Health Center
3833 Roswell Road,, Suite 110
Atlanta, GA 30342
404-841-0088

Epstein, David, D.O.
427 Moreland Ave, Suite 100
Atlanta, GA 30307
404-525-7333

Gunter, O.L., M.D.
24 North Ellis St.
P.O. Box 347
Camilla, GA 31730
912-336-7343

Woodard Jr., O. Jack, M.D.
The Wellness Center
1304 Whispering Pines
Albany, GA 31707
912-436-9535

ILLINOIS

Dunn, Paul J., M.D.
715 Lake Street, #106
Oak Park, IL 60301
708-383-3800

Elsasser, Stephen K., D.O.
Family Practice Center
205 S. Englewood Drive
Metamoa, IL 61548
309-367-2321

Hesselink, Thomas, M.D.
888 S. Edgelawn Suite 1735
Aurora, IL 60506
708-844-0011

Hrdlicka, Richard, M.D.
302 Randall
Geneva, IL 60134
708-232-1900

Mauer, William J., D.O.
Kingsley Medical Center
3401 N. Kennicutt Avenue
Arlington Heights, IL 60004
800-255-7030

Stone, Thomas L., M.D.
Center for Bio Energetic
Medicine
1811 Hicks Road
Rolling Meadows, IL 60008
708-934-1100

Tambone, John R., M.D.
Northwest Clinic
102 E. South St.
Woodstock, IL 60098
815-338-2345

Waters, Robert S., M.D.
Waters Preventive Medical
Center
739 Roosevelt Rd., Bldg. 8
Ste.314
Glen Ellyn, IL 60137
708-790-8100

INDIANA

Brasovan, S.N., M.D.
Health Realities Menopause
Center
310 E. 90th Drive, Suite 100
Merrillville, IN 46410
219-736-4099

Darbro, David A., M.D.
Indianapolis Medical Center Inc.
2124 E. Hanna
Indianapolis, IN 46227
317-787-7221

Sparks, Harold T., D.O.
3001 Washighton Avenue
Evansville, IN 47714
812-479-8228

Trufler, David E., D.O.
336 W. Navarre Street
South Bend, IN 46616
219-233-3840

Wolverton, George M., M.D.
647 Eastern Blvd.
Clarksville, IN 47129
812-282-4309

IOWA

Nebbeling, David P., D.O.
Osteopathic Health Center
622 E. 38th Street
Davenport, IA 52807
319-391-0321

KANSAS

Neil, Roy, M.D.
105 W. 13th Street
Hays, KS 67601
913-628-3215

Riordan, Hugh, M.D.
Center For Healing Arts
3100 N. Hillside Ave.
Wichita, KS 67219
316-682-3100

KENTUCKY

Morgan, Kirk D. M.D.
Morgan Medical Clinic
9105 U.S.42
Prospect, KY 40059
502-228-0156

Stoll, Walt, M.D.
Wellness Medicine
6801 Danville Road
Nicholasville, KY 40356
606-233-4273

Tapp, John C., M.D.
Tapp Medical Clinic
414 Old Morgantown Road
Bowling Green, KY 42101
502-781-1483

LOUISIANA

Montalband, Roy M., M.D.
Family Medical Clinic
4408 Hwy. 22
Mandeville, LA 70448
504-626-1985

MARYLAND

Beals, Paul, M.D.
1901 Cherryland
Laurel, MD 20708
301-490-9911

Goodman, Harold, D.O.
8609 Second Avenue
Suite 405B
Silver Springs, MD 20910
301-565-2494

Keeler III, George E., M.D.
5 Oxford Street
Chevy Chase, MD 20815
301-986-9447

MASSACHUSETTS

Janson, Michael, M.D.
Cambridge Center For
Holistic Health
2557 Massachusetts Avenue
Cambridge, MA 02140
617-661-6225

Kaufman, Svetlana, M.D.
24 Merrimack Street, #323
Lowell, MA 01852
508-851-7321

La Cava, Thomas, M.D.
360 West Boylston Street, #107
West Boylston, MA 01583
508-854-1380

MICHIGAN

Agbabian, Vahagn, D.O.
28 North Saginaw Street
Pontiace State Bank Bldg., #1105
Pontiac, MI 48342-2144
313-334-2424

Born, Grant, D.O.
2687 44th Street S.E.

Grand Rapids, MI 49512
(616) 455-3550

Downing, Nedra, D. O.
6300 Sashabaw Dr., Suite #C
Clarkston, MI 48346
313-625-6677

Leventer, Mark, M.D.
375 Lakeside
Grass Lake, MI 49240
517-522-8403

Nutt, James M., D.O.,
Longevity Centers of W.
Michigan
420 S. Layfayette
Greenville, MI 48838
616-754-3679

Parente, Paul A., D.O.
Farmington Medical Center
30275 W. Thirteen Mile Road
Farmington Hills, MI 48334
313-626-7544

Penwell, Marvin D. D.O.
Linden Medical Center
319 Bridge Street
Linden, MI 48451
313-735-7809

Scarchilli, Albert J., D.O.
Farmington Medical Center
30275 W. Thirteen Mile Road

Farmington Hills, MI 48334
313-626-7544

Tapert, Richard E., D.O.
Family Health Clinic
23550 Harper
St. Clair Shores, MI 48080
313-779-5700

MINNESOTA

Cady, Roger K., M.D.
Shealy Institute for
Comprehensive Health Care
1328 E. Evergreen Street
Springfield, MO 65803
417-865-5940

Eckerly, Jean R., M.D.
Preventive Medicine Associate
10700 Old County Rd., #350
Plymouth, MN 55441
612-593-9458

MISSISSIPPI

Evans, Walter C., M.D.
102 Midway Drive
Clinton, MS 39056
601-924-5605

MISSOURI

Dorman, L.E., D.O.,
Applewood Medical Center

9120 E. 35th Street
Independence, MO 64052
816-358-2712

Hayes Jr., Clinton C., D.O.
Union Medical Center
100 West Main
Union, MO 63084
314-583-8911

McDonagh, E.W., D.O.
McDonagh Medical Center
2800 Kendalwood Pky.
Kansas City, MO 64119
816-453-5940

Rudolph, Charles, D.O., Ph.D.
Mc Donagh Medical Center
2800A Kendalwood
Kansas City, MO 64119
816-453-5940

Schwent, John T., D.O.
MediPlex, Inc.
1400 Truman Blvd.
Festus, MO 63028
314-937-8688

Shealy, C. Norman, M.D.
Shealy Institute for
Comprehensive Health Care
1328 E. Evergreen Street
Springfield, MO 65803
417-865-5940

Sultan, Tipu, M.D.
Allergy Treatment Center
P.C., 11585 W. Florissant Ave.
Florissant, MO 63033
314-921-5600

Walker Jr., Harvey, M.D., Ph.D
Preventive Medicine, Inc.
138 North Meramec Avenue
St. Louis, MO 631053704
314-721-7227

Wilmes, Gerald W., M.D.
Wellness Institute of
Northwest Missouri
RR1 Box 105
Maryville, MO 64468
816--562-2290

NEBRASKA

Miller, Otis W., M.D.
408 South 14th Street
Ord, NE 68862

NEW JERSEY

Ali, Majid, M.D.
Institute of Preventive Medicine
95 East Main Street
Denville, NJ 07834
201-586-4111

Burnstein, Walter, D.O.
308-728-3251

3 Whitman Drive
Denville, NJ 07834
201-625-3111

Harris, Charles, M.D.
1 Ortley Playa
Ortley Beach, NJ 08751
908-793-6464

Holder, Kevin D. M.D.
5 Stanley Road
South Orange, NJ 07079
201-762-6077

Magaziner, Allan, D.O.
Magaziner Center
1907 Rain Tree Road
Cherry Hill, NJ 08003
609-424-8222

Menashe, Richard B., D.O.
Edison Medical Nutrition Center
15 South Main Street
Edison, NJ 08837
908-906-8866

Munits, Faina, M.D.
Essex Center for Preventive
Medicine
51 Pleasant Valley Way
West Orange, NJ 07052
201-736-3743

Panjwani, Harry K., M.D., Ph.D.
141 Dayton Street

P.O. Box 398
Ridgewood, NJ 07451
201-447-2033

NEW MEXICO

Cohen, Harold A., M.D.
Six Wind N.W.
Albuquerque, NM 87120
505-898-7115

Dean, Willard H., M.D.
Center For Self Healing
1320 Agua Fria
Santa Fe, NM 87501
505-983-1120

Khalsa, Dharma Singh, M.D.
SUPER Health Longevity Center
3939 Rio Grande NW
Albuquerque, NM 87102
505-345-5098

Luciani, Ralph J., D.O.
Albuquerque Clinic
2301 San Pedro NE, Suite G
Albuquerque, NM 87110
505-888-5995

Scott, Shirley B., M.D.
P.O. Box 2670
Santa Fe, NM 87504
505-986-9960

Stoesser, Annette, M.D.

122 So. Kentucky Ave.
Roswell, NM 88201
505-623-2444

NEVADA

McGuff, Paul, M.D. Ph.D.
McGuff Clinic West
3930 Swenson Street, #903
Las Vegas, NV 89119
702-733-7499

Milne, Robert D. M.D.
Omni Medical Center
502 S. Rancho, #44G
Las Vegas, NV 89106
702-385-1999

Vance, Robert B., D.O., H., M.D.
Center of Advanced Medicine
801 So. Rancho Drive F2
Las Vegas, NV 89106-3814

NEW YORK

Alboum, Lionel D. M.D. P.C.
Two Executive Boulevard
Suite 202
Suffren, NY 10901

Block, Neil L., M.D.
60 Dutch Hill Road
Orangeburg, NY 10962
914-359-3300

Bock, Kenneth, M.D.
Rhinebeck Health Center
108 Montgomery Street
Rhinebeck, NY 12572
914-876-7082

Corsello, Serfina, M.D.
175 E. Main St.
Huntington, NY 11743
516-271-0222

Corsello, Serfina, M.D.
The Corsello Center
200 West 57th Street
New York, NY 10019

Gunsberger, Maurice, M.D.
2920 Hempstead Turnpike
Levittown, NY 11766
516-735-4949

Hoffman, Ronald L., M.D.
Hoffman Center of Holistic
Medicine
40 East 30th Street
New York, NY 10016
212-779-1744

Kurk, Mitchell, M.D.
310 Broadway
Lawrence, NY 11559
516-239-5540

Levin, Warren M., M.D.
World Health Medical Group

444 Park Avenue South
New York, NY 100167350
212-696-1900

Nochmison, Frank, M.D.
416 74th Street
New York, NY 11209
718-833-5197

Ribner, Richard, M.D.
25 Central Park West
New York, NY 10023
212-246-7010

Schachter, Michael B., M.D., P.C.
Two Executive Boulevard
Suite 202
Suffren, NY 10901

Siebert, Majorie, D.O.
Queens Institue for
Complementary Medicine
7309 Myrtle Avenue
Glendale, NY 11385
718-386-2020

Snider, Robert W., M.D.
The Wellness Institute
Andrew Street Road HC61
Box 43D
Massena, NY 13662
315-764-7328

Weiss, Harold, M.D.
8002 19th Ave.
Brooklyn, NY 11214
718-236-2202

NORTH CAROLINA

Laird, John, M.D.
Great Smokies Medical Center
Route 63
Leicester, NC 28748
704-876-1617

OHIO

Aronica, Josephine C., M.D.
1867 W. Market Street
Akron, OH 44313
216-867-7361

Baron, John M., D.O.
Baron Clinic, Inc. & Associates
4807 Rockside Road, # 100
Cleveland, OH 44131
216-642-0082

Chappell, L. Terry, M.D.
Celebration of Health Center Inc.
122 Thurman Street
P.O. Box 248
Bluffton, OH 45817
419-358-4627

2227 W. Lindsey
Norman, OK 73069
405-329-4457

Gorges, Denis E., M.D.
Meta Brain/Mind Biomedical
Research Foundation
457476 Broadview Road
Cleveland, OH 44109-4602
216-749-1133

Taylor, Charles, M.D.
3715 N. Classen
Oklahoma City, OK 73118
405-525-7751

Lonsdale, Derrick, M.D.
Preventative Medicine Group
24700 Center Ridge Road
Westlake, OH 44145
216-835-0104

Lipovitch, Fred B., M.D.
1602 S.W. 82nd Street
Lawton, OK 73505
405-536-0077

Anderson, Leon, D.O.
Anderson Clinic Inc.
121 So. Second St.
Jenks, OK 74037
918-299-5038

Snyder, Don K., M.D.
11573 SR 111
Paulding, OH 45879
419-399-2045

Ventresco Jr., James, D.O.
3848 Tippecanoe Road
Youngstown, OH 44511
216-792-2349

OREGON

Fitzsimmons, J.W., M.D.
591 Hidden Valley Road
Grants Pass, OR 97527
503-474-2166

OKLAHOMA

Farr, Charles H., M.D., Ph.D.
Genesis Medical Center
8524 S. Western, #107
Oklahoma City, OK 73139
405-632-886

Gambee, John, M.D.
66 Club Drive, #140
Eugene, OR 97401
503-686-2536

Moser, Isabelle, M.D.
27402 State Hwy 38
Elkton, OR 97436

Hagglund, Howard E., M.D.
Hagglund Clinic

503-584-2325

Peters, Ronald, M.D.
1607 Siskiyou Blvd.
Ashland, OR 97520
503-482-7007

PENNSYLVANIA

Burton, Frederick D. M.D.
69 Schoolhouse Lane
Phildelphia, PA 19144
215-844-4660

Buttram, Harold E., M.D.
Woodland Medical Center
5724 Clymer Road
Quakertown, PA 18951
215-536-1890

Ellis, Leander T., M.D.
Beekman Place
2746 Belmont Ave.
Philadelphia, PA 19131
215-477-6444

Galperin, Mura, M.D.
824 Hendrix Street
Philadelphia, PA 19116
215-677-2337

Gilbert, Dennis L., D.O.
Walmer and Gilbert Associates
50 N. Market Street
Elizabethtown, PA 17022

717-367-1345

Goldstein, David M., M.D.
Harmarville Rehabilitation
Center
P.O. Box 11460 Guys Run Rd.
Pittsburgh, PA 15238
412-828-1300

Jayalakshmi, P., M.D.
New Life Center
6366 Sherwood Road
Philadelphia, PA 19151
215-473-4226

Koch, Arthur, D.O.,
57 W. Juniper Street
Hazleton, PA 18201

Maulfair Jr., Conrad G., D.O.
Maulfair Medical Center
RR2 Box 71
Mertztown, PA 19539
215-682-2104

Miranda, Ralph A., M.D.
Wholistic Health Center
Rd. #12, Box 108
Greensburg, PA 15601
412-838-7632

Peterson, Robert J., D.O.
64 Magnolia Drive
Newton, PA 18940
717-455-4747

215-579-0330

Posner, Howard, M.D.
Center for Preventative Medicine
111 Bala Ave.
Bala Cynwyd, PA 19004
215-66-7292

Rex, Sally Ann, D.O.
Health Dimensions
1343 Easton Ave.
Bethlehem, PA 18018
215-866-0900

Schmidt, Robert H., M.D.
1227 Liberty Street, #303
Allentown, PA 18102
215-437-1959

Shay, W., D.O.
407 E. Philadelphia
Boyertown, PA 19512122
215-367-5505

Sinha, Chandrika P., M.D.
Sinha Clinic
1177 South 6th Street
Indiana, PA 15701
412-349-1414

Wright, Lance S., M.D.
Box 1952 3901 Market St.
Phildelphia, PA 19104-3133
215-387-1200

SOUTH CAROLINA

Rozema, Ted, M.D.
Bio Genesis Medical Center
1000 East Rutherford Road
Landrum, SC 29356
803-457-4141

TENNESSEE

Thompson, Donald C., M.D.
1121 West 1st North St.
Morristown, TN 37816-2088
615-581-6367

TEXAS

Archer, Jim P., D.O.
North West Medical Center
8434 Fredricksberg Road
San Antonio, TX 78229
512-615-8445

Battle, Robert M., M.D.
McRee Medical Center
9910 Long Point Rd.
Houston, TX 77055
713-932-0552

Constant, George A., M.D.

Constant Clinic
115 Medical Drive, #201
Victoria, TX 77904
512-576-4182

Ettl, Edward John, M.D.
3500 N.Piedras
El Paso, TX 79930
915-566-9361

Fox, William, M.D.
1227 N. Mockingbird Lane
Abilene, TX 79603
915-672-7863

Huff, John D. M.D.
14859 Southwest Freeway
Houston, TX 77478
713-242-8300

Noble, R.W., M.D.
6757 Arapaho Rd., # 757
Dallas, TX 75248
214-458-9944

Parker, Gerald, D.O.
Doctors Clinic
6053 Ward
Amarillo, TX 79110
806-355-8263

Rea, William S., M.D.
Environmental Health Center
of Dallas
8345 Walnut Hill Lane, #205

Dallas, TX 75231
214-368-7132

Rizov, Vladimir, M.D.
8235 Shoal Creek Blvd.
Austin, TX 78758
512-451-8149

Samuels, Michael G., D.O.
Osteopathic Consultant of Dallas
7616 L.B.J. Fwy., #230
Dallas, TX 75251
214-991-3977

Soto, Francisoco, M.D.
Internnational Medical Center
1420 Geronimo D2
El Paso, TX 79925

Tan, Ricardo B., M.D.
423 S. Palm
Pecos, TX 79772
423-445-9090

Trowbridge, John Parks, M.D.
The Center For Health
Enhancement
9816 Memorial Blvd., #205
Houston, TX 77338
713-540-2329

UTAH

Remington, Dennis W., M.D.
800-621-8924

1765 No. Freedom Blvd., #11E
Provo, UT 84604
801-373-8500

VERMONT

Anderson, Charles E., M.D.
175 Pearl Street
Essex Junction, VT 05452
802-879-6544

VIRGINIA

Patel, Sohini P., M.D.
7023 Little River Turnpike
Annandale, VA 22003
703-941-3606

WASHINGTON

Anderson, Robert A., M.D.
The Center For Couseling &
Health Resources
611 Main Steet
Edmonds, WA 98020
206-771-5166

Bakken, Kenneth L., D.O.
St. Luke Medical Center
2285 116th Ave. NE
Bellevue, WA 98004
206-455-5515

Black, Murray L., D.O.
609 S. 48th Ave.
Yakima, WA 98908
509-966-1780

Bolles, Leo J., M.D.
The Bolles Clinic
15611 BelRed Rd.
Bellevue, WA 98008
206-881-2224

Buscher, David, M.D.
1603 116th Ave. NE
Bellevue, WA 98004
206-453-0288

Collin, Jonathan, M.D.
12911 120th Ave. N.E., #A50
Kirkland, WA 98034
206-820-0547

Corell, William F., M.D.
Corell & Associates
S. 3424 Grand Blvd.
Spokane, WA 99203
509-838-5800

Lane, Jeff, M.D.
3202 Colby Ave.
Everett, WA 98201
206-252-7113

McCabe, Donald Lee, D.O.
Freeland Medical Center
1689 E. Main St., Suite 1

P.O. Box 1086
Freeland, WA 98249
206-321-4424

Vesselago, Michael G., M.D.
217 N. 125th Street
Seattle, WA 98133
206-367-0760

Warner, Glenn A., M.D.
901 Boren Ave., #901
Seattle, WA 98104
206-292-2277

Wilkinson, Richard S., M.D.
Yakima Allergy Clinic
302 S. 12th Avenue
Yakima, WA 98902
509-453-5506

Wright, Jonathan V., M.D.
24030 132nd S.E.
Kent, WA 98042
206-631-8920

WEST VIRGINIA

Kostenko, Michael M., D.O.
The Clinic
114 East Main Street
Beckley, WV 25801
304-253-0591

Webb III, D.H., M.D.
Area Psychiatric Psychotherapy
Group
611 7th Avenue
Huntington, WV 25701
304-525-9355

Zekan, Steve, M.D.
1208 Kanawha Blvd. E
Charleston, WV 25301
304-343-7559

WISCONSIN

Alwa, Rathna, M.D.
717 Geneva Street
Lake Geneva, WI 53147
414-248-1430

Kadile, Eleazar M., M.D.
1538 Bellevue Street
Green Bay, WI 54311
414-468-9442

Royal, Dan, D.O.
Madison Oxygen Center
15 Bayside Drive
Madison, WI 53704
800-522-4279

Waters, Robert S., M.D.
Waters Preventive Medical Center
320 Race Street
Wisconsin Dells, WI 53965
608-254-7178

Acknowledgements

We wish to thank the following people for their invaluable assistance in the preparation of this book: Dr. Richard Passwater for the invaluable work he presented in *The New Supernutrition* which is available at book stores throughout the nation, and journalists Ronald Kotulak and Peter Gorner of the *Chicago Tribune* whose 1991 series on stopping the aging clock is the standard of reporting in the field of longevity research and must reading for anybody who wishes to pursue investigation into this fascinating area of science. (The series is available as an excellent book directly from the *Chicago Tribune.*) Finally, we wish to thank the many physicians and medical researchers who have contributed their thoughts, writing and editorial advice, including Drs. Linus Pauling, Denham Harman, Emanuel Cheraskin, Hans Kugler, Megan Shields, Earl Mindell, Cynthia Watson, Joan Priestley, Kaj Alvestrand, Benjamin Friedrich, Richard Cutler, Murray Susser, Ronald Peters, Ronald DiSalvo and Ronald Peters. Our goal, like theirs, has been to educate the public and extend the gift of a vital, long life to everybody.

INDEX

DISEASES AND THEIR NATURAL REMEDIES: A CROSS REFERENCE

YOU DON'T HAVE TO SUFFER FROM ARTHRITIS

Are You In Pain Too Much Of The Time?

About one-seventh of the U.S population is affected by arthritis. Are you in crippling pain night and day from joint discomfort? Are you losing mobility and the ability to get around the way you used to? Have your younger friends stopped calling? *If so, take action now.*

For years, the medical establishment has been telling people they just have to live with their arthritis and patients are given a prescription for anti-inflammatory medicine to ease the pain. The problem is this course of action only treats symptoms. It's not a cure. Besides, scientific study has begun to reveal that anti-inflammatory medicine takes a heavy long-term toll on the body by weakening the immune system.

You Can Get Arthritis Relief

Why not try a solid, well planned nutrition strategy? Dr. Robert Bingham, M.D., wrote in the *Journal of the Academy of Rheumatoid Disease* that more than 250,000 people have used supplements in arthritis treatment with a 80 to 90 % cure rate. It may sound too simple, but you should join the ranks of thousands who have spared themselves the ordeal of life-crippling arthritis.

Doctors' Report FREE As A Special Service

You can learn more about arthritis from current research from leading medical journals. Learn how women, men, and children of all ages can protect themselves from arthritis. Remember, an ounce of prevention is worth a pound of cure!

The author of this booklet is a respected doctor who takes the Hippocratic Oath seriously and wants you to get prompt relief from this crippling disease.

Get your free report on a painless approach to arthritis. Just simply send your name and address along with $2.00 for postage and handling to: Arthritis Research Center, 2532 Lincoln Blvd., Marina del Rey, CA 90291. Use the coupon below for your convenience.

FREE ARTHRITIS REPORT

ALTERNATIVE MEDICINE UPDATES

2532 Lincoln Blvd., Ste. 98, Dept. LE01

Marina del Rey, CA 90291

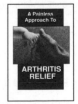

Please rush your free report detailing a painless approach to arthritis relief to me by return mail. I'm enclosing $2.00 for shipping and handling costs.

Mr. or Ms. _____

Address _____

City _____

State _____ Zip _____

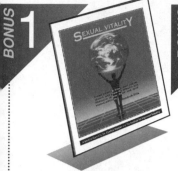
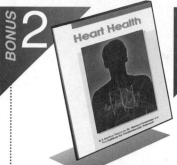
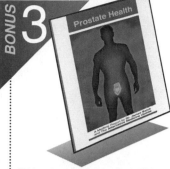

NOTES

NOTES

NOTES